Artificial Intelligence and Machine Learning in Spine Research

Artificial Intelligence and Machine Learning in Spine Research

Guest Editor

Min Cheol Chang

MDPI

Basel • Beijing • Wuhan • Barcelona • Belgrade • Novi Sad • Cluj • Manchester

Guest Editor
Min Cheol Chang
Department of Physical
Medicine & Rehabilitation
Yeungnam University
Taegu
Republic of Korea

Editorial Office
MDPI AG
Grosspeteranlage 5
4052 Basel, Switzerland

This is a reprint of the Special Issue, published open access by the journal *Bioengineering* (ISSN 2306-5354), freely accessible at: https://www.mdpi.com/journal/bioengineering/special_issues/QWLY156R35.

For citation purposes, cite each article independently as indicated on the article page online and as indicated below:

Lastname, A.A.; Lastname, B.B. Article Title. *Journal Name* **Year**, *Volume Number*, Page Range.

ISBN 978-3-7258-6089-0 (Hbk)
ISBN 978-3-7258-6090-6 (PDF)
https://doi.org/10.3390/books978-3-7258-6090-6

Contents

About the Editor . . . vii

Min Cheol Chang
Artificial Intelligence and Machine Learning in Spine Research: A New Frontier
Reprinted from: *Bioengineering* **2024**, *11*, 915, https://doi.org/10.3390/bioengineering11090915 . 1

Rahul Kumar, Conor Dougherty, Kyle Sporn, Akshay Khanna, Puja Ravi, Pranay Prabhakar and Nasif Zaman
Intelligence Architectures and Machine Learning Applications in Contemporary Spine Care
Reprinted from: *Bioengineering* **2025**, *12*, 967, https://doi.org/10.3390/bioengineering12090967 . 5

Christian Quinones, Deepak Kumbhare, Bharat Guthikonda and Stanley Hoang
Scoping Review of Machine Learning and Patient-Reported Outcomes in Spine Surgery
Reprinted from: *Bioengineering* **2025**, *12*, 125, https://doi.org/10.3390/bioengineering12020125 . 44

Aric Lee, Wilson Ong, Andrew Makmur, Yong Han Ting, Wei Chuan Tan, Shi Wei Desmond Lim, et al.
Applications of Artificial Intelligence and Machine Learning in Spine MRI
Reprinted from: *Bioengineering* **2024**, *11*, 894, https://doi.org/10.3390/bioengineering11090894 . 57

Yusuke Ohashi, Tomohiro Shimizu, Hidenori Koyano, Yumejiro Nakamura, Daisuke Takahashi, Katsuhisa Yamada and Norimasa Iwasaki
Evaluation of Operator Variability and Validation of an AI-Assisted α-Angle Measurement System for DDH Using a Phantom Model
Reprinted from: *Bioengineering* **2025**, *12*, 1004, https://doi.org/10.3390/bioengineering12091004 87

Jeoung Kun Kim, Donghwi Park and Min Cheol Chang
Automated Risser Grade Assessment of Pelvic Bones Using Deep Learning
Reprinted from: *Bioengineering* **2025**, *12*, 589, https://doi.org/10.3390/bioengineering12060589 . 98

Hyung Rae Lee, Wounsuk Rhee, Sam Yeol Chang, Bong-Soon Chang and Hyoungmin Kim
Deep Learning in Spinal Endoscopy: U-Net Models for Neural Tissue Detection
Reprinted from: *Bioengineering* **2024**, *11*, 1082, https://doi.org/10.3390/bioengineering11111082 107

Tatsuya Sugimoto, Nobuhito Taniguchi, Ryoto Yoshikura, Hiroshi Kawaguchi and Shintaro Izumi
Evaluation of Patients' Levels of Walking Independence Using Inertial Sensors and Neural Networks in an Acute-Care Hospital
Reprinted from: *Bioengineering* **2024**, *11*, 544, https://doi.org/10.3390/bioengineering11060544 . 120

Sung Hyun Noh, Gaeun Lee, Hyun-Jin Bae, Ju Yeon Han, Su Jeong Son, Deok Kim, et al.
Deep Learning Method for Precise Landmark Identification and Structural Assessment of Whole-Spine Radiographs
Reprinted from: *Bioengineering* **2024**, *11*, 481, https://doi.org/10.3390/bioengineering11050481 . 135

Xiaoyu Tong, Shigeng Wang, Jingyi Zhang, Yong Fan, Yijun Liu and Wei Wei
Automatic Osteoporosis Screening System Using Radiomics and Deep Learning from Low-Dose Chest CT Images
Reprinted from: *Bioengineering* **2024**, *11*, 50, https://doi.org/10.3390/bioengineering11010050 . 148

About the Editor

Min Cheol Chang

Min Cheol Chang is a professor in the Department of Physical Medicine and Rehabilitation at Yeungnam University College of Medicine, Daegu, Republic of Korea. His research focuses on neurorehabilitation, pain medicine, and the application of advanced technologies such as artificial intelligence and machine learning in musculoskeletal and neurological disorders. He has led numerous clinical and translational research projects investigating the mechanisms of neuropathic pain, motor recovery after stroke or spinal cord injury, and the development of innovative therapeutic interventions using neurostimulation and imaging-based prediction models. Professor Chang has published extensively in international peer-reviewed journals and has contributed significantly to advancing precision rehabilitation through data-driven approaches. His recent work explores the integration of AI into spine research, aiming to enhance diagnostic accuracy, optimize treatment planning, and improve patient outcomes. Through his research and academic leadership, he continues to promote the translation of emerging technologies into clinical practice to improve quality of life for patients with neurological and musculoskeletal conditions.

bioengineering

MDPI

Editorial

Artificial Intelligence and Machine Learning in Spine Research: A New Frontier

Min Cheol Chang

Department of Physical Medicine and Rehabilitation, College of Medicine, Yeungnam University, 42415, Daemyungdong, Namku, Taegu 705-717, Republic of Korea; wheel633@gmail.com

1. Introduction

Artificial Intelligence (AI) refers to the creation of computer systems capable of performing tasks typically requiring human intelligence [1], such as problem-solving, decision-making, language comprehension, perception, and learning. Different from systems that merely execute predefined commands, AI systems can learn directly from vast datasets and make autonomous decisions [1]. AI aims to simulate human cognitive functions, enabling machines to learn from data, adapt to new information, and make predictions or decisions without explicit programming for specific tasks. Machine Learning (ML)—a subset of AI—focuses on developing algorithms that allow computers to learn from data and improve their performance over time without being explicitly programmed [2]. ML models identify patterns in data and make predictions or decisions based on those patterns, enabling machines to learn and generalize from examples and increase their accuracy with more exposure to information.

AI and ML are transforming numerous industries, and healthcare is no exception [3]. In spine research, AI and ML are proving to be powerful tools for improving diagnostics, optimizing treatment plans, and enhancing patient outcomes. These technologies can analyze large quantities of data quickly and accurately, revealing patterns that are often imperceptible to humans [4]. This editorial presents some examples of how AI or ML is being applied in spine research.

2. The Role of AI and ML in Spine Research

Traditionally, spine research depends on manual and time-consuming methods for data collection, analysis, and interpretation. Moreover, using traditional statistical methods limits the ability to analyze and process imaging data effectively [1,2]. However, the emergence of AI and ML has revolutionized these processes [1,2]. Researchers can now leverage algorithms to analyze imaging data, recommend personalized treatment strategies, and even predict patient outcomes [5–8]. This advancement is especially significant in spine research, where the complexity of spinal disorders and variability in patient responses often complicate treatment planning.

3. AI and ML in Analyzing Imaging Data

AI and ML are making significant advances in the analysis of medical imaging within spine research. Imaging technologies, such as magnetic resonance imaging (MRI), computed tomography (CT), and X-rays, are essential for evaluating spinal conditions and guiding treatment plans for patients with spinal disorders [9]. However, interpreting these images can be subjective, time-consuming, and susceptible to human error.

AI and ML algorithms enhance image analysis by identifying subtle patterns and abnormalities that may be overlooked by the human eye. These technologies not only improve diagnostic accuracy but also accelerate the process. For instance, AI models can automatically segment spinal structures from imaging data, aiding clinicians in detecting spinal pathologies such as spinal stenosis, herniated discs, or spinal tumors with greater precision [7,10,11]. Hallinan et al. developed an AI model for the automated detection and classification of lumbar central canal, lateral recess, and foraminal stenosis [11]. They showed significant agreement between their AI model and radiologists in classifying stenosis severity, achieving kappa values of 0.98, 0.98, and 0.96 for the central canal stenosis, 0.92, 0.95, and 0.92 for lateral recess stenosis, and 0.94, 0.95, and 0.89 for foraminal stenosis. Gilberg et al. developed an AI algorithm to detect metastatic lesions in abdominal and thoracic CT scans [10]. In their study, the AI algorithm exhibited a sensitivity of 75.0% in identifying potentially malignant spinal bone lesions. Moreover, it improves the sensitivity of the radiologist in detecting metastasis by 20.8 percentage points.

Additionally, AI and ML algorithms could predict disease progression [12]. For example, by analyzing historical imaging and clinical data, algorithms can predict the likelihood of spinal degeneration or scoliosis progression. This predictive capability enables clinicians to make more informed treatment decisions for each patient and potentially prevent conditions from worsening before they become critical.

4. AI and ML in Personalized Treatment Planning

Personalized medicine is one of the most promising applications of AI and ML in spine research. The spine of each patient and their response to different treatments is unique. AI-driven models can analyze extensive datasets, including demographics, clinical history, genetic information, and imaging data, to predict how a patient might respond to specific treatments.

ML algorithms can determine which surgical techniques are most likely to succeed based on the unique profile of a patient [13]. Factors influencing spine surgery outcomes include the type of spinal disorder, patient anatomy, and surgeon experience [14,15]. AI-based systems can provide surgeons with a comprehensive analysis of these factors, helping them to select the most appropriate surgical approach. This can lead to fewer complications, faster recovery times, and improved patient satisfaction.

Furthermore, robotic-assisted spine surgery is another area where AI and ML are advancing rapidly [16]. These systems can improve the precision of surgical procedures by providing real-time feedback based on preoperative imaging and predictive models [16]. Although fully autonomous surgeries remain experimental, the ongoing evolution of AI may allow this capability in the future.

5. AI and ML in Predicting Therapeutic Outcomes

Another significant advantage of AI and ML in spine research is their ability to predict patient outcomes. ML models can forecast recovery times, potential complications, and therapeutic outcomes for different treatment approaches by analyzing clinical and imaging data from patients with spinal disorders [17–21]. These insights enable clinicians and patients to make more informed decisions regarding treatment options.

For instance, in spinal surgery, ML algorithms can predict the likelihood of reoperation or complications such as infections or hardware failure. These predictive tools are essential for preoperative planning, helping surgeons mitigate risks and tailor interventions to individual patients [17,18,20]. Beyond surgical outcomes, AI and ML can also predict the effectiveness of nonsurgical outcomes such as spine intervention [19,21]. Kim et al. developed an AI algorithm that predicts therapeutic outcomes following transforaminal epidural stenosis injection (TFESI) for managing chronic lumbosacral radicular pain caused by herniated lumbar discs, using T2-weighted sagittal lumbar spine MRI data [19]. A "good outcome" was defined as a $\geq$50% reduction in pretreatment pain after 2 months, while a "poor outcome" was defined as a <50% pain reduction after the same duration. In the prediction of therapeutic outcomes (good outcome vs. poor outcome) after TFESI on the validation dataset, the area under the curve was 0.827. Similarly, Wang et al. created an AI algorithm to predict the therapeutic outcome of cervical TFESI in patients with cervical foraminal stenosis using cervical axial MRI data [21]. The area under the curve of our developed model for predicting the therapeutic outcome of cervical TFESI in patients with cervical foraminal stenosis was 0.801.

AI-powered predictive analytics can help clinicians choose the most appropriate treatment paths, ultimately improving patient satisfaction and quality of life.

6. Challenges and Ethical Considerations

AI and ML hold great promise in spine research; however, they also present significant challenges. A major concern is the quality and quantity of data used to train these algorithms. In many cases, spine research involves small datasets, which can reduce the accuracy and generalizability of AI models. Furthermore, data bias presents a serious risk as certain populations may be underrepresented in clinical trials and studies. Training AI models on biased data may result in biased outcomes.

Another challenge is the integration of AI into clinical practice. Although AI can assist in decision-making, clinicians should maintain oversight and responsibility for patient care. AI should complement, not replace, human expertise. To ensure safe implementation, AI systems should be transparent and explainable, allowing clinicians to understand the rationale behind AI-generated recommendations.

Ethical issues should be considered, particularly regarding patient privacy and data security [22]. AI and ML rely on large amounts of patient data, raising concerns about how these data are collected, stored, and used. Regulatory frameworks need to evolve to address these issues and safeguard patient rights in AI-driven healthcare.

7. The Future of AI and ML in Spine Research

The future of AI and ML in spine research is promising. As these technologies evolve, we can anticipate increasingly sophisticated applications in diagnostics, treatment planning, and outcome prediction. Advances in deep learning, natural language processing, and computer vision will possibly lead to further breakthroughs in this field.

Moreover, the integration of AI and ML with other emerging technologies, such as wearable devices and telemedicine, may transform how spine conditions are monitored and managed. For instance, wearable sensors could continuously track the posture and movement of a patient, feeding this information into AI algorithms to deliver real-time feedback and personalized interventions. Telemedicine allows physicians to access AI-generated analysis and feedback, enabling patients to receive care without meeting physicians in person.

In the future, AI and ML may pave the way for more proactive and preventive spine care. These technologies could facilitate earlier interventions by identifying early signs of spinal degeneration or injury, reducing the need for invasive procedures, and improving overall patient outcomes.

8. Conclusions

AI and ML are transforming spine research in unprecedented ways. These technologies are enhancing diagnostics, personalizing treatments, and predicting outcomes, creating new opportunities for clinicians and researchers. However, their integration into clinical practice requires careful consideration of ethical issues, data quality, and clinician oversight. Undoubtedly, these technologies will play a pivotal role in shaping the future of spine research and care. In this Special Issue, "Artificial Intelligence and Machine Learning in Spine Research," we explore the current applications of AI and ML in this field. This issue may advance spinal research and assist researchers in identifying promising new avenues for investigation.

Conflicts of Interest: The author declares no conflict of interest.

References

1. Janiesch, C.; Zschech, P.; Heinrich, K. Machine learning and deep learning. *Electron. Mark.* **2021**, *31*, 685–695. [CrossRef]
2. Jovel, J.; Greiner, R. An Introduction to Machine Learning Approaches for Biomedical Research. *Front. Med.* **2021**, *8*, 771607. [CrossRef] [PubMed]

3. Bajwa, J.; Munir, U.; Nori, A.; Williams, B. Artificial intelligence in healthcare: Transforming the practice of medicine. *Future Healthc. J.* **2021**, *8*, e188–e194. [CrossRef] [PubMed]
4. Farzan, R. Artificial intelligence in Immuno-genetics. *Bioinformation* **2024**, *20*, 29–35. [CrossRef]
5. Fathi, M.; Eshraghi, R.; Behzad, S.; Tavasol, A.; Bahrami, A.; Tafazolimoghadam, A.; Bhatt, V.; Ghadimi, D.; Gholamrezanezhad, A. Potential strength and weakness of artificial intelligence integration in emergency radiology: A review of diagnostic utilizations and applications in patient care optimization. *Emerg. Radiol.* **2024**. [CrossRef]
6. Huang, J.; Shlobin, N.A.; DeCuypere, M.; Lam, S.K. Deep Learning for Outcome Prediction in Neurosurgery: A Systematic Review of Design, Reporting, and Reproducibility. *Neurosurgery* **2022**, *90*, 16–38. [CrossRef]
7. Lee, S.; Jung, J.Y.; Mahatthanatrakul, A.; Kim, J.S. Artificial Intelligence in Spinal Imaging and Patient Care: A Review of Recent Advances. *Neurospine* **2024**, *21*, 474–486. [CrossRef]
8. Zhang, Y.; Xing, Z.; Deng, A. Prediction of treatment outcome for branch retinal vein occlusion using convolutional neural network-based retinal fluorescein angiography. *Sci. Rep.* **2024**, *14*, 20018. [CrossRef] [PubMed]
9. Ruiz Santiago, F.; Láinez Ramos-Bossini, A.J.; Wáng, Y.X.J.; Martínez Barbero, J.P.; García Espinosa, J.; Martínez Martínez, A. The value of magnetic resonance imaging and computed tomography in the study of spinal disorders. *Quant. Imaging Med. Surg.* **2022**, *12*, 3947–3986. [CrossRef]
10. Gilberg, L.; Teodorescu, B.; Maerkisch, L.; Baumgart, A.; Ramaesh, R.; Gomes Ataide, E.J.; Koç, A.M. Deep Learning Enhances Radiologists' Detection of Potential Spinal Malignancies in CT Scans. *Appl. Sci.* **2023**, *13*, 8140. [CrossRef]
11. Hallinan, J.T.P.D.; Zhu, L.; Yang, K.; Makmur, A.; Algazwi, D.A.R.; Thian, Y.L.; Lau, S.; Choo, Y.S.; Eide, S.E.; Yap, Q.V.; et al. Deep Learning Model for Automated Detection and Classification of Central Canal, Lateral Recess, and Neural Foraminal Stenosis at Lumbar Spine MRI. *Radiology* **2021**, *300*, 130–138. [CrossRef] [PubMed]
12. Ren, G.; Yu, K.; Xie, Z.; Wang, P.; Zhang, W.; Huang, Y.; Wang, Y.; Wu, X. Current Applications of Machine Learning in Spine: From Clinical View. *Glob. Spine J.* **2022**, *12*, 1827–1840. [CrossRef] [PubMed]
13. Charles, Y.P.; Lamas, V.; Ntilikina, Y. Artificial intelligence and treatment algorithms in spine surgery. *Orthop. Traumatol. Surg. Res.* **2023**, *109*, 103456. [CrossRef] [PubMed]
14. Chin-Hung Chen, V.; Yang, Y.H.; Chen, P.Y.; Yang, J.T.; Chen, C.P.C.; Chen, C.J.; Lu, M.L.; Lee, Y.; McIntyre, R.S.; Huang, Y.C. Factors affecting lumbar surgery outcome: A nation-wide, population-based retrospective study. *J. Affect. Disord.* **2017**, *222*, 98–102. [CrossRef]
15. Finkelstein, J.A.; Stark, R.B.; Lee, J.; Schwartz, C.E. Patient factors that matter in predicting spine surgery outcomes: A machine learning approach. *J. Neurosurg. Spine* **2021**, *35*, 127–136. [CrossRef]
16. Rasouli, J.J.; Shao, J.; Neifert, S.; Gibbs, W.N.; Habboub, G.; Steinmetz, M.P.; Benzel, E.; Mroz, T.E. Artificial Intelligence and Robotics in Spine Surgery. *Glob. Spine J.* **2021**, *11*, 556–564. [CrossRef]
17. Arvind, V.; Kim, J.S.; Oermann, E.K.; Kaji, D.; Cho, S.K. Predicting Surgical Complications in Adult Patients Undergoing Anterior Cervical Discectomy and Fusion Using Machine Learning. *Neurospine* **2018**, *15*, 329–337. [CrossRef]
18. Habibi, M.A.; NaseriAlavi, S.A.; SoltaniFarsani, A.; MousaviNasab, M.M.; Tajabadi, Z.; Kobets, A.J. Predicting the Outcome and Survival of Patients with Spinal Cord Injury Using Machine Learning Algorithms: A Systematic Review. *World Neurosurg.* **2024**, *188*, 150–160. [CrossRef]
19. Kim, J.K.; Wang, M.X.; Chang, M.C. Deep Learning Algorithm Trained on Lumbar Magnetic Resonance Imaging to Predict Outcomes of Transforaminal Epidural Steroid Injection for Chronic Lumbosacral Radicular Pain. *Pain Physician* **2022**, *25*, 587–592.
20. Tragaris, T.; Benetos, I.S.; Vlamis, J.; Pneumaticos, S. Machine Learning Applications in Spine Surgery. *Cureus* **2023**, *15*, e48078. [CrossRef]
21. Wang, M.X.; Kim, J.K.; Chang, M.C. Deep Learning Algorithm Trained on Cervical Magnetic Resonance Imaging to Predict Outcomes of Transforaminal Epidural Steroid Injection for Radicular Pain from Cervical Foraminal Stenosis. *J. Pain Res.* **2023**, *16*, 2587–2594. [CrossRef] [PubMed]
22. Chiruvella, V.; Guddati, A.K. Ethical Issues in Patient Data Ownership. *Interact. J. Med. Res.* **2021**, *10*, e22269. [CrossRef] [PubMed]

bioengineering

MDPI

Review

Intelligence Architectures and Machine Learning Applications in Contemporary Spine Care

Rahul Kumar [1], Conor Dougherty [2], Kyle Sporn [3], Akshay Khanna [2], Puja Ravi [4], Pranay Prabhakar [5] and Nasif Zaman [6,*]

1 Department of Biochemistry and Molecular Biology, University of Miami Miller School of Medicine, 1600 NW 10th Ave, Miami, FL 33136, USA; rxk641@miami.edu
2 Sidney Kimmel Medical College, Thomas Jefferson University, 1025 Walnut St., Philadelphia, PA 19107, USA; cjd127@students.jefferson.edu (C.D.); aya156@students.jefferson.edu (A.K.)
3 Norton College of Medicine, Upstate Medical University, Syracuse, NY 13210, USA; spornk@upstate.edu
4 Department of Biology, University of Michigan, 500 S State St., Ann Arbor, MI 48109, USA; puja.mi.us@gmail.com
5 Albany Medical College, 43 New Scotland Ave, Albany, NY 12208, USA; prabhap@amc.edu
6 Human-Machine Perception Laboratory, Department of Computer Science, University of Nevada Reno, 1664 N. Virginia St. LME 314, Reno, NV 89557, USA
* Correspondence: zaman@nevada.unr.edu

Abstract

The rapid evolution of artificial intelligence (AI) and machine learning (ML) technologies has initiated a paradigm shift in contemporary spine care. This narrative review synthesizes advances across imaging-based diagnostics, surgical planning, genomic risk stratification, and post-operative outcome prediction. We critically assess high-performing AI tools, such as convolutional neural networks for vertebral fracture detection, robotic guidance platforms like Mazor X and ExcelsiusGPS, and deep learning-based morphometric analysis systems. In parallel, we examine the emergence of ambient clinical intelligence and precision pharmacogenomics as enablers of personalized spine care. Notably, genome-wide association studies (GWAS) and polygenic risk scores are enabling a shift from reactive to predictive management models in spine surgery. We also highlight multi-omics platforms and federated learning frameworks that support integrative, privacy-preserving analytics at scale. Despite these advances, challenges remain—including algorithmic opacity, regulatory fragmentation, data heterogeneity, and limited generalizability across populations and clinical settings. Through a multidimensional lens, this review outlines not only current capabilities but also future directions to ensure safe, equitable, and high-fidelity AI deployment in spine care delivery.

Keywords: spine surgery; artificial intelligence; machine learning; predictive modeling; neural networks; spinal diagnostics; computer vision; surgical robotics; clinical decision support; biomedical informatics; musculoskeletal imaging; outcome prediction; precision medicine

1. Introduction

In this comprehensive narrative review, we analyze how artificial intelligence (AI) and machine learning (ML) technologies are shaping contemporary spine surgery and spine care. By examining advanced applications from diagnostic imaging to predictive genomics, we take an in-depth look at how sophisticated AI algorithms are revolutionizing multiple domains of orthopedic and spine-focused medicine, including automated radiological

 https://doi.org/10.3390/bioengineering12090967

interpretation, surgical planning optimization, robotic-assisted procedures, and personalized risk stratification through genomic analysis. Current evidence demonstrates that AI-powered systems such as Aidoc's cervical spine fracture detection [1], Zebra Medical Vision's vertebral compression fracture identification [2], and SpineNet's comprehensive spinal pathology analysis [3], among other systems and software, achieve diagnostic accuracies comparable to or exceeding specialist radiologists. In essence, we strongly believe that at the very least, these tools can be used alongside clinician practice as a secondary guide. Furthermore, emerging clinical decision support platforms, including Suki AI, Nuance Dragon Ambient eXperience (DAX), and Ambience Healthcare, are streamlining documentation workflows and enhancing physician-patient interactions through ambient intelligence capabilities [4]. In a similar vein, as many robotic systems like the Mazor X Stealth Edition, ExcelsiusGPS, and ROSA Spine with AI-driven surgical planning are being increasingly tested and even taught to incoming residents [5], we believe there is an ongoing shift toward precision-guided interventions that minimize invasive approaches while maximizing surgical accuracy. Genomics is also finding its role in risk prediction and stratification, as genome-wide association studies (GWAS) and deep learning models are enabling new insights into genetic predispositions for pathologies and outcomes alike, thus allowing clinicians to now factor in patient-specific risk profiles [6]. In this review, we synthesize current evidence across these diverse applications while addressing implementation challenges, regulatory considerations, and future directions for AI integration in spine care.

2. Methodology

This narrative review was conducted as a structured narrative synthesis of peer-reviewed literature, regulatory reports, and industry documentation related to artificial intelligence (AI) and machine learning (ML) applications in spine care. The aim was to provide a comprehensive overview of validated AI tools, clinical decision support systems, genomic integration models, and robotic surgical platforms in contemporary spinal diagnostics and intervention; it does not present original experimental data.

2.1. Literature Search Strategy

The literature search was conducted between January 2024 and May 2025 across PubMed, Scopus, IEEE Xplore, and Google Scholar. Search terms included "artificial intelligence AND spine surgery," "machine learning AND spinal imaging," "robotic spine systems," "spinal genomics," "polygenic risk score AND spine," "ambient clinical intelligence," and "federated learning in healthcare." Boolean operators were used to refine the scope. References were also drawn from FDA medical device databases and reports (e.g., HealthVCF 510(k) clearance, 2020 [7,8]), corporate white papers, and open-access AI repositories.

Only English-language sources published between 2007 and 2025 were considered. Priority was given to high-impact clinical studies, FDA-approved systems, externally validated models, and articles published in peer-reviewed journals with known impact factors. Foundational studies on algorithm development and AI architectures dating back to 2007 (e.g., Gstoettner et al. on Cobb angle measurement accuracy [9]) were included to provide historical context.

2.2. Inclusion and Exclusion Criteria

Studies were included if they met at least one of the following criteria:

- Described AI/ML systems used in spine diagnostics, surgical planning, or outcome prediction (e.g., SpineNetV2 2017 [3,10–12], Aidoc Cervical Spine AI Version 1, 2021 [1,13–15], ExcelsiusGPS, 2024 [5,16,17]).
- Reported external validation results of AI-based tools in spinal imaging (e.g., Yeh et al., 2021 [18]; Nigru et al., 2024 [3]).
- Detailed FDA-cleared robotic systems with spine-specific capabilities (e.g., Mazor X, 2021 [3,5,16,19], VELYS, 2024 [10,20]).
- Investigated genomic risk stratification or pharmacogenomic frameworks applied to spinal pathologies (e.g., Sigala et al., 2023 [6]; Salo et al., 2024 [21]).
- Described ambient clinical intelligence or documentation automation tools with demonstrated implementation in spine-related clinical settings (e.g., Nuance DAX, 2024 [22]; Ambience Healthcare, 2025 [23]).

Excluded were unpublished conference abstracts, non-peer-reviewed preprints (unless containing novel datasets or architectures), non-English publications, and studies lacking clear methodological description or validation metrics.

2.3. Data Extraction and Synthesis

Key information extracted included the following: system/tool name, validation methodology (e.g., peer-reviewed study, FDA clearance, or real-world data), clinical domain of application (diagnostic imaging, robotics, genomics, etc.), performance metrics (e.g., AUC, sensitivity/specificity, error rates), and year of publication. Data were synthesized into thematic domains including (1) diagnostic imaging and automated classification; (2) morphometric and functional analysis; (3) surgical robotics and navigation; (4) genomic and pharmacogenomic personalization; (5) documentation and decision support; and (6) cost-effectiveness and health systems modeling.

The extracted data were organized into summary tables (e.g., Table 1: AI application overview; Table 2: implementation barriers) and visualized across domains to highlight clinical utility, limitations, and translational gaps.

Table 1. Overview of AI applications in spine surgery and diagnostic workflows. This table categorizes current AI-driven technologies across various domains of spine care, including diagnostic imaging, surgical planning, intraoperative navigation, functional outcome prediction, and economic modeling. Each entry outlines the specific AI tools or systems in use, their validation status, clinical benefits, and known limitations. The table is designed to offer clinicians, researchers, and health policymakers a concise reference for evaluating the maturity, clinical utility, and future development needs of spine-focused AI systems.

AI/ML Application Area	Key Tools/Systems	Validation Status	Clinical Benefit	Limitations
Fracture Detection and Classification	Zebra HealthJOINT [24,25], Aidoc Cervical Spine AI [1,26–28]	FDA Approved; Real-world validation	Reduced under-detection; Improved triage accuracy	Limited chronic fracture detection; Sensitivity varies
Spinal Segmentation and Grading	SpineNetV2 [3,29–31], Multimodal Segmentation Platforms	External validation across modalities	Automated grading of stenosis, disk degeneration	Performance may vary across demographics
Morphometric Analysis	CobbAngle Pro Version 1 [32–34], Yeh et al. Ensemble Model [35]	Validated vs. clinical experts	Reduced measurement error; Field-applicable	Dependence on image quality

Table 1. *Cont.*

AI/ML Application Area	Key Tools/Systems	Validation Status	Clinical Benefit	Limitations
Ultrasound-based Imaging	UGBNet [36], Attention-Unet [7]	Peer-reviewed feasibility studies	Segmentation of low-contrast images	Noise sensitivity in complex anatomy
Muscle Quality Quantification	CTSpine1K [37,38], TrinetX [38]	Open-source annotated datasets	Cross-sectional muscle area and fat infiltration	Need for standardized protocols
Preoperative Planning	Mazor X [3,5,39,40], ExcelsiusGPS [5,39,41]	Clinical integration with robotic systems	Optimized screw trajectory, virtual planning	Variable accuracy in deformed anatomy
Robotic Execution	VELYS [10,20], ROSA Spine [5,42], Mazor Robotics [10]	FDA-cleared, commercial use	Real-time trajectory correction; Error reduction	Cost and infrastructure requirements
Navigation and Guidance	Brainlab Curve [43], Medtronic StealthStation [10]	Integrated AI + imaging validation	Adaptive navigation; Improved pedicle accuracy	Setup complexity; Intraoperative variability
Outcome Prediction	GNNs, Transformers, Sentiment NLP [44–47]	Ongoing studies; Cross-disciplinary use	Predict functional recovery, mental health monitoring	Integration of heterogeneous data types
Cost-Effectiveness and QOL Modeling	Dynamic Simulations, Complexity Economics	Emerging models; Not yet widespread	Forecasting long-term impact; Behavioral insights	Lack of spine-specific QOL instruments

Table 2. Technical limitations and implementation barriers to clinical integration. This table delineates key challenges impeding the widespread adoption of AI in spine diagnostics and surgery, categorized across imaging variability, algorithmic brittleness, dataset bias, explainability deficits, regulatory complexity, infrastructure costs, and clinical integration issues. Each barrier is described in detail, along with its technical considerations, and paired with its practical clinical or operational consequences. The table aims to guide researchers, developers, and healthcare administrators in identifying systemic vulnerabilities and prioritizing translational improvements necessary for safe and scalable AI deployment in spinal healthcare.

Category	Barrier	Technical Detail	Clinical/Operational Consequence
Imaging and Model Generalizability	Cross-Vendor Imaging Variability	Heterogeneity in scanner vendor output (e.g., GE vs. Siemens vs. Philips) causes domain shift in AI models; non-uniform slice thickness and FOV distort CNN feature extraction layers.	Decreased classification precision for compression fractures; high false-negative rates in under-standardized imaging environments.
Hardware-Induced Artifacts	Metallic Implant Interference	Titanium-induced susceptibility artifacts in T1/T2 MRI sequences disrupt segmentation accuracy in deep neural networks like SpineNet and V-Net variants.	Invalidated predictions in post-fusion patients; potential for underestimation of central canal and foraminal compromise.
Pathological Heterogeneity	Low Representation of Rare Tumors	Model sensitivity drops when exposed to rare presentations (e.g., sacral chordomas, extradural myxopapillary ependymomas) due to weak class priors and minimal edge-case training data.	False negatives in tumor surveillance; unreliable outputs for oncological follow-up assessments.
Training Data Bias	Geographic and Socioeconomic Overfitting	Training sets skewed toward tertiary care centers cause latent space misalignment for rural/underserved demographics; manifests as calibration drift in diagnostic AI systems.	Inaccurate prioritization in triage algorithms; potential exacerbation of healthcare disparities.

Table 2. *Cont.*

Category	Barrier	Technical Detail	Clinical/Operational Consequence
Model Explainability	Opacity in Neural Attribution Maps	Lack of saliency map interpretability or explainable AI (XAI) frameworks in real-time decision support; attention-based models still fall short in spine-specific pathologies.	Limited clinician trust in AI output; inability to validate or refute system recommendations during multidisciplinary rounds.
Infrastructure and Cost	High-Cost HPC Requirements	Inference latency optimization via GPU clusters (e.g., NVIDIA A100) requires capital investment exceeding $500k; suboptimal throughput without federated inference pipelines.	Barriers to adoption in rural and small private clinics; delayed implementation in mid-tier health systems.
Regulatory and Legal Complexity	Validation of Continuous Learning Systems	Regulatory frameworks not equipped for post-deployment model drift; challenge in validating self-updating AI modules under FDA's Good Machine Learning Practice (GMLP) guidelines.	Post-market liability ambiguity; disincentivizes procurement by risk-averse hospital administrators.
Workflow and Physician Engagement	Non-Interoperability with Legacy EHRs	Lack of native HL7/FHIR compliance in AI tools (e.g., DeepScribe); interface incompatibility leads to fragmented data workflows and redundancy in documentation.	Cognitive overload and duplication of work; rejection by high-volume providers.
Patient-Centric Barriers	Privacy Anxiety from Data Breaches	2024 cyberattack exposure of biometric and imaging datasets undermines patient confidence in AI-driven diagnostics; hesitancy persists even with federated learning protocols.	Consent withdrawal and decreased utilization of AI-assisted care; limits scalability of patient-facing applications.

2.4. Risk of Bias and Validation Considerations

To assess generalizability and real-world relevance, we prioritized studies that included external validation cohorts (e.g., SpineNetV2, validated in 2022–2024), FDA-approved platforms (e.g., HealthVCF, 2020 [7,8]; Aidoc, 2021 [1,13,14,48]), or independent cross-institutional replication. Risk of bias was addressed by identifying overfitting to synthetic datasets, geographic underrepresentation (e.g., urban-biased cohorts in CT-Spine1K [49,50]), and algorithmic opacity (e.g., black-box decision-making in sentiment analysis tools). Studies were cross-referenced with regulatory databases and critical evaluations (e.g., Clark et al., 2023 [20]; Chouffani El Fassi et al., 2024 [51]) to ensure proper documentation of clinical applicability.

3. Current Applications of AI in Imaging and Radiological Analysis

3.1. Automated Detection and Classification of Spinal Pathologies

AI, and more importantly, the resultant sophisticated deep learning algorithms, are increasingly capable of detecting and classifying complex pathological conditions, largely changing clinical practice. Convolutional neural networks (CNNs) are a class of deep learning models designed to process images by automatically learning which visual features matter for a task (for example, detecting lesions on an X-ray or classifying a scan). Rather than requiring manually engineered image descriptors, CNNs ingest large, labeled imaging datasets and build a hierarchy of spatial features: early processing emphasizes simple patterns (edges, textures), while deeper processing combines those elements into organ- or pathology-level representations. This hierarchical, data-driven feature learning is a practical reason CNNs have advanced diagnostic image analysis. [24]

In clinical practice CNNs are applied to both image-level tasks (e.g., classification such as "tumor present/absent") and pixel-level tasks (e.g., segmentation or localization), and they can produce auxiliary outputs such as heatmaps that help indicate influential regions. Their performance depends strongly on the quality and quantity of annotated training data and on robust validation, but when well-trained, they achieve high sensitivity and specificity across many imaging tasks [25,26,52–55]. (See Appendix A for technical details.)

Convolutional neural networks (CNNs) are increasingly integrated into routine radiographic evaluation of the spine. They can automate the detection, localization, and characterization of fractures and other pathologies across modalities, thereby reducing missed injuries and accelerating diagnosis. Research studies across radiography, CT, and dual-energy X-ray absorptiometry (DXA) demonstrate the breadth and performance of modern CNN approaches. On plain thoracolumbar radiographs, a deep convolutional neural network achieved an accuracy of 86.0%, sensitivity of 84.7%, and specificity of 87.3% for vertebral fracture detection; a performance that was non-inferior to orthopedic and spine surgeons [29]. On CT, a multistage system combining U-Net segmentation with graph convolutional networks (U-GCN) for detection, localization, and AO classification of acute thoracolumbar vertebral body fractures demonstrated vertebra-level sensitivity of 95.23%, accuracy of 97.93%, and specificity of 98.35% [56]. In DXA-based vertebral fracture assessment, an ensemble of CNNs achieved an area under the curve (AUC) of 0.94 with a sensitivity of 87.4% and a specificity of 88.4% for vertebral fracture identification; importantly, fractures identified by the CNNs predicted future nonvertebral and hip fractures comparably to expert readers, underscoring prognostic as well as diagnostic utility [30]. Recent reviews confirm that these AI models achieve very high diagnostic accuracy, especially for vertebral fractures. In one 2024 meta-analysis of 40 studies, AI tools yielded AUROC $\approx$ 0.92 for osteoporotic vertebral fracture diagnosis (and AUROC $\approx$ 0.87 overall for vertebral compression fractures) [36]. These pooled results reinforce that CNNs routinely approach or exceed expert radiologist performance in spine imaging.

Cervical spine findings mirror these advances. A hybrid transfer-learning approach that combined Inception-ResNet-v2 with U-Net for CT-based cervical vertebra fracture detection reported an overall accuracy of 98.44% on a large test set, outperforming radiologist predictions [31]. Likewise, a U-Net–based segmentation pipeline detected 87.2% of cervical spine fractures with a low false-positive rate, supporting its deployment in trauma workflows where rapid, reliable triage is critical [32]. Similarly, CNNs have shown excellent accuracy on cervical spine X-rays. Liawrungrueang et al. (2024) trained a CNN on lateral C-spine radiographs and achieved 92.1% overall accuracy for fracture detection (sensitivity $\approx$ 88.6%, specificity $\approx$ 95.7%), demonstrating that deep learning can reliably flag cervical fractures even on standard X-ray films [57]. Together, these modality-spanning results show that CNNs can match or exceed clinician performance for many spine-imaging tasks, offering standardized, fast screening and level-by-level characterization that augment radiologist interpretation and improve the timeliness of care. While some studies highlight limitations in generalizability, scan mode sensitivity, or reduced performance in certain clinical scenarios, the overall body of evidence supports the diagnostic utility of CNNs for this application [35,58–60]. Multiple systematic reviews and meta-analyses, as well as large cohort studies, consistently report that CNNs achieve high accuracy, sensitivity, and specificity for vertebral fracture detection on radiographs and related imaging modalities, often matching or approaching expert clinician performance [30,33,34,36,61].

Given their effectiveness, there has been a push for creation of commercial CNNs aimed at being implemented in hospital workflow, such as the Zebra Medical Vision's FDA-cleared HealthVCF. HealthVCF version 5.1.1 is a CNN based software that accurately detects moderate-to-severe vertebral compression fractures (VCFs), which seamlessly integrates into the existing hospital Picture Archive and Communication (PAC) infrastructures [7], thus enabling the automatic transfer and analysis of CT scans without manual intervention [7]. In the detection of moderate-to-severe (Grade 2–3) VCFs, HealthVCF has demonstrated strong performance. A study focusing on incidental fracture detection using HealthVCF on chest and abdominal CT scans reported an overall diagnostic accuracy of 89.6% (95% CI: 87.4–91.5%) for moderate-to-severe VCFs [62]. This study detailed a sensitivity of 73.8%, a specificity of 92.7%, and an NPV of 94.8% [62].

Beyond its general accuracy, HealthVCF was able to identify fractures that radiologists failed to report in 42.8% of positive scans, and it identified 38 additional ones from the scans [62]. These findings highlight HealthVCF's ability to achieve diagnostic performance non-inferior to human specialists and, sometimes, even detect fractures missed by human radiologists. Given these findings, AI can become a crucial safety net in clinical practice, helping to reduce human error, enhancing diagnostic completeness. Its integration into radiological workflow for fracture identification can help improve overall patient safety and quality of care. This augmentation of human capabilities is particularly valuable in high-volume settings where subtle findings might otherwise be overlooked.

In practice, these AI accuracies have been translated into clinical tools. For example, an FDA-cleared CNN triage system (Aidoc) for acute cervical spine fractures reported ~94.8% overall diagnostic accuracy (sensitivity $\approx$ 89.8%, specificity $\approx$ 95.3%) in one large study [63]. However, a subsequent real-world evaluation of the same Aidoc algorithm showed lower sensitivity (~54.9%) [63], highlighting that performance can vary across settings. Nonetheless, these results illustrate that modern AI platforms can achieve radiologist-level accuracy in spine fracture detection, though careful validation in diverse populations is needed.

Besides fractures, CNNs have been applied extensively in lumbar spine MRI to identify degenerative disk diseases. For example, herniated disks on axial T2 MRI can be detected and graded by deep learning models. Zhang et al. developed a two-stage deep model (Faster R-CNN for detection + ResNeXt101 for classification) to identify and grade lumbar disk herniation according to the Michigan State University (MSU) classification [64]. Their model achieved high detection accuracy (mean intersection over union $\approx$0.82 internally and 0.70 on an external set) and correctly classified herniation grade in about 87.7% of cases (internal test) [64]. In other words, the CNN could rapidly draw bounding boxes around disks and assign a herniation grade with "high consistency" to expert radiologists [64]. This illustrates a general workflow: a CNN first finds the disk (or region of interest) and then classifies its pathology. Since the MSU grading in this study was more objective than some older schemes, the model's agreement with surgeons was high, indicating such systems could standardize interpretations and even potentially flag cases needing surgery.

CNNs can also grade disk degeneration (e.g., Pfirrmann grades). For instance, a recent YOLOv5-based model simultaneously detected and graded disk degeneration, herniation, and high-intensity zones on lumbar MRI [65]. It achieved precisions in the range of ~0.80–0.90 and recall ~0.84–0.94 for detecting disk herniations and degeneration (with Cohen's kappa ~0.84 between the model and a senior surgeon) [65]. Such multi-task models integrate several classification steps into one network, improving efficiency. The study supports the notion that CNNs can automatically identify disk pathology on MRI (i.e., locating the affected disk and providing an objective severity grade) with performance rivaling human readers.

Lumbar spinal stenosis (LSS) is another area where CNNs have shown promise. Tumko et al. (2024) designed a three-stage CNN: one stage segments relevant anatomy, and two stages separately classify stenosis for central canal, lateral recess, and foraminal regions [66]. On an external test set of 150 MRI studies, their model's detection of any stenosis and its grading (normal/mild/moderate/severe) was comparable to a panel of radiologists. In fact, the model's sensitivity and specificity for detecting each subtype were very high, e.g., for central stenosis the CNN achieved sensitivity of 0.971 and area under the receiving operating chrematistics curve of 0.963, exceeding the average radiologist (0.786 and 0.842, respectively) [66]. This study suggests that CNNs can detect and classify LSS comparable to radiologists. Likewise, Hallinan et al. (2021) [37] trained a CNN to identify central canal, lateral recess, and foraminal stenosis in lumbar MRI. Their deep model's agreement (κ ~0.92–0.96) with subspecialist radiologists was "almost perfect" for dichotomous classification of stenosis (normal/mild vs. moderate/severe). In other words, whether for assigning a grade or simply flagging significant stenosis, CNN-based tools can match the accuracy of experienced neuroradiologists in lumbar spine MRI [37]. These studies suggest that automated lumbar stenosis detection could improve efficiency and consistency in MRI reporting. AI has similarly excelled in other spine diagnostic tasks. For example, deep learning pipelines can estimate scoliosis Cobb angles with error $\lesssim 3.5^{\circ}$ [67] matching human variability, and recent YOLOv8-based models for lumbar disk herniation detection achieved mAP $\approx$ 0.78 in validation sets [67]. These results confirm that AI tools now rival experts across a broad range of spine imaging diagnoses.

While some AI models are focused on detecting pathologies traditionally identified by radiologists, radiomics focuses on capturing patterns on radiographical images that are not visible to the human eye [38]. Radiomic models extract hundreds of features (e.g., intensity histograms, shape descriptors, texture matrices) from standard medical images (e.g., MRI, CT, X-ray). They then apply mathematical algorithms to quantify the spatial distribution of voxel intensities and their interrelationships, turning visual cues (e.g., differences in intensity, shape, texture) into numeric biomarkers [38]. In practice, a region of interest (e.g., a spinal disk or vertebra) is segmented by first-order (e.g., intensity), second-order (e.g., texture), and higher-order (e.g., wavelet or LoG-filtered) features [38]. These features are then compounded and fed into machine-learning models, augmenting standard radiology with objective indicators of subtle pathology.

The application of radiomics in spine relation pathologies ranges from grading spinal degeneration to determining ideologies of infectious spondylitis. For example, Xie et al. (2024) developed an MRI radiomics workflow to automatically classify cervical disk degeneration [68]. They extracted ~924 features from segmented disks on T1- and T2-weighted MRI and trained a random forest classifier. The combined T1–T2 model achieved a test AUC $\approx$ 0.95 for distinguishing low-grade from high-grade degeneration [68]. Crucially, higher-order texture features accounted for ~80% of the model's predictive power [68], implying that subtle textural heterogeneity in the disk (imperceptible on routine MRI) drove the diagnosis. In other words, radiomics quantified microscopic variations in nucleus pulposus signal and annular appearance that are only qualitatively appreciated on standard images. This automated approach could standardize disk degeneration assessment, reducing dependence on subjective Pfirrmann grading.

Radiomics also enhances tumor characterization and prognostication in the spine. For instance, spinal multiple myeloma and metastatic lesions often look similar on MRI, but Cao et al. (2024) showed that a radiomics model using T2 and contrast-enhanced T1 MRI could distinguish myeloma from metastasis with a ~86% accuracy (AUC $\approx$ 0.87) [39]. In this study hundreds of texture and shape features were combined in a classifier, yielding good differential performance that would be difficult by eye alone. Beyond diagnosis, radiomics can predict treatment response; in spinal metastases treated with stereotactic radiotherapy, Chen et al. (2023) [41] found that radiomic features from pre-treatment

MRI improved outcome prediction. Their combined radiomics–clinical model achieved AUC ≈ 0.83 for local control (versus AUC ≈ 0.73 using clinical factors alone). In other words, radiomic signatures on baseline MRI (e.g., reflecting tumor heterogeneity, edema, etc.) carried prognostic information inaccessible by conventional review. These examples illustrate that radiomics encodes latent biologic information in tumors (e.g., cell density, angiogenesis, necrosis) into quantifiable metrics, sharpening diagnostic and predictive accuracy in spine oncology.

Radiomics has likewise revealed hidden cues in non-neoplastic spine disorders. In infectious spondylitis, MRI radiomic signatures can differentiate etiologies that overlap with imaging. Qin et al. (2025) [69] extracted hundreds of radiomic features from spine MRIs in patients with tuberculous, brucellar, or pyogenic spondylitis and built a classifier model. The resulting nomogram achieved AUC ≈ 0.92 in training and ≈0.87 in testing, effectively distinguishing the three infection types. The authors concluded that their radiomics model could "gradually differentiate tuberculous spondylitis, brucellosis spondylitis, and pyogenic spondylitis", a level of detail beyond routine MRI interpretation [69]. In a different domain, CT radiomics has been used to predict osteoporotic fracture risk. For example, Yang et al. (2025) analyzed postoperative spine CT scans of patients treated with vertebroplasty and found that a model combining CT-radiomic features with clinical factors predicted adjacent-level fracture (AUC ≈ 0.86) [40]. This suggests that radiomics can capture minute bone texture and density variations (microarchitecture deterioration) not apparent on standard images, flagging patients at high fracture risk.

Overall, these studies demonstrate that radiomics systematically uncovers image features (e.g., texture, shape, intensity patterns) that are usually imperceivable by the naked eye. By transforming subtle imaging heterogeneity into quantitative biomarkers, radiomics augments conventional spine imaging and enhances diagnostic precision in conditions ranging from degenerative disk disease to tumors, infections, and fractures. In essence, radiomics provides additional data beyond visual inspection, enabling earlier detection and more accurate characterization of spine pathology.

Despite their promise, current AI tools in spine imaging still require rigorous validation across diverse patient populations, careful integration into clinical workflows, and demonstration of consistent performance, as they are not yet universally equivalent to expert clinicians. Evidence from real-world evaluations highlights this concern. For example, researchers who processed approximately 10,000 CT scans with HealthVCF at a Danish hospital reported a sensitivity of 0.68 (68%, 95% CI 0.581–0.776) and a specificity of 0.91 (91%, 95% CI 0.89–0.928) [42]. The investigators noted that the algorithm's performance was "poorer than expected" and concluded that the tested version was "not generalizable to the Danish population," highlighting potential variability in real-world clinical settings [42]. While initial studies on HealthVCF have shown robust metrics, the observed lack of generalizability in a real-world setting underscores a critical challenge for all AI models: their consistent effectiveness across diverse patient populations and varied clinical environments.

The urgency of addressing this limitation is amplified by the fact that numerous AI systems entered clinical practice without undergoing thorough validation by the U.S. Food and Drug Administration (FDA) prior to 2025. Clark et al. examined 119 medical devices marketed as AI- or ML-enabled and found that 23 (19.3%) displayed discrepancies or ambiguities between their advertised capabilities and actual FDA clearance [20]. Moreover, many AI/ML tools undergo validation using synthetic or "phantom" datasets, such as Generative Adversarial Networks (GANs), which often fail to capture the complexity of real-world clinical conditions. Supporting this concern, Chouffani El Fassi et al. reported that

226 of 521 FDA-approved AI-enabled clinical devices lacked peer-reviewed validation and were not trained on genuine patient data [51]. These findings emphasize the critical need for strengthened regulatory oversight, stricter validation requirements, and mechanisms for continuous post-market monitoring. Without clinically representative training data and real-time performance auditing, so-called "shadow" AI systems risk perpetuating bias, jeopardizing patient safety, and obscuring liability.

3.2. Advanced Morphometric Analysis and Quantitative Assessment

AI-driven segmentation is rapidly transforming spinal radiographic imaging by automating the precise delineation and labeling of vertebral bodies, intervertebral disks, neural foramina, and other anatomical landmarks. Automated segmentation and labeling remove much of the repetitive manual workload, reduce inter-observer variability, and create the consistent regions of interest required for downstream quantification (e.g., Cobb angles, Pfirrmann grading, canal cross-sectional area). By converting anatomy into structured, pixel-accurate masks, these tools enable reproducible measurements, longitudinal monitoring, and the reliable extraction of radiomic features that feed diagnostic and prognostic models.

New tools, such as SpineNet by Jamaludin et al., represent a landmark achievement in comprehensive spinal analysis, as they can automate segmentation and label spinal structures across various imaging modalities (e.g., CT, MRI) [10,70]. This automated process allows for the one unified system to grade disk degeneration (e.g., Pfirrmann grades), endplate defects, bone marrow changes, foraminal stenosis, and spondylolisthesis [10,70]. Fortunately, many similar platforms are emerging, and external validation studies have confirmed that these platforms are beginning to show consistent performance across different institutional, socioeconomic, and patient settings (e.g., rural, urban, etc.) [9,11].

Other networks such as *Spine-GAN* have extended this approach by performing semantic segmentation of spinal anatomy: it segments intervertebral disks, vertebral bodies, and neural foramina on MRI to aid in diagnosing foraminal stenosis and degeneration [71]. More recent multi-stage pipelines combine diverse inputs: for instance, Windsor et al. (2024) describe an AI that first detects and labels vertebral bodies across T1, T2, and STIR MRI sequences and then applies Transformer-based networks to diagnose disk pathology, cord compression, metastases, and vertebral fractures [43]. Such end-to-end systems effectively replicate an expert reader by linking image registration and diagnosis in one workflow.

Critically, these advanced AI platforms are beginning to prove robust across settings. Open-source models like SpineNetV2, an updated second-generation version of SpinNet, have undergone external validation in independent datasets. In one study, SpineNetV2 showed "strong performance" in predicting disk pathologies: Cohen's κ and related metrics exceeded 0.7 for most evaluated features, although foraminal stenosis and herniation were somewhat harder [3]. These results demonstrate that a model trained at one site can generalize with high reliability elsewhere. The availability of large, annotated datasets is accelerating progress: for example, the CTSpine1K resource contains over 11,000 labeled vertebrae (healthy and diseased), providing a rich training ground for segmentation algorithms [49]. When such algorithms are open-sourced or deployed via federated networks (e.g., TriNetX), researchers worldwide can contribute to and refine AI models, improving their performance across patient populations.

These AI automated segmentation advances are also opening new modality frontiers. Ultrasound spine images are notoriously difficult for analysis given their low contrast and speckled noise, but attention-based deep networks have made segmentation feasible. Jiang et al. (2022) introduced the ultrasound global guidance block network (UGBNet), which incorporates spatial and channel attention to segment vertebral landmarks in noisy ultrasound scans [72]. In their scoliosis study, UGBNet significantly outperformed baseline models, achieving a Dice segmentation score of 0.742 [72]. By focusing on long-range spatial context and feature channels, UGBNet can reliably trace bone contours that were previously hard to see. With such tools, clinicians can use portable ultrasound to visualize spine curvature in real time. In effect, attention-augmented U-Nets turn ultrasounds into more interpretable images, expanding AI spine analysis into new modalities.

AI is similarly transforming quantitative measurements of spinal alignment. Conventional manual Cobb angle measurements have 95% confidence intervals on the order of 4–8°, while deep learning has markedly improved consistency with mean absolute errors consistently below 3° (Figure 1) [18]. Galbusera et al. demonstrated that a CNN can automatically measure lumbar lordosis, thoracic kyphosis, sagittal vertical alignment, coronal Cobb angle, and pelvic parameters (e.g., frontal pelvic asymmetry, sacral slope, pelvic tilt, and pelvic incidence) on whole-spine radiographs with accuracy parallel to human evaluators (Figure 2) [73]. In other words, AI can quickly replicate the full battery of clinical angles that a spine surgeon would manually compute, but in a fraction of the time and with less variability. Subsequent studies have extended these models to very large cohorts, showing that AI can process thousands of archived spine films to derive alignment statistics that would otherwise take months of manual work [44].

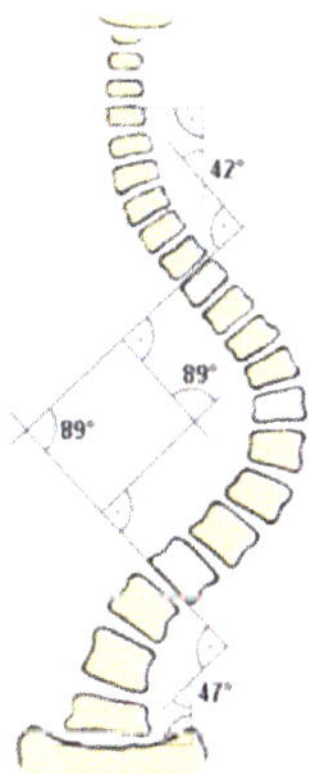

Figure 1. Cobb angle measurement in scoliosis. Permission is granted to copy, distribute and/or modify this document under the terms of the GNU Free Documentation License, Version 1.2 or any later version published by the Free Software Foundation, with no Invariant Sections, no Front-Cover Texts, and no Back-Cover Texts. This file is licensed under the Creative Commons Attribution-Share Alike 3.0 Unported license with permission from Wikimedia Commons [74].

Deep networks have also been developed specifically for landmark localization. Yeh et al. (2021) trained models on 2,210 lateral spine X-rays of diverse pathology to detect 45 anatomical landmarks and automatically compute 18 key sagittal parameters (e.g., C2–C7 angle, SVA, pelvic tilt) [18]. Their ensemble model's measurements were highly correlated with expert annotations; in fact, they matched clinician reliability in 15 of the 18 parameters [18]. This approach, first localizing landmarks, then calculating angles, means AI can handle even off-center or suboptimal films by focusing on consistent internal references. In practice, this yields near-expert performance on tasks like Cobb angle measurement, even if the X-ray is rotated or partially cut off.

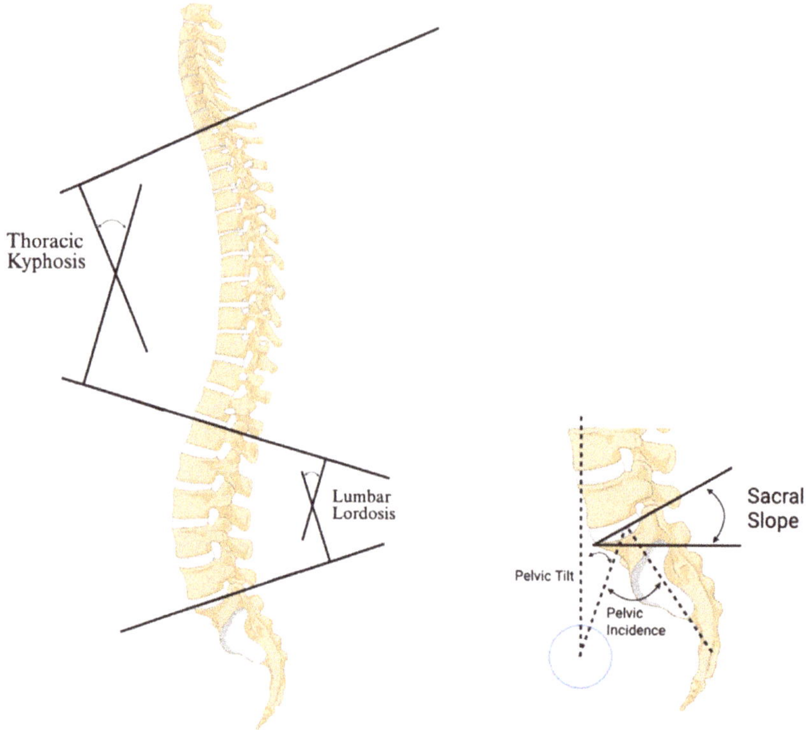

Figure 2. Graphical representation of spinal and pelvic alignment parameters that convolutional neural networks (CNNs) can automatically extract from whole-spine radiographs. Shown here are thoracic kyphosis, lumbar lordosis, sacral slope, pelvic tilt, and pelvic incidence. CNN models have also been demonstrated to measure additional parameters such as sagittal vertical alignment, coronal Cobb angles, and frontal pelvic asymmetry with accuracy comparable to human evaluators. Figure created with BioRender.com.

These capabilities are being packaged into practical tools. For instance, CobbAngle Pro is a smartphone app that employs deep learning to analyze mobile photos of spine X-rays and output scoliosis curvature. Field users (e.g., combat medics or rural clinicians) can simply photograph the radiograph, and the app will identify vertebral endplates and draw Cobb angles automatically. Published reports indicate this app's measurements agree closely with expert readers across mild, moderate, and severe scoliosis [45,46]. Since it is commercially available and designed for ease of use, CobbAngle Pro exemplifies how AI-driven morphometry is reaching frontline practice: it allows clinicians to perform reliable alignment analysis at the bedside or in austere settings, freeing them from tedious manual angle calculations [45,46].

Another advanced development is tissue segmentation. Models are now demonstrating automated quantification of paravertebral muscle characteristics, including cross-sectional areas and fatty infiltration patterns that correlate with functional outcomes and disability measures. A primary example of this is the CTSpine1K dataset, which has annotations for over 11,000 vertebrae including both healthy and pathological specimens [47]. The main benefit of CTSpine1k and related datasets, especially open-source datasets such as those available on TrinetX [47,50], is that they can objectively measure muscle quality and quantity on a large scale, thus enabling smaller research groups to study pathology and incidence without necessarily needed an IRB-dictated patient cohort.

Another significant application is AI-enabled image reconstruction and enhancement. Modern imaging modalities, such as MRI and CT, often face trade-offs between image resolution, signal-to-noise ratio, and scan time. AI tools, such as those developed by NVIDIA Clara Imaging, use deep learning to reconstruct clearer, higher-resolution images from lower-quality raw data [50]. This not only improves diagnostic confidence but also allows for faster scans, reducing patient discomfort and motion artifacts, which is particularly useful for spinal imaging where movement can compromise image quality.

Modern spine MRI and CT scans face inherent trade-offs between scan time, resolution, and noise. Recent deep learning (DL) methods have begun to overcome these limits by reconstructing high-quality images from undersampled or noisy data. In spine MRI, DL reconstruction can dramatically speed up exams while maintaining (or improving) image quality. For example, a prospective study of lumbar spine MRI found that a DL-reconstructed turbo spin-echo protocol (TSE-DL) cut scan time by ~45% (i.e., 2:55 vs. 5:17 min) versus standard imaging, without compromising overall image quality or pathology detection [75]. Similarly, another clinical series reported a ~61% reduction in exam time with DL reconstruction, with the accelerated MRI showing significantly less noise and artifacts, higher sharpness, and even greater diagnostic confidence than the standard scans [76,77]. In short, these DL-MRI techniques allow faster spine scans (reducing patient discomfort and motion blur) while preserving or boosting image clarity.

DL is also used to generate or enhance MRI sequences that would otherwise require extra scan time. For instance, a synthetic STIR (Short Tau Inversion Recovery) image can be generated by a neural network from routine T1/T2 images. One study showed that synthetic STIR reduced the dedicated STIR acquisition by ~3 min, yet yielded significantly higher signal-to-noise ratio (SNR) and contrast-to-noise ratio (CNR) than a standard STIR; radiologists found the synthetic STIR images diagnostically interchangeable with the real STIR [78]. Likewise, in cervical spine imaging, applying DL reconstruction to zero-echo-time (ZTE) MRI, a CT-like sequence, greatly improved bone detail. Blinded readers rated the DL-enhanced ZTE images as having "superior image quality and bone visualization" compared to conventional ZTE, making it easier to evaluate osseous stenosis [79]. These examples show that AI can synthesize or enhance MRI contrasts, speeding protocols and improving visualization of both soft tissue and bone, without losing diagnostic information [78,79].

In spine CT, AI-powered reconstruction mainly targets noise reduction and dose savings. Modern scanners already use iterative reconstruction, but DL reconstruction (e.g., GE's TrueFidelity or ClariCT.AI) can push quality further. In one 2025 clinical study, lumbar CT scans were processed with a DL denoising algorithm, ClariCT.AI, and compared to standard filtered back-projection [80]. The DL-reconstructed CT showed a much higher sensitivity for detecting disk herniations (60% vs. 44%) and higher specificity for stenosis than standard CT; radiologists rated the DL-reconstructed CT images as having superior image quality and diagnostic confidence [80]. In other words, the AI denoising made subtle soft tissue findings on CT more conspicuous, improving clinical performance. Phantom studies echo these benefits: an experiment using GE Healthcare's DL image reconstruction model, TrueFidelity, showed that deep learning reconstruction dramatically reduces noise and boosts spatial resolution and lesion detectability compared to hybrid iterative methods [81]. This implies that for a given image quality, radiation dose could be substantially lowered using DL image reconstruction techniques.

AI can also fuse modalities to enhance spine evaluation. A striking example is MRI-based synthetic CT (sCT) of the spine. In a multicenter study of acute cervical spine trauma, an AI algorithm generated CT-like bone images from routine MRI. The sCT images detected 97.3% of fractures (sensitivity) and showed near-perfect agreement with actual CT in measuring vertebral heights and alignment [82]. The authors concluded that sCT is a "promising, radiation-free" approach with accuracy comparable to CT [82]. In practice, this means a patient could undergo one MRI exam and obtain both soft tissue and CT-like bone information, reducing the need for a separate CT.

Together, these studies illustrate the real-world clinical value of AI reconstructions. DL-enhanced MRI protocols allow substantially shorter spine exams (often 40–60% faster) while maintaining or improving image quality [76,77]. DL-denoised CT scans enable a lower radiation dose with equal or better disease detection [80,81]. Synthesized sequences like STIR or ZTE-DL maintain full diagnostic content with far less scan time [81]. Additionally, multimodal tools like sCT combine the strengths of MRI and CT in one step [82]. Many of these AI reconstructions are now integrated into commercial systems (for example, FDA-cleared software like SubtleMR uses DL back-projection networks trained on millions of MRI images) so that radiology departments can apply them in routine spine imaging [76].

3.3. AI's Ability to Enhance Workflow

AI is increasingly being applied to optimize clinical workflow in spinal imaging. One key frontier is scanning triage, where AI algorithms automatically prioritize studies that show critical or urgent findings, ensuring that radiologists review these cases first and reducing delays in time-sensitive diagnoses [83,84].

AI triage tools are increasingly deployed to flag urgent spinal pathologies and streamline radiology workflow. For example, Aidoc's FDA-cleared cervical-spine fracture algorithm automatically analyzes trauma CT scans and prioritizes patients with potential fractures by sending them to the top of the radiologist's patient list [13]. In practice this means the radiologist is alerted to subtle C-spine fractures within minutes.

This quick alert helps reduce diagnostic time; researchers found a 16 min (46%) reduction in time to diagnosis for positive cases of cervical spine fractures when using Aidoc compared to traditional methods [63]. These spine-imaging triage systems that automatically detect acute findings (e.g., cord compression or vertebral fractures) and push those studies up the queue can substantially improve radiologist efficiency. Faster turnaround for urgent cases not only speeds diagnosis but can improve outcomes: the American College of Radiology notes that AI detection of acute cord compression could "reduce turnaround time and improve quality of care," potentially averting paralysis or other deficits [85].

In sum, AI triage in spine imaging ensures that critical findings are recognized and reported more rapidly. Systems like Aidoc's C-spine algorithm platform illustrate how deep learning can flag urgent pathology and automatically notify clinicians. This process improves overall workflow by focusing radiologist attention on high-priority cases first, reducing the risk of missed injuries, and shortening diagnostic delays. Early clinical results suggest that these tools can significantly cut report wait times and length of stay for patients. Moreover, opportunistic AI screening (e.g., algorithms that detect vertebral fragility fractures on routine CT) can identify otherwise undetected spine injuries in thousands of patients. By integrating AI alerts into the PACS and reporting system, radiology departments can achieve faster turnaround, more consistent detection of acute spine findings, and more efficient communication with treating teams. However, recent external validation studies have highlighted important limitations, particularly in detecting chronic fractures and subtle pathological changes amid varying fracture characteristics and imaging quality [86,87]. This is a cautionary tale to developers and hospital administration alike: all parties must ensure continuous model refinement and, if needed, failure mode analysis to optimize clinical performance.

Large language models (LLMs) and Natural Language Processing-driven (NLP-driven) tools are beginning to automate the creation of radiology reports from spine imaging data. Many current systems combine image analysis (e.g., segmentation, detection, measurements) with templated language output. For example, SmartSoft's FDA-cleared CoLumbo software Version 3 analyzes lumbar spine MRIs, identifying and measuring vertebral structures and pathologies, and then creates a detailed draft report with the findings that clinicians can edit [88]. Similarly, RemedyLogic's Radiology AI platform creates concise summaries on its findings after identifying abnormalities and incidental findings [89]. In practice, these systems pre-populate structured report templates with key observations (e.g., levels of stenosis, disk degeneration) and draft language, which the radiologist can then review and finalize. These reports in turn should help improve workflow and save radiologists' time. Studies have shown that LLM-assisted reporting can significantly reduce reporting time compared to conventional methods, with one study demonstrating a reduction from 8.95 to 6.76 min per report using summary-based workflows and LLM-generated templates, without compromising report quality [90]. Another study found that multimodal LLMs using minimal audio input reduced reporting time and corrections compared to conventional speech recognition workflows, while maintaining or improving report quality [91] LLMs also support multilingual and personalized reporting, further streamlining the process [92].

Beyond rule-based reporting, generative AI is also being introduced into radiology workflows. For instance, Nuance/Microsoft's PowerScribe Smart Impression uses an LLM to automatically draft the impression section of a report from the imaging findings that are highly rated for scientific terminology, coherence, and comprehensiveness; these reports either matched or exceeded human performance in clarity and completeness [93]. In a similar spirit, one study fine-tuned an 8-billion-parameter Llama-3 model on thousands of MRI and CT reports and found that the LLM could generate clinically accurate descriptions for new imaging exams [94]. These proof-of-concept systems illustrate how an LLM can ingest structured findings and output clinically sensible narrative text, thereby lightening the radiologist's workload and improving report uniformity.

Importantly, integrating AI outputs into the reporting workflow has proven efficiency benefits. For example, an "AI-to-structured-report" pipeline was developed for chest X-rays, in which AI findings automatically populate a structured report template. Reports generated with this pipeline were completed in significantly less time (mean ~67 s) than traditional free-text reports (~86 s) and were rated as higher quality [95]. Translating this to spine imaging, a similar workflow could automatically fill out a spine MRI or CT report with measurement values and descriptions (e.g., disk height, neural foramina size), vastly reducing administrative burden. In practice, these tools not only accelerate reporting but also standardize reports. Consistent language and structured output ensure that referring clinicians (e.g., surgeons, pain specialists, etc.) receive clear, comparable information across patients. By reducing repetitive transcription and variability, AI-generated preliminary reports help radiologists focus on complex interpretation and ensure that key findings are communicated efficiently and uniformly to the clinical team.

4. Surgical Planning and Robotic-Assisted Interventions

4.1. Advanced Preoperative Planning and Simulation

Artificial intelligence (AI) has transformed preoperative planning in spinal surgery, shifting the paradigm from generalized heuristics toward patient-specific, data-driven optimization. Traditional imaging review and surgeon experience remain foundational, but modern AI-powered platforms now extract detailed biomechanical and anatomical features from CT and MRI to build 3D reconstructions tailored to each patient [16]. These reconstructions are not static visual aids; they increasingly integrate predictive analytics, offering simulations of surgical trajectories, guide implant selection, and anticipated biomechanical stresses.

One significant development is the incorporation of finite element analysis (FEA) into AI-driven platforms. By simulating load-bearing mechanics under various conditions, FEA helps forecast implant longevity, risk of hardware failure, and the distribution of spinal stresses post-fusion [96]. Such modeling has direct clinical relevance, especially in osteoporotic patients or those undergoing multilevel fusions where the interaction between native bone and implants can be unpredictable.

Robotic platforms are embedding these tools into their workflows. The Mazor X Stealth Edition integrates predictive planning with robotic navigation, enabling surgeons to simulate screw placement in virtual environments before transferring the plan intraoperatively [17]. Similarly, the ExcelsiusGPS provides real-time feedback during execution, linking preoperative CT-based models with intraoperative adjustments that account for cortical thickness and bone mineral density. These features are particularly valuable in deformity or revision surgeries, where conventional anatomic landmarks are unreliable [17,19,97].

Peer-reviewed validation studies highlight the accuracy of such systems. Jia et al. demonstrated that an AI-driven planning algorithm designed screws that were not only larger and longer than those chosen manually, but also safer: 85.1% of AI-suggested screws achieved a Grade A accuracy (i.e., no cortical breach) compared to 64.9% in freehand techniques [98]. Similarly, a DL-based planning system using the nnU-Net architecture successfully segmented spinal anatomy and recommended trajectories on par with human experts, although its robustness across highly variable pathologies remains an open question [99].

Imaging innovation is extending planning into radiation-conscious domains. A study by Levi Chazen et al. showed that deep learning-reconstructed 3D MRI could mimic CT for pedicle screw planning, achieving nearly identical geometric accuracy [100]. This approach could significantly reduce patient exposure to ionizing radiation, especially in young or revision-prone populations.

The next frontier lies in adaptive, intelligent planning frameworks. The SafeRPlan model exemplifies this evolution, applying deep reinforcement learning (DRL) to refine screw trajectories intraoperatively. Importantly, it integrates safety filters to mitigate errors, representing a step toward autonomous yet surgeon-supervised planning systems [101]. Such "learning-in-action" methodologies mark a shift away from static preoperative designs toward continuously adaptive surgical strategies.

4.2. Robotic-Assisted Surgical Execution

Robotics in spine surgery is evolving from navigational assistance toward true AI-driven co-surgeons. Early systems like ROSA Spine or da Vinci SP functioned primarily as stabilizers for surgeon-guided trajectories, but modern platforms increasingly incorporate AI for dynamic adjustment and real-time control [102].

The VELYS™ Active Robotic-Assisted System, developed by DePuy Synthes with eCential Robotics, exemplifies this shift. FDA-cleared for use across cervical, thoracolumbar, and sacroiliac fusions, VELYS employs active robotics with independent navigation that recalibrates in response to intraoperative imaging and even subtle patient movement [102,103]. This millimeter-level adaptability is particularly critical in revision and deformity surgeries where unexpected tissue shifts or hardware interference often derail traditional navigation.

Medtronic has also advanced robotic intelligence by linking its Mazor platform with real-time analytics. The system integrates intraoperative CT, fluoroscopy, and

MRI, dynamically updating trajectories when deviations occur [104]. This "closed-loop" design reduces cumulative error, a limitation often cited in earlier-generation systems. Likewise, the eCential Robotics Spine Suite consolidates planning, navigation, and execution into one environment, enabling continuous recalibration across modalities and surgical phases [105–107].

Importantly, the trend is toward self-improving systems. Cloud-based federated learning allows robotic platforms to assimilate global datasets, tracking outcomes across institutions, while maintaining patient privacy [108]. This collective intelligence could eventually normalize performance across centers, reducing variability that currently depends heavily on surgeon skill and institutional resources.

Early experimental work suggests where this is heading: DRL-driven robotic frameworks that autonomously adjust trajectories in real time. These models learn to adapt to intraoperative conditions such as tissue deformation, with built-in safeguards to ensure error containment [101]. While still investigational, their translation into clinical robotics could herald a new era of semi-autonomous intraoperative adaptation.

4.3. Integration with Advanced Navigation and Guidance Systems

Navigation technologies remain the backbone of precision in spine surgery, but AI is fundamentally reshaping how guidance is achieved. Brainlab Curve Navigation, for example, now couples intraoperative CT and fluoroscopy with AI-based registration to accelerate setup and improve accuracy in pedicle screw placement [109]. This reduces not only operative time but also the radiation burden from repeated imaging.

Stryker's NAV3i expands this model through automatic landmark recognition, which simplifies registration in anatomically complex cases such as scoliosis [27]. Medtronic's StealthStation S8 similarly enhances adaptability by continuously correcting navigation drift using AI-driven error modeling [28]. These advances address one of the most persistent problems in spine navigation: progressive misalignment during surgery.

Zimmer Biomet's ROSA ONE Spine and NuVasive's Pulse platforms add further layers with AI-enabled augmented reality (AR) overlays. These overlays visualize planned screw paths directly in the surgical field, while feedback systems dynamically warn surgeons of deviation from optimal parameters [110–112]. Such human–machine synergy enables surgeons to anticipate complications in real time rather than respond reactively.

Emerging techniques now bypass traditional markers altogether. A deep neural network was recently used to segment the lumbar spine directly from RGB-D camera input, enabling AR-guided navigation with registration errors averaging ~1.2 mm and 100% pedicle screw accuracy in ex vivo testing [113]. Similarly, a modular hybrid system achieved ~1.1 mm accuracy using as few as three C-arm images per screw, underscoring the feasibility of combining AI-guided efficiency with reduced radiation exposure [114].

Together, these approaches illustrate the convergence of AI, robotics, and AR/VR into fully integrated surgical ecosystems, where each component strengthens the accuracy and safety of the others.

4.4. Functional Outcome Prediction and Treatment Optimization

Beyond intraoperative execution, AI is increasingly applied to predicting recovery and optimizing long-term outcomes. This is particularly relevant in spine surgery, where radiographic success does not always correlate with patient satisfaction or functional improvement.

Recent work with Graph Neural Networks (GNNs), GAN, and Transformer models demonstrates the potential of integrating diverse datasets, ranging from imaging biomarkers to psychosocial indices, to predict complications, pain persistence, or quality-of-life outcomes [115–118]. These models extend beyond statistical regression, uncovering nonlinear patterns invisible to conventional analytics.

NLP represents another frontier. By mining clinical notes, postoperative journals, or patient-reported text, NLP algorithms can quantify subtle psychological factors such as anxiety, resilience, or depressive sentiment that heavily influence recovery (Figure 3) [119–121]. Such insights could individualize rehabilitation strategies in ways radiographic assessment cannot.

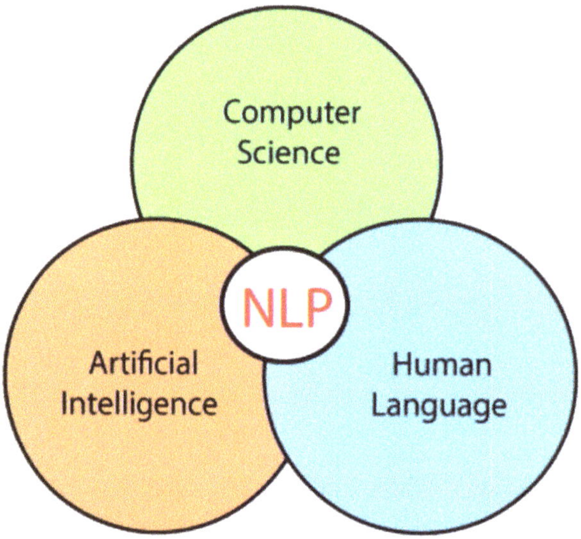

Figure 3. Diagram showing the hierarchy of Natural Language Processing. The depicted text is ineligible for copyright and therefore in the public domain because it is not a "literary work" or other protected type in sense of the local copyright law [122].

Wearable technology provides the data backbone for these predictive frameworks. Devices such as ActiGraph GT9X and WHOOP Strap 4.0 generate continuous physiological, activity, and sleep data [123,124]. When analyzed through AI models, these datasets create dynamic recovery profiles, guiding interventions like physiotherapy intensity or pain management titration. Edge AI and federated learning approaches allow such analyses while preserving patient privacy, enabling multicenter datasets to inform global predictive models [125].

Early pilot studies suggest that integrating intraoperative robotic performance metrics (e.g., screw placement accuracy, time to completion) with postoperative wearable-derived physiology may produce holistic predictions of recovery trajectories. Such models could ultimately drive adaptive, individualized rehabilitation regimens, optimizing both functional outcomes and patient satisfaction.

4.5. Cost-Effectiveness Analysis

Despite these technical advances, the sustainability of AI in spine surgery depends on its economic justification. Health systems operating under value-based care frameworks increasingly demand demonstration that technology improves outcomes relative to costs [126]. Yet, spine surgery lacks disease-specific quality-of-life (QOL) instruments that adequately capture its unique blend of functional, neurological, and psychosocial outcomes [74,127,128].

Cost-effectiveness studies of navigation and robotics generally report improved accuracy, shorter operating times, and reduced complication rates. However, high acquisition and maintenance costs, coupled with steep training curves, remain major barriers to adoption [129]. These findings underscore the need for comprehensive cost models that incorporate both direct (equipment, training, OR time) and indirect (rehabilitation, reoperation avoidance) variables.

Future frameworks may need to incorporate behavioral economics and complexity theory, assessing not just cost per procedure but how surgeon learning, institutional adoption, and interdisciplinary workflows evolve in response to AI integration [9,129]. Coupling these models with predictive outcome analytics could allow reimbursement structures that tie financial incentives directly to demonstrated patient-centered improvements.

5. Genomic Applications and Precision Medicine

5.1. Genome-Wide Association Studies in Spine Surgery Risk Assessment

Large-scale genome-wide association studies (GWAS) leveraging national biobanks (e.g., UK Biobank, FinnGen) are beginning to clarify the heritable architecture of spinal disease and perioperative risk. In surgically managed adult spinal deformity (ASD), a study of 540 patients identified 21 single-nucleotide polymorphisms (SNPs) associated with surgical risk, with the LDB2 variant (rs12913832) showing the most robust signal and implicating ectodermal differentiation pathways in spinal morphogenesis and repair [21,130–134]. Parallel meta-analyses for lumbar disk herniation (LDH) across three biobank cohorts reported 41 novel loci, implicating genes central to inflammatory signaling (IL6R), extracellular matrix composition (COL11A1), and Wnt/β-catenin regulation (DKK1)—pathways that mechanistically influence disk integrity and biomechanical behavior. For lumbar spinal stenosis (LSS), replicated associations near GFPT1 and AAK1 point to roles for glycosylation and synaptic vesicle trafficking in modulating neural vulnerability to compressive forces [132–136].

Translating these associations into clinical utility requires aggregation and contextualization. Polygenic risk scores (PRS) that combine genome-wide variant weights with clinical covariates (body-mass index, radiographic severity, comorbidity indices) now permit probabilistic stratification of patients for adverse outcomes, examples include heightened predicted risk for pseudarthrosis tied to SMAD3-related signaling and elevated reoperation probability in certain genetic strata [137,138]. Importantly, integrating GWAS signals with phenotypic features using machine learning models, where genomic data are fused with radiomics and clinician notes parsed by large language models, has improved prediction of early neurological deterioration and postoperative sepsis in ASD cohorts, enabling earlier, preemptive resource allocation [139]. Clinically actionable findings are emerging: carriers of CHST3 variants, which associate with degenerative disk phenotypes, may be prioritized for intensified rehabilitation or considered for targeted biologic strategies (e.g., matrix metalloproteinase inhibitors in MMP2-linked stenotic disease). These represent early but concrete instances of genomics informing individualized perioperative plans.

Beyond risk assessment, the field is exploring interventional genomics. Ongoing translational efforts and early-phase trials investigate gene-editing (e.g., CRISPR-Cas9) and small-molecule modulation of GWAS-implicated targets such as NFU1 in stenosis and GSDMC in inflammatory disk degeneration, highlighting a therapeutic horizon where genotype guides targeted molecular therapy in conjunction with surgical management [140].

5.2. Pharmacogenomics and Personalized Pain Management

Pharmacogenomics is increasingly relevant to postoperative analgesia and medication safety in spine surgery. Allelic variation in cytochrome P450 enzymes—principally CYP2D6 and CYP3A4—substantially influences opioid pharmacokinetics and clinical response: CYP2D6 poor metabolizers risk inadequate conversion of prodrugs such as codeine, whereas ultra-rapid metabolizers face overdose risk from active metabolites, a nuance critical for perioperative prescribing [141]. Clinical decision support systems (e.g., PharmCAT) and consensus resources from CPIC translate genotype (including OPRM1 rs1799971) into EHR-integrated prescribing guidance, enabling clinicians to tailor opioid selection or choose alternatives such as tapentadol or non-opioid adjuncts (e.g., duloxetine for COMT Val158Met carriers) [142–144]. Similarly, polymorphisms in inflammatory mediators, IL6 rs1800795 and TNF-α rs1800629, have been associated with differential NSAID efficacy and adverse-event profiles, informing safer anti-inflammatory choices in at-risk patients [145]. For bone healing, genetic variation in BMP2 (rs235768) and the vitamin D receptor (VDR rs731236) have been used to triage patients who may benefit from anabolic agents such as teriparatide to reduce nonunion risk following fusion [146,147]. Commercial pharmacogenomic panels (e.g., OneOme RightMed) are broadening their gene coverage and are increasingly incorporated into pre- and postoperative workflows to mitigate adverse events and optimize analgesic efficacy. Together with the shift toward non-addictive agents (gabapentin for neuropathic pain; SNRIs for centralized pain syndromes), these genomic tools support individualized, safer multimodal pain regimens in the post-opioid-epidemic era [148,149].

5.3. Multi-Omics Analysis

Integrative multi-omics platforms operationalize complex molecular datasets to delineate pathobiology and predict therapeutic response. Cloud-enabled pipelines (Seven Bridges, DNAnexus) now permit the harmonized analysis of genomics (GWAS/PheWAS), proteomics (e.g., Olink Target 96 inflammation assays), metabolomics (Metabolon HD4), and single-cell transcriptomics (10× Genomics) to map dysregulated pathways in spinal disease [150]. Proteomic profiling by proximity–extension assays has repeatedly identified elevations in IL-6 and COMP in degenerative disk disease, while high-throughput proteomics (Somalogic SomaScan 7K) has associated increased MMP-3 expression with subsequent pseudarthrosis, suggesting candidate biomarkers for failed fusion risk [151]. Machine learning frameworks such as DeepOmics now integrate these modalities, linking specific genomic variants (e.g., COL1A1 mutations) to downstream collagen dysregulation and ACAN variants to proteoglycan depletion and disk desiccation, thereby predicting which molecular phenotypes may respond to particular biologic or regenerative interventions [22]. As these multiomic signatures are validated longitudinally and embedded into clinical decision pipelines, they will enable precision stratification of patients for targeted biologics, optimized surgical timing, and personalized rehabilitation regimens.

6. Clinical Decision Support and Documentation Systems

6.1. Ambient Clinical Intelligence and Documentation Automation

Ambient clinical intelligence (ACI) platforms have substantially reconfigured documentation workflows in contemporary practice. Systems such as Nuance Dragon Ambient eXperience (DAX) and Suki AI combine advanced speech recognition with natural language processing to generate clinical notes directly from physician–patient conversations [23]. These platforms can diarize encounters, identify salient clinical findings, and structure documentation according to specialty-specific templates and guideline-driven frameworks. When integrated with electronic health records (EHRs), ACI tools enable scribes, nurses, and physician assistants to document more efficiently and with greater consistency, reducing duplication of effort across the care team.

Specialty-focused charting solutions further extend these capabilities. For example, Ambience Healthcare provides co-pilot functionality for pre-charting, real-time scribing, and automated post-visit summaries [48]. Its connectivity with major EHR vendors supports bidirectional data exchange and richer secondary analysis of clinical information [48]. Similarly, DeepScribe and Notable Health illustrate how deep learning-based systems can be tailored for orthopedics and spine care. These platforms are trained on large, domain-specific datasets so that their output reflects spine anatomy and pathology in addition to surface linguistic features; this allows for more clinically relevant error detection and correction than grammar-only dictation tools.

Across implementations, the principal reported benefit is a reduction in after-hours documentation and associated clerical burden, which can improve clinician work–life balance and reduce the risk of burnout. Importantly, these technologies are positioned as augmentative rather than replacement tools: clinicians retain supervisory control, reviewing and validating algorithm-generated content. This human–AI collaboration functions as a check-and-balance that both streamlines documentation and mitigates charting errors, while preserving clinician accountability and the integrity of the medical record.

6.2. Clinical Decision Support Systems

AI-enabled clinical decision support systems (CDSS) deliver real-time, evidence-based guidance to assist diagnosis, therapeutic selection, and management optimization in spine care. IBM Watson for Clinical Decision Support exemplifies the marriage of cognitive computing and clinical expertise, mining large bodies of medical literature together with patient-level data to produce tailored treatment recommendations [14,152]. Such systems can synthesize complex presentations to generate differential diagnoses, suggest treatment options, and estimate prognoses that reflect both current best evidence and individual patient characteristics.

Critical to their utility is the ability to integrate heterogeneous data streams (e.g., imaging features, demographics, comorbidities, and operative variables) to perform comprehensive risk stratification and outcome prediction. Continuous learning mechanisms permit these systems to incorporate new research findings and real-world outcomes, progressively refining their recommendations. Moreover, real-time analytics deliver dynamic risk updates as a patient's status evolves or as intraoperative information becomes available, enabling proactive adjustments to management plans that aim to optimize clinical outcomes.

7. Current Challenges, Limitations, and Implementation Barriers

7.1. Technical and Algorithmic Limitations

The adoption of novel AI technologies into routine spine care remains constrained by several interrelated technical and algorithmic limitations. Prominent examples illustrate limited generalizability: systems developed for cervical spine fracture detection (e.g., Aidoc) and joint assessment (e.g., Zebra Medical Vision's HealthVCF) have demonstrated performance drops when applied to imaging produced under different protocols or scanner vendors. Variations in slice thickness, field of view, and contrast administration commonly degrade model performance when these algorithms encounter unfamiliar datasets. In practice, complete harmonization across major vendors (e.g., GE, Siemens, Philips) is unrealistic, and algorithm robustness must therefore be addressed through design and deployment strategies rather than idealized standardization [15,153,154].

Hardware-related artifacts further complicate reliable performance. Metallic implants, frequent in revision spine surgery, produce signal distortions that have led to segmentation failures in systems such as SpineNet when processing MRI scans with titanium hardware [155]. These fragilities raise both patient-safety and economic concerns, because models require ongoing surveillance, periodic retraining, and software maintenance to remain clinically useful, increasing implementation and lifecycle costs.

Algorithmic limitations also arise from the intrinsic heterogeneity and rarity of certain pathologies. SpineNet and similar tools exhibit weaker performance in grading disk degeneration and quantifying spondylolisthesis for less common conditions; examples include sacral chordomas, which present atypical anatomy, histopathology, and metastatic patterns that are poorly represented in training sets [156–158]. Although enlarging and diversifying training datasets can mitigate some failures, it is neither practical nor feasible to expect any system to achieve perfect sensitivity and specificity across every rare presentation.

Dataset bias and representativeness are additional, persistent problems. Publicly available collections (e.g., CTSpine1K) and many institutional repositories disproportionately reflect urban, academic practice populations, leaving rural and underserved patient presentations underrepresented. Geographic, linguistic, and practice-pattern variations therefore create sampling biases that limit external validity. Retrospective curation further compounds the issue through selection effects. Consequently, no training corpus can be entirely comprehensive or error-free, an unavoidable constraint that must be acknowledged during model evaluation and clinical deployment.

Longitudinal assessment poses yet another technical challenge. Many current models are cross-sectional by design, inhibiting consistent tracking of disease progression across pre- and postoperative intervals. This limitation is particularly consequential for practices without access to high-performance computing resources. Smaller private groups and many community hospitals may be unable to bear the USD 500,000–USD 1 million capital costs associated with real-time processing infrastructure, a disparity that persists alongside the closure of over 140 U.S. hospitals since 2010 [159–161]. Finally, limited model interpretability, the so-called "black box" problem, can obscure decision rationale, impairing clinician trust and complicating the translation of algorithmic outputs into patient-centered care [162].

7.2. Regulatory and Validation Challenges

Regulatory pathways and validation requirements introduce additional barriers. The FDA's evolving framework struggles to accommodate continuous learning systems, such as those embedded in platforms like Mazor X Stealth Edition, where post-market performance may change as algorithms adapt. Worryingly, a 2022 analysis found that 226 of 521 FDA-cleared AI devices lacked peer-reviewed clinical validation, raising questions about the evidence base supporting many deployed tools and the potential risks to patient safety [51].

Robust, multi-institutional validation, necessary to demonstrate generalizability across heterogeneous care settings, is logistically and financially demanding. Collaborative validation efforts that coordinate datasets across rural and urban hospitals have been estimated to cost on the order of USD 250,000 annually, limiting participation by resource-constrained centers and slowing generation of high-quality external evidence [163]. The ALIGNMENT study provides a cautionary precedent: despite guideline dissemination, uptake of short-course radiotherapy did not increase substantially, illustrating how dissemination alone cannot substitute for practical validation and institution-specific implementation work [164].

Physician skepticism compounds these challenges. Concerns about workflow disruption, loss of autonomy, and uncertain reimbursement influence adoption decisions, small practices are particularly sensitive to economic pressures, and recent Medicare payment reductions for spine procedures (2024) have further constrained capital investments such as robotic platforms (e.g., ExcelsiusGPS) [165]. Regulatory and documentation burdens, reporting requirements that can add an estimated 10–15 administrative hours per week, further disincentivize adoption in understaffed clinics. Collectively, these forces create a conservative adoption environment where only well-validated, cost-effective, and workflow-friendly solutions are likely to gain traction.

7.3. Clinical Integration and Workflow Challenges

Finally, integrating AI into the clinical ecosystem challenges established workflows and cultural norms. Intergenerational differences shape expectations: some senior clinicians view tools like automated scribes (e.g., DeepScribe) as encroachments on clinical autonomy, while newer clinicians expect seamless EHR integration and interoperability to reduce clerical burden [166]. Patient acceptance is equally critical and increasingly fragile; high-profile healthcare data breaches in 2024 have heightened privacy concerns and made patients more cautious about the use of AI/ML tools, especially those that perform sentiment analysis or rely on extensive, linked datasets. Addressing these integration barriers requires not only technical robustness and regulatory clarity but also transparent governance, clear communication about data stewardship, and implementation strategies co-designed with clinicians and patients to preserve trust and clinical utility.

7.4. Data Quality, Generalization, and Statistical Stability

Despite promising diagnostic accuracy in controlled research settings, AI-driven spine imaging tools remain fundamentally constrained by data quality and representativeness. Convolutional neural networks (CNNs) implicitly assume that training and clinical images share the same statistical properties; any distribution shift (e.g., different scanner vendors, acquisition protocols, or patient populations) can markedly degrade performance [167,168]. Studies consistently report that models trained at one center often underperform on external data, with accuracy drops when applied to images from unfamiliar sites or devices [167,168]. In short, the "garbage in, garbage out" principle holds: CNNs learn superficial statistical cues in the training set and therefore rely critically on high-quality, well-curated data [24,167]. If data are noisy, biased, or limited in scope, model outputs become unreliable; for instance, mislabeled cases or subtle imaging artifacts in the training set will propagate directly to model errors, since CNNs are not inherently robust to annotation errors [24,167]. Additionally, large-scale datasets can increase statistical power but also introduce distinct risks when data provenance, sampling biases, or measurement semantics are not explicitly handled. Roccetti et al. describe a useful cautionary example: training an RNN on $\approx$15 million water-meter readings from >1 million meters initially produced non-positive results until the authors defined a clear "semantics of validity" and curated a representative subset, at which point model accuracy rose from roughly 60% to the 80–90% range [169]. This work illustrates a practical paradox: more data does not automatically resolve bias, and indiscriminate upscaling can amplify noise or confounders rather than improve real-world performance. Consequently, we emphasize the need for (i) careful data provenance reporting, (ii) explicit criteria for inclusion/exclusion and semantic validation of records, and (iii) external validation across heterogeneous cohorts before asserting clinical or operational generalizability [169].

Typical medical datasets are often small, imbalanced, and collected under narrow conditions. High-quality labels require expert effort and are expensive, so many available datasets contain annotation errors, ambiguity, or limited case diversity [24,170]. Rare spine pathologies and uncommon patient demographics may be underrepresented, causing CNNs to overfit common patterns and miss atypical cases. This problem has been highlighted by Alizadehsani et al. and others, who show that data scarcity and class imbalance significantly impair CNN robustness and generalizability [167,170]. Ensuring statistical stability and that training data truly reflect real-world variability is therefore a major obstacle. Practical remedies include continuous external validation, assembling multicenter training cohorts, and applying domain-adaptation techniques to maintain performance across diverse clinical settings [168,170]. Without such rigorous data curation and ongoing model refinement, AI systems risk failing in non-ideal conditions and should be applied with caution.

Training data should be expertly annotated to cover the full spectrum of disease presentations and patient demographics to ensure reliability and clinical relevance. In reality, datasets vary widely in annotation quality and scope: multi-site collections can suffer from inconsistent protocols and labeling conventions, and retrospective curation often favors easily obtainable cases (e.g., urban hospitals or clear-cut pathology), thereby omitting rare presentations or underrepresented populations [171]. This dataset bias, when training data do not fully reflect the target patient population, produces models that perform well on familiar cases but degrade on new scenarios [171]. Recent reviews therefore emphasize the need to standardize data collection and annotation across institutions and to explicitly document dataset provenance (e.g., imaging vendor and patient mix) so users can assess generalizability [171].

Beyond data composition, statistical rigor in model evaluation is essential for stability and trust. Models trained on small or narrow datasets are prone to overfitting, and a number of systematic reviews have found that many published AI studies rely solely on cross-validation with small samples and omit sample-size calculations, a significant methodological shortcoming [171]. Without proper power analysis or independent test sets, reported accuracies may be inflated or highly variable. Developers should therefore compute confidence intervals for performance metrics and, whenever possible, reserve a held-out test set or perform external split-validation. Larger, multi-institutional datasets are also needed: empirical evidence suggests that increasing sample size often yields lower, but more realistic, accuracy estimates, implying that some earlier small-sample reports were over-optimistic [171]. Reporting only a single metric (e.g., a solitary AUC) without confidence bounds obscures the potential range of true performance and can undermine clinical trust.

Finally, AI systems must remain statistically stable over time. After deployment, data distributions commonly drift because of changes in equipment, protocols, or patient populations; even well-calibrated models can misbehave on shifted inputs. Responsible implementations therefore include ongoing data monitoring and drift detection (e.g., checking input histograms or outcome rates), with retraining or recalibration triggered as needed. Regulatory guidance is beginning to address these concerns: for adaptive or continuous learning systems, an Algorithm Change Protocol is advised to specify retraining criteria and requisite validation steps after any update [24]. In sum, ensuring high data quality (i.e., comprehensive, consistently annotated training sets), applying rigorous statistical validation, and explicitly quantifying uncertainty (e.g., with confidence intervals and external testing) are cornerstones of robust, generalizable AI in healthcare.

7.5. Bias, Fairness, and Subgroup Performance

AI tools can unintentionally perpetuate or worsen healthcare disparities when training data reflects historical biases. Experts caution that deployment must assess not just overall accuracy but performance across demographic subgroups [172]. For example, recent studies have found that chest X-ray classifiers tend to systematically underdiagnose disease in Black patients [172]. Deep learning models have even been shown to infer sensitive attributes (race, gender, age) from imaging data, using them as "shortcuts" [172], learning correlations that exist in the data but have no true causal basis. If unaddressed, such biases can lead to unequal care (e.g., delayed treatment for one group), defeating the equitable intent of AI.

To uncover and mitigate these biases, subgroup performance must be reported explicitly. Recent reporting guidelines (i.e., TRIPOD-AI) now require that model evaluations include metrics with confidence intervals for each key subgroup (e.g., race, sex, age, or other clinically relevant categories) [173]. In practice, this means a developer should present, say, the sensitivity and specificity separately for men vs. women or for different racial groups. This can reveal hidden failures: for instance, a model with 90% sensitivity overall might have only 75% sensitivity in a minority subgroup. Encouragingly, TRIPOD-AI explicitly embeds fairness in its checklist with the "issues of fairness" in the interpretation section and advises the use of subgroup plots or heterogeneity analyses [173]. By contrast, many older studies omitted such details, making it impossible to know if an algorithm is safe for all populations. Demanding transparent subgroup reporting is thus a practical step toward fairness in spine imaging and beyond.

When biases are identified, steps should be taken to mitigate them. These steps might include rebalancing training data (e.g., adding more examples from underrepresented groups) or incorporating fairness-aware algorithms that penalize disparate error rates. Importantly, even good fairness performance in the training context is not guaranteed to hold after deployment: models must also be tested for bias under distribution shifts [172]. Ultimately, ensuring equitable AI in medicine requires both (a) rigorous measurement of subgroup outcomes and (b) thoughtful adjustment of models and workflows to correct any unfairness.

7.6. External Validation, Robustness, and Failure-Mode Testing

Demonstrating an AI model's robustness requires testing beyond its own training environment. Numerous systematic reviews have found that radiology AI algorithms suffer performance drops when tested on external data. In one review, fully 81% of published external validations showed a decline in accuracy on new datasets, with about a quarter showing large ($\geq$0.10) drops in AUC [174]. This drop is strong evidence that models often "overfit" to the specifics of one site. For this reason, current best practice is to perform multi-center external validation before deployment. Ideally, developers should evaluate their model on data from several hospitals or vendors that were not used in training, to ensure it generalizes across scanners and patient populations. Indeed, experts urge a shift from single-center studies to multi-center trials and prospective evaluations [29,56]. Such validation might include, for example, scanning new MR images from a partner institution to see if the AI's performance holds steady.

Robustness to edge cases and data shifts is also critical. AI systems should be explicitly stress-tested with challenging cases. A concrete illustration of the pitfalls of scale comes from Roccetti et al. (2019), who found that training on a very large, uncurated time-series initially produced poor results until the dataset's "semantics of validity" and inclusion criteria were defined and a representative subset curated, after which performance improved substantially [169]. This example highlights that stress-testing should include checks for dataset validity and semantic consistency in addition to the usual perturbation/failure-mode analyses. Domain experts recommend failure-mode analysis by identifying scenarios where the model fails and why as part of validation [29]. For instance, specialized testing of a spine fracture detection model revealed that false negatives clustered in patients with severe degenerative changes or metallic hardware, common in spine surgery [30]. These were "stress tests" the model had not seen. By systematically generating or collecting such cases, teams can quantify how performance degrades. Similarly, models should be checked for sensitivity to common perturbations (e.g., motion artifact, different slice thicknesses, etc.), since real-world images are often noisier than textbook examples. Reporting robustness measures (e.g., worst-case error or uncertainty estimates on outlier inputs) provides critical context for safe use.

A further layer of validation comes from shadow deployments. Before entrusting AI with patient care, many institutions run it in parallel: the model receives real imaging data and makes predictions, but clinicians do not act on them. This "shadow mode" allows observation of the AI's real-time performance and failure modes without any risk to patients [31]. During this phase, developers can monitor for calibration drift (i.e., changes in accuracy over time) and gather user feedback. Regulatory experts suggest that even low-risk automation tools undergo shadow evaluation, while higher-risk systems (like autonomous decision-making) ultimately need prospective trials [31, 32]. In practice, this staged rollout (i.e., silent shadowing to supervised testing to live use) has been a common feature of successful AI integrations, as it catches issues that retrospective tests may miss.

7.7. The Gap Between Promising Research and Clinical Reality

Despite promising results on curated datasets, AI models have inherent limitations that temper their clinical utility. First, most AI algorithms do not truly "understand" disease the way humans do; they learn statistical patterns, which may not hold outside the training context [171]. In medical imaging, this is manifested as dataset bias: available data often do not fully represent the clinical spectrum of patients. For example, one review notes that common practice is to train on convenience samples (e.g., cases from academic centers) that only partially reflect real patient populations [171]. In consequence, a model that performs well on a benchmark can "fail catastrophically" when faced with a new hospital's images [171]. In fact, a systematic review of COVID-19 imaging AI found none of 62 studies had demonstrable readiness for clinical use [35], illustrating how overfit solutions on limited data may not translate to practice. These findings underscore that AI is not a panacea; models should always be seen as supporting, not replacing, clinical judgment, especially in novel scenarios. More broadly, scale cannot substitute for semantic validation: studies found that increasing dataset size without explicit semantics of validity can amplify noise and confounders rather than improve real-world performance [171]. Therefore, practical deployment strategies should pair dataset expansion with rigorous semantic curation and transparent inclusion/exclusion rules.

Second, many technical challenges remain. Deep learning models are often "black boxes" with limited interpretability. This opacity can hinder trust and obscure failure modes; currently there is no guarantee that a given model will behave sensibly on a rare case or under adversarial perturbations. Relatedly, most AI studies focus on single-timepoint classification and do not model patient longitudinally or causally; they lack an understanding of progression over time. There is also the issue of calibration: AI confidence scores can be poorly calibrated, giving a misleading sense of certainty. Handling domain shifts and adversarial examples, intentional or not, remains an active research problem. In short, current models do not self-correct when facing truly new challenges.

Finally, practical deployment limitations cannot be ignored. Regulatory pathways for AI are still evolving, and most models enter the clinic with limited evidence: few have randomized trial validation or real-world outcome studies. Even with validation, implementation requires robust IT infrastructure, privacy safeguards, and user training, which are obstacles that many hospitals struggle with. Economic and workflow factors (e.g., cost of hardware, integration into PACS, clinician workload) often become rate-limiting. In the spine imaging domain in particular, the relatively small volume of cases and the diversity of pathologies mean that algorithmic improvements have to overcome a high bar of cost and complexity. In sum, AI promises much but also has real constraints:

its outputs must be interpreted in the context of clinical judgment, sound data practice, and ongoing surveillance. Only through acknowledging and addressing these limitations can safe, effective AI tools be realized.

8. Discussion

The body of evidence synthesized in this review demonstrates that artificial intelligence (AI) and machine learning (ML) are no longer exploratory curiosities in spine care; they are operational technologies that touch imaging pipelines, preoperative planning, intraoperative navigation, postoperative monitoring, and even early translational genomics [3,9–11,13,16,17,19,43,63,70,71,83–85,96,97]. Across these domains, the recurring theme is one of tremendous potential tempered by real-world limits: algorithmic brittleness when exposed to heterogeneous data, infrastructural and economic barriers to equitable deployment, gaps in external validation and regulatory oversight, and non-trivial cultural and workflow frictions among clinicians, patients, and institutions. Below we synthesize the clinical implications of the evidence, examine mechanistic reasons for persistent performance gaps, and propose a pragmatic translational roadmap that aligns technical priorities with regulatory and health-system realities.

From a practical standpoint, AI has already demonstrated clinically meaningful benefits where tasks are structured, repetitive, and well-defined. Automated fracture and acute-pathology triage systems shorten time-to-diagnosis in emergent settings [29–32,56], opportunistic screening algorithms identify otherwise-missed fragility fractures [63], and segmentation/morphometric pipelines markedly reduce measurement variability for alignment metrics such as Cobb angle and sagittal vertical axis (SVA) [13,44,63,83–85]. In preoperative planning and robotics, predictive modeling and finite-element-assisted planning improve the precision and reproducibility of screw trajectories and implant selection [88–95]. Meanwhile, emerging multimodal prognostic models that integrate imaging, wearable data, and genomic signals offer a new avenue to personalize perioperative risk-reduction strategies, rehabilitation intensity, and pharmacologic plans [3,9–11,43,70,71]. Collectively, these capabilities point to a hybrid clinical model in which AI augments clinician judgment, automates low-value work, and provides earlier, finer-grained signals to inform decision-making.

However, these practical benefits are often undermined by persistent performance gaps, particularly when models are deployed beyond their development environments. Recent reports showing markedly higher diagnostic accuracies than older studies likely reflect multiple converging factors, not solely algorithmic breakthroughs. Larger, better-curated training corpora, improved network architectures and transfer-learning methods, and more sophisticated image-reconstruction pipelines have raised retrospective test metrics. At the same time, reporting practices (e.g., use of internal test sets, selective case sampling, and the occasional presence of data leakage) and publication bias toward positive results can inflate apparent performance. Crucially, prospective and external evaluations frequently reveal lower, more clinically realistic performance (see, e.g., external evaluations of triage algorithms), underscoring that headline accuracy numbers should be interpreted in the context of dataset provenance, validation methodology, and deployment environment. For deployment decisions and regulatory assessment, emphasis should be placed on multi-center prospective validation, calibration reporting, and transparent failure-mode analysis.

Additionally, several interlocking technical realities explain the recurring drop in performance when models leave their development environments. First, domain shift is pervasive: scanner vendors, slice thickness, acquisition protocols, contrast timing, and local reporting conventions create distributional differences that degrade generalizability [15,153,154]. Second, the presence of metallic hardware or unusual anatomy produces imaging artifacts and edge cases that were underrepresented in training sets, generating catastrophic failure modes in segmentation and measurement algorithms [155]. Third, many current models are trained on retrospective, single-center cohorts that overrepresent tertiary-care populations; the result is geographic and socio-economic selection bias that erodes external validity [156–158]. Fourth, cross-sectional model designs hamper longitudinal monitoring; a model trained for single-timepoint classification struggles to track progression or the effects of serial interventions [159–161]. Finally, opaque model explanations, the "black box" problem, hamper clinician trust and obstruct effective failure-mode analysis [162]. These technical deficits are compounded by human and organizational factors: clinicians resist workflows that feel unstable or require substantial retooling, administrators balk at high upfront capital costs for compute and devices [163], and patients worry about privacy and data misuse [164–166].

Beyond these technical and human challenges, current regulatory pathways were not designed for adaptive, continuously learning systems deployed across thousands of variable clinical contexts. Analyses show that many AI devices entered the clinical domain with limited peer-reviewed validation and that post-market performance monitoring is inconsistent [20,51]. For safe, equitable scaling, regulators and clinical stakeholders must converge on practical expectations for premarket evidence (external, multi-institutional validation), transparent reporting, and robust post-market surveillance. A key step in this modernization is for the FDA to mandate several guidance upgrades for spine AI. A risk-stratified evidence model is needed: low-risk tools such as automated measurements should demonstrate analytic validity across multiple sites and undergo a supervised "shadow mode" deployment before approval. Moderate-risk systems, like diagnostic triage and surgical planning assistants, should be required to prove external validity across diverse patient groups, include calibration analyses by demographic and technical subgroups, and report at least one prospective clinical impact study. High-risk tools, particularly autonomous or closed-loop robotic systems, must meet the most stringent standards, such as randomized or controlled prospective trials paired with robust post-market surveillance. Beyond these evidentiary thresholds, guidance should mandate disclosure of dataset provenance, including geographic distribution, vendor diversity, and patient demographics, so that reviewers can gauge generalizability. For adaptive systems, an Algorithm Change Protocol should be required, specifying retraining conditions, validation steps after updates, rollback procedures, and clinician/end-user notifications when performance shifts occur. To safeguard clinical use, vendors should also provide regular real-world performance dashboards, including sensitivity, specificity, and calibration metrics broken down by demographic categories, and be subject to mandatory adverse-event reporting when misclassification leads to harm or near-miss events.

While governance is critical, evidence also suggests that requiring a technology to be clinically useful is not the same as designing it to be deployable. Successful implementations share several features: native interoperability with EHRs (FHIR/HL7 compliance), minimal workflow disruption (e.g., integration that populates structured report fields rather than forcing transcription changes), clinician-facing explainability (clear, concise model outputs with uncertainty estimates), and a staged roll-out with shadow mode, supervised use, and then live deployment [14,23,48,152]. Change management also matters: clinician champions, multidisciplinary AI governance committees, and clear metrics of clinical utility (turnaround time, diagnostic yield, patient-centered outcomes) accelerate adoption. Economic models that account for total cost of ownership, including retraining, maintenance, and regulatory reporting, better predict institutional willingness to adopt [163].

To address the issue of equitable access, the promise of AI magnifies existing inequities if models are trained and validated on narrow cohorts. Federated learning and privacy-preserving analytics provide technical pathways to broaden training datasets while minimizing raw data movement, but these must be paired with deliberate inclusion strategies (such as incentives for rural/underserved centers to participate in consortia) and prospective audits of model calibration across demographic strata [47]. Patient trust hinges on transparent data governance, explicit consent for secondary uses, auditable data lineage, and rigorous cybersecurity measures; the high-profile breaches of recent years have demonstrably eroded public confidence and must guide any implementation strategy [164–166].

Ultimately, to move the field forward, research must shift from single-center optimization to multi-center external validation and prospective impact trials. Priority areas include robustness engineering (domain-adaptation methods, uncertainty quantification, and explicit failure-mode detection for edge cases such as metal hardware and severe deformity); longitudinal modeling frameworks for consistent tracking of disease state across serial imaging and clinic visits; explainability and human–AI interaction studies that produce clinically meaningful visualizations of model reasoning; federated and distributed learning initiatives to improve representativeness without compromising privacy; cost-effectiveness and outcomes research that couples clinical outcomes, quality-of-life instruments, and economic impact; and open benchmark datasets with reporting checklists (e.g., TRIPOD-AI, CONSORT-AI adaptations) [159–161].

The FDA should also emphasize transparency and explainability: models should disclose interpretability methods, provide standardized uncertainty metrics, and include clinician-facing output templates that clearly distinguish prediction, confidence, and suggested action. Interoperability standards (e.g., HL7/FHIR compliance, standardized labeling) must be enforced to reduce integration costs and ensure comparability across platforms. Finally, equity and cybersecurity must be central. Systems should report subgroup-level performance, incentivize validation that includes underrepresented populations, and adhere to rigorous encryption, penetration testing, and vendor transparency standards. Through these measures, FDA guidance can both protect patients and accelerate innovation in AI for spine care [51,163].

9. Conclusions

AI and ML technologies have reached a point of clinical maturity in specific, high-value tasks within spine care: emergent triage, standardized morphometrics, surgical planning assistance, and nascent prognostic modeling [3,9–11,13,16,17,19,43,63,70,71,83–85,96,97]. These technologies promise measurable improvements in diagnostic speed, reproducibility, and personalization of perioperative care. However, the translation of algorithmic promise into broad, safe clinical benefit is not automatic. Persistent technical fragilities, including domain shift, hardware artifacts, limited longitudinal modeling, and underrepresentation of diverse populations, combined with unequal access to infrastructure, insufficient external validation, and regulatory gaps, constrain equitable deployment [15,51,153–159,162].

To move from demonstration to durable clinical impact, the field requires aligned action on three fronts. First, technical innovation must prioritize robustness, explainability, and longitudinal fidelity, not just peak accuracy on curated datasets. Second, implementation science must make AI a practical clinical collaborator through seamless interoperability, clinician-centered interfaces, staged rollouts, and careful change management [14,23,48,152,163]. Third, regulators and health systems must modernize governance frameworks with risk-proportionate evidentiary requirements, transparent dataset reporting, algorithm-change protocols, mandatory post-market surveillance, and equity safeguards [51].

Concretely, an upgraded FDA approach, one that combines stratified premarket standards, adaptive system governance, enforced external validation, ongoing real-world performance auditing, and interoperability mandates, will both protect patients and accelerate clinically meaningful adoption. Parallel investments in federated learning, subsidized computational infrastructure for resource-limited centers, and incentives for multi-center prospective validation studies will prevent a two-tiered system in which AI-enhanced care is only accessible in well-resourced institutions [159–161].

In sum, AI is poised to become an integral, augmentative element of contemporary spine care. Yet the pathway to safe, equitable, and effective scale depends as much on governance, workflow design, and economic strategy as it does on algorithmic advances. A coordinated effort among developers, clinicians, regulators, payers, and patients, guided by transparent validation, robust monitoring, and explicit equity goals, will be essential to realize AI's promise while minimizing foreseeable harm.

Author Contributions: All authors contributed to the conception and design of this review manuscript. Conceptualization: R.K. and N.Z.; Methodology: R.K., A.K., P.R. and N.Z.; Investigation: R.K., C.D., K.S. and P.P.; Resources: N.Z.; Writing—Original Draft Preparation: R.K.; Writing—Review and Editing: C.D., K.S., A.K., P.R., P.P. and N.Z.; Visualization: R.K., C.D. and K.S.; Supervision: N.Z.; Project Administration: R.K. All authors have read and agreed to the published version of the manuscript.

Funding: This research did not receive any funding.

Institutional Review Board Statement: Not applicable. This study did not involve human participants or animals.

Conflicts of Interest: The authors declare no conflicts of interest.

Appendix A. Technical Background on CNNs

Appendix A.1. Rationale and Overview

At the core of many of these applications are Convolutional Neural Networks (CNNs), a class of deep learning models specially designed to mimic the human visual cortex in how they process and analyze visual data. They can ingest large image datasets and automatically extract spatial features from raw pixels to hierarchically learn subtle patterns of disease [24].

Appendix A.2. Architecture, Layers and Feature Hierarchy

CNNs are built from repeating blocks of convolutional and pooling layers, often followed by one or more fully connected, dense layers [24,25]. To start, each convolutional layer applies a set of trainable filters across the image, producing feature maps that highlight where certain patterns (e.g., an edge, texture, shape) occur. Pooling layers then downsample these feature maps, reducing spatial resolution while preserving the strongest signals. This pooling confers spatial invariance: small shifts in the image do not drastically change the pooled characteristics [25]. By alternating convolution and pooling layers, the network builds a hierarchy of features; early layers capture simple structures (e.g., lines or edges) while deeper layers combine them into complex shapes or pathology-specific patterns [24,52]. In practical terms, low-level convolutional filters might respond to simple edges or blobs, whereas higher-level filters in deeper layers respond to organs or lesions. Finally, one or more fully connected layers aggregate these features to produce a prediction [24,25]. In summary, CNNs automatically learn to detect and synthesize the relevant spatial features in an image, mimicking the brain's hierarchical visual processing [24].

Appendix A.3. Training, Tasks, and Outputs

CNN models are trained on large, annotated imaging datasets (e.g., MRI, CT or X-ray scans labeled by experts) split into training and test sets (e.g., an 80:20 training–test split) [53]. During training, the network's filter weights are iteratively adjusted via backpropagation and gradient descent to minimize the difference between the network's predictions and the ground-truth labels [24]. For classification tasks, the final output of the CNN is a categorical label (e.g., "tumor present" vs. "absent," or disease severity grading); the network learns to output class probabilities. In localization or detection tasks, the network produces spatial outputs. For example, object-detection CNNs (e.g., Faster R-CNN) regress bounding-box coordinates to surround each abnormality, while segmentation CNNs (e.g., U-Net) output pixel-wise masks delineating the lesion [26,54]. Some networks also produce heatmaps that highlight the image regions most influential for the decision [55]. In practice, CNNs excel at both pixel-level tasks (e.g., identifying the exact region of a tumor) and image-level tasks (e.g., classifying an entire scan), often achieving high sensitivity and specificity once well-trained. Their fully connected layers effectively translate the hierarchical features into final predictions, enabling breakthroughs in diagnostic accuracy and patient care [25,52].

References

1. Voter, A.F.; Larson, M.E.; Garrett, J.W.; Yu, J.J. Diagnostic Accuracy and Failure Mode Analysis of a Deep-Learning Algorithm for the Detection of Cervical Spine Fractures. *AJNR. Am. J. Neuroradiol.* **2021**, *42*, 1550–1556. [CrossRef]
2. Page, J.H.; Moser, F.G.; Maya, M.M.; Prasad, R.; Pressman, B.D. Opportunistic CT Screening-Machine Learning Algorithm Identifies Majority of Vertebral Compression Fractures: A Cohort Study. *JBMR Plus* **2023**, *7*, e10778. [CrossRef]
3. Nigru, A.S.; Benini, S.; Bonetti, M.; Bragaglio, G.; Frigerio, M.; Maffezzoni, F.; Leonardi, R. External validation of SpineNetV2 on a comprehensive set of radiological features for grading lumbosacral disc pathologies. *N. Am. Spine Soc. J.* **2024**, *20*, 100564. [CrossRef]
4. Elhaddad, M.; Hamam, S. AI-Driven Clinical Decision Support Systems: An Ongoing Pursuit of Potential. *Cureus* **2024**, *16*, e57728. [CrossRef]
5. O'Connor, T.E.; O'Hehir, M.M.; Khan, A.; Mao, J.Z.; Levy, L.C.; Mullin, J.P.; Pollina, J. Mazor X Stealth Robotic Technology: A Technical Note. *World Neurosurg.* **2021**, *145*, 435–442. [CrossRef]
6. Sigala, R.E.; Lagou, V.; Shmeliov, A.; Atito, S.; Kouchaki, S.; Awais, M.; Prokopenko, I.; Mahdi, A.; Demirkan, A. Machine Learning to Advance Human Genome-Wide Association Studies. *Genes* **2023**, *15*, 34. [CrossRef] [PubMed]
7. U.S. Food and Drug Administration. *510(k) Summary: HealthVCF (K192901)*; U.S. Food and Drug Administration: Silver Spring, MD, USA, 2020. Available online: https://www.accessdata.fda.gov/cdrh_docs/pdf19/K192901.pdf (accessed on 20 August 2025).
8. Monchka, B.A.; Schousboe, J.T.; Davidson, M.J.; Kimelman, D.; Hans, D.; Raina, P.; Leslie, W.D. Development of a manufacturer-independent convolutional neural network for the automated identification of vertebral compression fractures in vertebral fracture assessment images using active learning. *Bone* **2022**, *161*, 116427. [CrossRef] [PubMed]
9. Gstoettner, M.; Sekyra, K.; Walochnik, N.; Winter, P.; Wachter, R.; Bach, C.M. Inter- and intraobserver reliability assessment of the Cobb angle: Manual versus digital measurement tools. *Eur. Spine J.* **2007**, *16*, 1587–1592. [CrossRef] [PubMed]
10. Jamaludin, A.; Kadir, T.; Zisserman, A. SpineNet: Automated classification and evidence visualization in spinal MRIs. *Med. Image Anal.* **2017**, *41*, 63–73. [CrossRef] [PubMed]
11. Grob, A.; Loibl, M.; Jamaludin, A.; Winklhofer, S.; Fairbank, J.C.T.; Fekete, T.; Porchet, F.; Mannion, A.F. External validation of the deep learning system "SpineNet" for grading radiological features of degeneration on MRIs of the lumbar spine. *Eur. Spine J.* **2022**, *31*, 2137–2148. [CrossRef]
12. McSweeney, T.P.; Tiulpin, A.; Saarakkala, S.; Niinimäki, J.; Windsor, R.; Jamaludin, A.; Kadir, T.; Karppinen, J.; Määttä, J. External Validation of SpineNet, an Open-Source Deep Learning Model for Grading Lumbar Disk Degeneration MRI Features, Using the Northern Finland Birth Cohort 1966. *Spine (Phila Pa 1976).* **2023**, *48*, 484–491. [CrossRef] [PubMed] [PubMed Central]

13. Small, J.E.; Osler, P.; Paul, A.B.; Kunst, M. CT Cervical Spine Fracture Detection Using a Convolutional Neural Network. *AJNR. Am. J. Neuroradiol.* **2021**, *42*, 1341–1347. [CrossRef] [PubMed]
14. van den Wittenboer, G.J.; van der Kolk, B.Y.M.; Nijholt, I.M.; Langius-Wiffen, E.; van Dijk, R.A.; van Hasselt, B.A.A.M.; Podlogar, M.; van den Brink, W.A.; Bouma, G.J.; Schep, N.W.L.; et al. Diagnostic accuracy of an artificial intelligence algorithm versus radiologists for fracture detection on cervical spine CT. *Eur. Radiol.* **2024**, *34*, 5041–5048. [CrossRef]
15. Kumar, R.; Gosain, A.; Saintyl, J.J.; Zheng, A.; Chima, K.; Cassagnol, R. Bridging gaps in orthopedic residency admissions: Embracing diversity beyond research metrics. *Can. Med. Educ. J.* **2025**, *16*, 68–70. [CrossRef]
16. Smith, A.; Picheca, L.; Mahood, Q. *Robotic Surgical Systems for Orthopedics: Emerging Health Technologies*; Canadian Agency for Drugs and Technologies in Health: Ottawa, ON, Canda, 2022. Available online: https://www.ncbi.nlm.nih.gov/books/NBK602663/ (accessed on 15 August 2025).
17. Bhimreddy, M.; Hersh, A.M.; Jiang, K.; Weber-Levine, C.; Davidar, A.D.; Menta, A.K.; Judy, B.F.; Lubelski, D.; Bydon, A.; Weingart, J.; et al. Accuracy of Pedicle Screw Placement Using the ExcelsiusGPS Robotic Navigation Platform: An Analysis of 728 Screws. *Int. J. Spine Surg.* **2024**, *18*, 712–720. [CrossRef]
18. Yeh, Y.C.; Weng, C.H.; Huang, Y.J.; Fu, C.J.; Tsai, T.T.; Yeh, C.Y. Deep learning approach for automatic landmark detection and alignment analysis in whole-spine lateral radiographs. *Sci. Rep.* **2021**, *11*, 7618. [CrossRef]
19. Ammarullah, M.I. Integrating finite element analysis in total hip arthroplasty for childhood hip disorders: Enhancing precision and outcomes. *World J. Orthop.* **2025**, *16*, 98871. [CrossRef]
20. Clark, P.; Kim, J.; Aphinyanaphongs, Y. Marketing and US Food and Drug Administration Clearance of Artificial Intelligence and Machine Learning Enabled Software in and as Medical Devices: A Systematic Review. *JAMA Netw. Open* **2023**, *6*, e2321792. [CrossRef] [PubMed]
21. Salo, V.; Määttä, J.; Sliz, E.; FinnGen; Reimann, E.; Mägi, R.; Estonian Biobank Research Team; Reis, K.; Elhanas, A.G.; Reigo, A.; et al. Genome-wide meta-analysis conducted in three large biobanks expands the genetic landscape of lumbar disc herniations. *Nat. Commun.* **2024**, *15*, 9424. [CrossRef]
22. Haberle, T.; Cleveland, C.; Snow, G.L.; Barber, C.; Stookey, N.; Thornock, C.; Younger, L.; Mullahkhel, B.; Ize-Ludlow, D. The impact of nuance DAX ambient listening AI documentation: A cohort study. *J. Am. Med. Inform. Assoc.* **2024**, *31*, 975–979. [CrossRef] [PubMed]
23. Shah, S.J.; Devon-Sand, A.; Ma, S.P.; Jeong, Y.; Crowell, T.; Smith, M.; Liang, A.S.; Delahaie, C.; Hsia, C.; Shanafelt, T.; et al. Ambient artificial intelligence scribes: Physician burnout and perspectives on usability and documentation burden. *J. Am. Med. Inform. Assoc.* **2025**, *32*, 375–380. [CrossRef]
24. Yamashita, R.; Nishio, M.; Do, R.K.G.; Togashi, K. Convolutional neural networks: An overview and application in radiology. *Insights Into Imaging* **2018**, *9*, 611–629. [CrossRef]
25. Lin, W.-C.; Tu, Y.-C.; Lin, H.-Y.; Tseng, M.-H. A Comparison of Deep Learning Techniques for Pose Recognition in Up-and-Go Pole Walking Exercises Using Skeleton Images and Feature Data. *Electronics* **2025**, *14*, 1075. [CrossRef]
26. Su, Z.; Adam, A.; Nasrudin, M.F.; Prabuwono, A.S. Proposal-Free Fully Convolutional Network: Object Detection Based on a Box Map. *Sensors* **2024**, *24*, 3529. [CrossRef] [PubMed]
27. Li, S.; Du, J.; Huang, Y.; Hao, D.; Zhao, Z.; Chang, Z.; Zhang, X.; Gao, S.; He, B. Comparison of the S8 navigation system and the TINAVI orthopaedic robot in the treatment of upper cervical instability. *Sci. Rep.* **2024**, *14*, 6487. [CrossRef] [PubMed]
28. Kirchner, G.J.; Kim, A.H.; Kwart, A.H.; Weddle, J.B.; Bible, J.E. Reported Events Associated With Spine Robots: An Analysis of the Food and Drug Administration's Manufacturer and User Facility Device Experience Database. *Glob. Spine J.* **2023**, *13*, 855–860. [CrossRef] [PubMed]
29. Murata, K.; Endo, K.; Aihara, T.; Suzuki, H.; Sawaji, Y.; Matsuoka, Y.; Nishimura, H.; Takamatsu, T.; Konishi, T.; Maekawa, A.; et al. Artificial intelligence for the detection of vertebral fractures on plain spinal radiography. *Sci. Rep.* **2020**, *10*, 20031. [CrossRef]
30. Derkatch, S.; Kirby, C.; Kimelman, D.; Jozani, M.J.; Davidson, J.M.; Leslie, W.D. Identification of Vertebral Fractures by Convolutional Neural Networks to Predict Nonvertebral and Hip Fractures: A Registry-based Cohort Study of Dual X-ray Absorptiometry. *Radiology* **2019**, *293*, 405–411. [CrossRef]
31. Singh, M.; Tripathi, U.; Patel, K.K.; Mohit, K.; Pathak, S. An efficient deep learning based approach for automated identification of cervical vertebrae fracture as a clinical support aid. *Sci. Rep.* **2025**, *15*, 25651. [CrossRef]
32. Golla, A.K.; Lorenz, C.; Buerger, C.; Lossau, T.; Klinder, T.; Mutze, S.; Arndt, H.; Spohn, F.; Mittmann, M.; Goelz, L. Cervical spine fracture detection in computed tomography using convolutional neural networks. *Phys. Med. Biol.* **2023**, *68*, 115010. [CrossRef]
33. Li, K.Y.; Ye, H.B.; Zhang, Y.L.; Huang, J.W.; Li, H.L.; Tian, N.F. Enhancing Diagnostic Accuracy of Fresh Vertebral Compression Fractures With Deep Learning Models. *Spine* **2025**, *50*, E330–E335. [CrossRef] [PubMed]
34. Kuo, R.Y.L.; Harrison, C.; Curran, T.A.; Jones, B.; Freethy, A.; Cussons, D.; Stewart, M.; Collins, G.S.; Furniss, D. Artificial Intelligence in Fracture Detection: A Systematic Review and Meta-Analysis. *Radiology* **2022**, *304*, 50–62. [CrossRef]

35. Chen, H.Y.; Hsu, B.W.; Yin, Y.K.; Lin, F.H.; Yang, T.H.; Yang, R.S.; Lee, C.K.; Tseng, V.S. Application of deep learning algorithm to detect and visualize vertebral fractures on plain frontal radiographs. *PLoS ONE* **2021**, *16*, e0245992. [CrossRef]
36. Namireddy, S.R.; Gill, S.S.; Peerbhai, A.; Kamath, A.G.; Ramsay, D.S.C.; Ponniah, H.S.; Salih, A.; Jankovic, D.; Kalasauskas, D.; Neuhoff, J.; et al. Artificial intelligence in risk prediction and diagnosis of vertebral fractures. *Sci. Rep.* **2024**, *14*, 30560. [CrossRef]
37. Hallinan, J.T.P.D.; Zhu, L.; Yang, K.; Makmur, A.; Algazwi, D.A.R.; Thian, Y.L.; Lau, S.; Choo, Y.S.; Eide, S.E.; Yap, Q.V.; et al. Deep Learning Model for Automated Detection and Classification of Central Canal, Lateral Recess, and Neural Foraminal Stenosis at Lumbar Spine MRI. *Radiology* **2021**, *300*, 130–138. [CrossRef]
38. Van Timmeren, J.E.; Cester, D.; Tanadini-Lang, S.; Alkadhi, H.; Baessler, B. Radiomics in medical imaging—"how-to" guide and critical reflection. *Insights Into Imaging* **2020**, *11*, 91. [CrossRef]
39. Cao, J.; Li, Q.; Zhang, H.; Wu, Y.; Wang, X.; Ding, S.; Chen, S.; Xu, S.; Duan, G.; Qiu, D.; et al. Radiomics model based on MRI to differentiate spinal multiple myeloma from metastases: A two-center study. *J. Bone Oncol.* **2024**, *45*, 100599. [CrossRef] [PubMed]
40. Yang, J.; Zhang, S.B.; Yang, S.; Ge, X.Y.; Ren, C.X.; Wang, S.J. CT-based radiomics predicts adjacent vertebral fracture after percutaneous vertebral augmentation. *Eur. Spine J.* **2025**, *34*, 528–536. [CrossRef] [PubMed]
41. Chen, Y.; Qin, S.; Zhao, W.; Wang, Q.; Liu, K.; Xin, P.; Yuan, H.; Zhuang, H.; Lang, N. MRI feature-based radiomics models to predict treatment outcome after stereotactic body radiotherapy for spinal metastases. *Insights Into Imaging* **2023**, *14*, 169. [CrossRef]
42. Bendtsen, M.G.; Hitz, M.F. Opportunistic Identification of Vertebral Compression Fractures on CT Scans of the Chest and Abdomen, Using an AI Algorithm, in a Real-Life Setting. *Calcif. Tissue Int.* **2024**, *114*, 468–479. [CrossRef]
43. Windsor, R.; Jamaludin, A.; Kadir, T.; Zisserman, A. Automated detection, labelling and radiological grading of clinical spinal MRIs. *Sci. Rep.* **2024**, *14*, 14993. [CrossRef]
44. Galbusera, F.; Bassani, T.; Panico, M.; Sconfienza, L.M.; Cina, A. A fresh look at spinal alignment and deformities: Automated analysis of a large database of 9832 biplanar radiographs. *Front. Bioeng. Biotechnol.* **2022**, *10*, 863054. [CrossRef]
45. Li, H.; Qian, C.; Yan, W.; Fu, D.; Zheng, Y.; Zhang, Z.; Meng, J.; Wang, D. Use of Artificial Intelligence in Cobb Angle Measurement for Scoliosis: Retrospective Reliability and Accuracy Study of a Mobile App. *J. Med. Internet Res.* **2024**, *26*, e50631. [CrossRef] [PubMed]
46. Chui, C.E.; He, Z.; Lam, T.P.; Mak, K.K.; Ng, H.R.; Fung, C.E.; Chan, M.S.; Law, S.W.; Lee, Y.W.; Hung, L.A.; et al. Deep Learning-Based Prediction Model for the Cobb Angle in Adolescent Idiopathic Scoliosis Patients. *Diagnostics* **2024**, *14*, 1263. [CrossRef]
47. Deng, Y.; Wang, C.; Hui, Y.; Li, Q.; Li, J.; Luo, S.; Sun, M.; Quan, Q.; Yang, S.; Hao, Y. Ctspine1k: A large-scale dataset for spinal vertebrae segmentation in computed tomography. *arXiv* **2021**, arXiv:2105.14711.
48. Lee, W.S.; Ahn, S.M.; Chung, J.W.; Kim, K.O.; Kwon, K.A.; Kim, Y.; Sym, S.; Shin, D.; Park, I.; Lee, U.; et al. Assessing Concordance With Watson for Oncology, a Cognitive Computing Decision Support System for Colon Cancer Treatment in Korea. *JCO Clin. Cancer Inform.* **2018**, *2*, 1–8. [CrossRef] [PubMed]
49. Cina, A.; Galbusera, F. Advancing spine care through AI and machine learning: Overview and applications. *EFORT Open Rev.* **2024**, *9*, 422–433. [CrossRef]
50. Leis, A.; Fradera, M.; Peña-Gómez, C.; Aguilera, P.; Hernandez, G.; Parralejo, A.; Ramírez-Anguita, J.M., Mayer, M.A. Real World Data and Real World Evidence Using TriNetX: The TauliMar Clinical Research Network. *Stud. Health Technol. Inform.* **2025**, *327*, 759–760. [CrossRef]
51. Chouffani El Fassi, S.; Abdullah, A.; Fang, Y.; Natarajan, S.; Masroor, A.B.; Kayali, N.; Prakash, S.; Henderson, G.E. Not all AI health tools with regulatory authorization are clinically validated. *Nat. Med.* **2024**, *30*, 2718–2720. [CrossRef]
52. Mienye, I.D.; Swart, T.G.; Obaido, G.; Jordan, M.; Ilono, P. Deep Convolutional Neural Networks in Medical Image Analysis: A Review. *Information* **2025**, *16*, 195. [CrossRef]
53. Baur, D.; Kroboth, K.; Heyde, C.E.; Voelker, A. Convolutional Neural Networks in Spinal Magnetic Resonance Imaging: A Systematic Review. *World Neurosurg.* **2022**, *166*, 60–70. [CrossRef]
54. Neha, F.; Bhati, D.; Shukla, D.K.; Dalvi, S.M.; Mantzou, N.; Shubbar, S. U-net in medical image segmentation: A review of its applications across modalities. *arXiv* **2024**, arXiv:2412.02242. [CrossRef]
55. Watanabe, A.; Ketabi, S.; Namdar, K.; Khalvati, F. Improving disease classification performance and explainability of deep learning models in radiology with heatmap generators. *Front. Radiol.* **2022**, *2*, 991683. [CrossRef]
56. Zhang, J.; Liu, F.; Xu, J.; Zhao, Q.; Huang, C.; Yu, Y.; Yuan, H. Automated detection and classification of acute vertebral body fractures using a convolutional neural network on computed tomography. *Front. Endocrinol.* **2023**, *14*, 1132725. [CrossRef] [PubMed]
57. Liawrungrueang, W.; Han, I.; Cholamjiak, W.; Sarasombath, P.; Riew, K.D. Artificial Intelligence Detection of Cervical Spine Fractures Using Convolutional Neural Network Models. *Neurospine* **2024**, *21*, 833–841. [CrossRef] [PubMed]

58. Monchka, B.A.; Kimelman, D.; Lix, L.M.; Leslie, W.D. Feasibility of a generalized convolutional neural network for automated identification of vertebral compression fractures: The Manitoba Bone Mineral Density Registry. *Bone* **2021**, *150*, 116017. [CrossRef]
59. Inoue, T.; Maki, S.; Furuya, T.; Mikami, Y.; Mizutani, M.; Takada, I.; Okimatsu, S.; Yunde, A.; Miura, M.; Shiratani, Y.; et al. Automated fracture screening using an object detection algorithm on whole-body trauma computed tomography. *Sci. Rep.* **2022**, *12*, 16549. [CrossRef]
60. Husarek, J.; Hess, S.; Razaeian, S.; Ruder, T.D.; Sehmisch, S.; Müller, M.; Liodakis, E. Artificial intelligence in commercial fracture detection products: A systematic review and meta-analysis of diagnostic test accuracy. *Sci. Rep.* **2024**, *14*, 23053. [CrossRef] [PubMed]
61. Paik, S.; Park, J.; Hong, J.Y.; Han, S.W. Deep learning application of vertebral compression fracture detection using mask R-CNN. *Sci. Rep.* **2024**, *14*, 16308. [CrossRef]
62. Pereira, R.F.B.; Helito, P.V.P.; Leão, R.V.; Rodrigues, M.B.; Correa, M.F.P.; Rodrigues, F.V. Accuracy of an artificial intelligence algorithm for detecting moderate-to-severe vertebral compression fractures on abdominal and thoracic computed tomography scans. *Radiol. Bras.* **2024**, *57*, e20230102. [CrossRef]
63. Ruitenbeek, H.C.; Oei, E.H.; Schmahl, B.L.; Bos, E.M.; Verdonschot, R.J.; Visser, J.J. Towards clinical implementation of an AI-algorithm for detection of cervical spine fractures on computed tomography. *Eur. J. Radiol.* **2024**, *173*, 111375. [CrossRef]
64. Zhang, W.; Chen, Z.; Su, Z.; Wang, Z.; Hai, J.; Huang, C.; Wang, Y.; Yan, B.; Lu, H. Deep learning-based detection and classification of lumbar disc herniation on magnetic resonance images. *JOR Spine* **2023**, *6*, e1276. [CrossRef]
65. Wang, A.; Wang, T.; Liu, X.; Fan, N.; Yuan, S.; Du, P.; Zang, L. Automated diagnosis and grading of lumbar intervertebral disc degeneration based on a modified YOLO framework. *Front. Bioeng. Biotechnol.* **2025**, *13*, 1526478. [CrossRef]
66. Tumko, V.; Kim, J.; Uspenskaia, N.; Honig, S.; Abel, F.; Lebl, D.R.; Hotalen, I.; Kolisnyk, S.; Kochnev, M.; Rusakov, A.; et al. A neural network model for detection and classification of lumbar spinal stenosis on MRI. *Eur. Spine J.* **2024**, *33*, 941–948. [CrossRef]
67. Shahid, A.; Kim, J.; Byon, S.S.; Hong, S.; Lee, I.; Lee, B.D. An end-to-end pipeline for automated scoliosis diagnosis with standardized clinical reporting using SNOMED CT. *Sci. Rep.* **2025**, *15*, 17274. [CrossRef]
68. Xie, J.; Yang, Y.; Jiang, Z.; Zhang, K.; Zhang, X.; Lin, Y.; Shen, Y.; Jia, X.; Liu, H.; Yang, S.; et al. MRI radiomics-based decision support tool for a personalized classification of cervical disc degeneration: A two-center study. *Front. Physiol.* **2024**, *14*, 1281506. [CrossRef] [PubMed]
69. Qin, C.; Dai, L.P.; Zhang, Y.L.; Wu, R.C.; Du, K.L.; Zhang, C.Q.; Liu, W.G. The value of MRI radiomics in distinguishing different types of spinal infections. *Comput. Methods Programs Biomed.* **2025**, *264*, 108719. [CrossRef]
70. Jamaludin, A.; Kadir, T.; Zisserman, A.; McCall, I.; Williams, F.M.K.; Lang, H.; Buchanan, E.; Urban, J.P.G.; Fairbank, J.C.T. ISSLS PRIZE in Clinical Science 2023: Comparison of degenerative MRI features of the intervertebral disc between those with and without chronic low back pain. An exploratory study of two large female populations using automated annotation. *Eur. Spine J.* **2023**, *32*, 1504–1516. [CrossRef] [PubMed]
71. Han, Z.; Wei, B.; Mercado, A.; Leung, S.; Li, S. Spine-GAN: Semantic segmentation of multiple spinal structures. *Med. Image Anal.* **2018**, *50*, 23–35. [CrossRef] [PubMed]
72. Jiang, W.; Mei, F.; Xie, Q. Novel automated spinal ultrasound segmentation approach for scoliosis visualization. *Front. Physiol.* **2022**, *13*, 1051808. [CrossRef]
73. Galbusera, F.; Niemeyer, F.; Wilke, H.J.; Bassani, T.; Casaroli, G.; Anania, C.; Costa, F.; Brayda-Bruno, M.; Sconfienza, L.M. Fully automated radiological analysis of spinal disorders and deformities: A deep learning approach. *Eur. Spine J.* **2019**, *28*, 951–960. [CrossRef]
74. Taphoorn, M.J.; Claassens, L.; Aaronson, N.K.; Coens, C.; Mauer, M.; Osoba, D.; Stupp, R.; Mirimanoff, R.O.; van den Bent, M.J.; Bottomley, A.; et al. An international validation study of the EORTC brain cancer module (EORTC QLQ-BN20) for assessing health-related quality of life and symptoms in brain cancer patients. *Eur. J. Cancer* **2010**, *46*, 1033–1040. [CrossRef] [PubMed]
75. Hawkins, J.R.; Olson, M.P.; Harouni, A.; Qin, M.M.; Hess, C.P.; Majumdar, S.; Crane, J.C. Implementation and prospective real-time evaluation of a generalized system for in-clinic deployment and validation of machine learning models in radiology. *PLOS Digit. Health* **2023**, *2*, e0000227. [CrossRef]
76. Tang, H.; Hong, M.; Yu, L.; Song, Y.; Cao, M.; Xiang, L.; Zhou, Y.; Suo, S. Deep learning reconstruction for lumbar spine MRI acceleration: A prospective study. *Eur. Radiol. Exp.* **2024**, *8*, 67. [CrossRef]
77. Estler, A.; Hauser, T.K.; Brunnée, M.; Zerweck, L.; Richter, V.; Knoppik, J.; Örgel, A.; Bürkle, E.; Adib, S.D.; Hengel, H.; et al. Deep learning-accelerated image reconstruction in back pain-MRI imaging: Reduction of acquisition time and improvement of image quality. *La Radiol. Medica* **2024**, *129*, 478–487. [CrossRef] [PubMed]

78. Li, J.; Xu, M.; Jiang, B.; Dong, Q.; Xia, Y.; Zhou, T.; Lin, X.; Ma, Y.; Jiang, S.; Zhang, Z.; et al. Diagnostic interchangeability of deep-learning based Synth-STIR images generated from T1 and T2 weighted spine images. *Eur. Radiol.* **2025**, 1–11. [CrossRef] [PubMed]
79. Kaniewska, M.; Zecca, F.; Obermüller, C.; Ensle, F.; Deininger-Czermak, E.; Lohezic, M.; Guggenberger, R. Deep learning reconstruction of zero-echo time sequences to improve visualization of osseous structures and associated pathologies in MRI of cervical spine. *Insights Into Imaging* **2025**, *16*, 29. [CrossRef]
80. Park, S.; Kang, J.H.; Moon, S.G. Diagnostic performance of lumbar spine CT using deep learning denoising to evaluate disc herniation and spinal stenosis. *Eur. Radiol.* **2025**, 1–10. [CrossRef]
81. Greffier, J.; Hamard, A.; Pereira, F.; Barrau, C.; Pasquier, H.; Beregi, J.P.; Frandon, J. Image quality and dose reduction opportunity of deep learning image reconstruction algorithm for CT: A phantom study. *Eur. Radiol.* **2020**, *30*, 3951–3959. [CrossRef]
82. Fischer, G.; Schlosser, T.P.C.; Dietrich, T.J.; Kim, O.C.-H.; Zdravkovic, V.; Martens, B.; Fehlings, M.G.; Jans, L.; Vereecke, E.; Stienen, M.N.; et al. Radiological evaluation and clinical implications of deep learning- and MRI-based synthetic CT for the assessment of cervical spine injuries. *Eur. Radiol.* **2025**, 1–13. [CrossRef]
83. Bousson, V.; Benoist, N.; Guetat, P.; Attané, G.; Salvat, C.; Perronne, L. Application of artificial intelligence to imaging interpretations in the musculoskeletal area: Where are we? Where are we going? *Jt. Bone Spine* **2023**, *90*, 105493. [CrossRef] [PubMed]
84. Bharadwaj, U.U.; Chin, C.T.; Majumdar, S. Practical applications of artificial intelligence in spine imaging: A review. *Radiol. Clin. N. Am.* **2024**, *62*, 355–370. [CrossRef]
85. American College of Radiology. Cord compression—AI in Your Practice: AI Use Cases; Creative Commons 4.0. Available online: https://www.acr.org/Data-Science-and-Informatics/AI-in-Your-Practice/AI-Use-Cases/Use-Cases/Cord-Compression (accessed on 20 August 2025).
86. Ramadanov, N.; John, P.; Hable, R.; Schreyer, A.G.; Shabo, S.; Prill, R.; Salzmann, M. Artificial intelligence-guided distal radius fracture detection on plain radiographs in comparison with human raters. *J. Orthop. Surg. Res.* **2025**, *20*, 468. [CrossRef]
87. Harper, J.P.; Lee, G.R.; Pan, I.; Nguyen, X.V.; Quails, N.; Prevedello, L.M. External Validation of a Winning AI-Algorithm from the RSNA 2022 Cervical Spine Fracture Detection Challenge. *AJNR. Am. J. Neuroradiol.* **2025**, *46*, 1852–1858. [CrossRef]
88. U.S. Food and Drug Administration. *K241211: CoLumbo—510(k) Premarket Notification Decision Summary*. Available online: https://www.accessdata.fda.gov/cdrh_docs/pdf24/K241211.pdf (accessed on 15 August 2024).
89. U.S. Food and Drug Administration. *K241108: RemedyLogic AI MRI Lumbar Spine Reader—510(k) Decision Summary*. Available online: https://www.accessdata.fda.gov/cdrh_docs/pdf24/K241108.pdf (accessed on 30 October 2024).
90. Gupta, A.; Hussain, M.; Nikhileshwar, K.; Rastogi, A.; Rangarajan, K. Integrating Large language models into radiology workflow: Impact of generating personalized report templates from summary. *Eur. J. Radiol.* **2025**, *189*, 112198. [CrossRef] [PubMed]
91. Gertz, R.J.; Beste, N.C.; Dratsch, T.; Lennartz, S.; Bremm, J.; Iuga, A.I.; Bunck, A.C.; Laukamp, K.R.; Schönfeld, M.; Kottlors, J. From dictation to diagnosis: Enhancing radiology reporting with integrated speech recognition in multimodal large language models. *Eur. Radiol.* **2025**, 1–9. [CrossRef]
92. Busch, F.; Hoffmann, L.; Dos Santos, D.P.; Makowski, M.R.; Saba, L.; Prucker, P.; Hadamitzky, M.; Navab, N.; Kather, J.N.; Truhn, D.; et al. Large language models for structured reporting in radiology: Past, present, and future. *Eur. Radiol.* **2025**, *35*, 2589–2602. [CrossRef]
93. Huang, J.; Wittbrodt, M.T.; Teague, C.N.; Karl, E.; Galal, G.; Thompson, M.; Chapa, A.; Chiu, M.L.; Herynk, B.; Linchangco, R.; et al. Efficiency and Quality of Generative AI–Assisted Radiograph Reporting. *JAMA Netw. Open* **2025**, *8*, e2513921. [CrossRef]
94. Voinea, Ș.V.; Mămuleanu, M.; Teică, R.V.; Florescu, L.M.; Selișteanu, D.; Gheonea, I.A. GPT-driven radiology report generation with fine-tuned llama 3. *Bioengineering* **2024**, *11*, 1043. [CrossRef]
95. Jorg, T.; Halfmann, M.C.; Stoehr, F.; Arnhold, G.; Theobald, A.; Mildenberger, P.; Müller, L. A novel reporting workflow for automated integration of artificial intelligence results into structured radiology reports. *Insights Into Imaging* **2024**, *15*, 80. [CrossRef]
96. Wang, J.; Miao, J.; Zhan, Y.; Duan, Y.; Wang, Y.; Hao, D.; Wang, B. Spine Surgical Robotics: Current Status and Recent Clinical Applications. *Neurospine* **2023**, *20*, 1256–1271. [CrossRef]
97. Anderson, P.A.; Kadri, A.; Hare, K.J.; Binkley, N. Preoperative bone health assessment and optimization in spine surgery. *Neurosurg. Focus* **2020**, *49*, E2. [CrossRef]
98. Jia, S.H.; Weng, Y.Z.; Wang, K.; Qi, H.; Yang, Y.; Ma, C.; Lu, W.W.; Wu, H. Performance evaluation of an AI-based preoperative planning software application for automatic selection of pedicle screws based on CT images. *Front. Surg.* **2023**, *10*, 1247527. [CrossRef]
99. Scherer, M.; Kausch, L.; Bajwa, A.; Neumann, J.-O.; Ishak, B.; Naser, P.; Vollmuth, P.; Kiening, K.; Maier-Hein, K.; Unterberg, A. Automatic Planning Tools for Lumbar Pedicle Screws: Comparison of DL vs atlas-based planning. *J. Clin. Med.* **2023**, *12*, 2646. [CrossRef]
100. Chazen, L.; Lim, E.; Li, Q.; Sneag, D.B.; Tan, E.T. Deep-learning reconstructed lumbar spine 3D MRI for surgical planning equivalency to CT. *Eur. Spine J.* **2023**, *33*, 4144–4154.

101. Ao, Y.; Esfandiari, H.; Carrillo, F.; Laux, C.J.; As, Y.; Li, R.; Van Assche, K.; Davoodi, A.; Cavalcanti, N.A.; Farshad, M.; et al. SafeRPlan: Safe Deep Reinforcement Learning for Intraoperative Planning of Pedicle Screw Placement. *Comput. Biol. Med.* **2024**, *99*, 103345. [CrossRef] [PubMed]
102. Johnson & Johnson MedTech. *DePuy Synthes Launches Its First Active Spine Robotics and Navigation Platform*; Johnson & Johnson Newsroom: Weehawken, NJ, USA, 2024.
103. Quiceno, E.; Soliman, M.A.R.; Khan, A.; Mullin, J.P.; Pollina, J. How Do Robotics and Navigation Facilitate Minimally Invasive Spine Surgery? A Case Series and Narrative Review. *Neurosurgery* **2025**, *96*, S84–S93. [CrossRef]
104. Khalsa, S.S.S.; Mummaneni, P.V.; Chou, D.; Park, P. Present and Future Spinal Robotic and Enabling Technologies. *Oper. Neurosurg.* **2021**, *21* (Suppl. S1), S48–S56. [CrossRef]
105. Haida, D.M.; Mohr, P.; Won, S.Y.; Möhlig, T.; Holl, M.; Enk, T.; Hanschen, M.; Huber-Wagner, S. Hybrid-3D robotic suite in spine and trauma surgery—Experiences in 210 patients. *J. Orthop. Surg. Res.* **2024**, *19*, 565. [CrossRef] [PubMed]
106. Judy, B.F.; Pennington, Z.; Botros, D.; Tsehay, Y.; Kopparapu, S.; Liu, A.; Theodore, N.; Zakaria, H.M. Spine Image Guidance and Robotics: Exposure, Education, Training, and the Learning Curve. *Int. J. Spine Surg.* **2021**, *15*, S28–S37. [CrossRef] [PubMed]
107. Ellis, C.A.; Gu, P.; Sendi, M.S.E.; Huddleston, D.; Mahmoudi, B. A Cloud-based Framework for Implementing Portable Machine Learning Pipelines for Neural Data Analysis. *Annu. Int. Conf. IEEE Eng. Med. Biol. Soc.* **2019**, *2019*, 4466–4469. [CrossRef]
108. Wood, J.S.; Purzycki, A.; Thompson, J.; David, L.R.; Argenta, L.C. The Use of Brainlab Navigation in Le Fort III Osteotomy. *J. Craniofacial Surg.* **2015**, *26*, 616–619. [CrossRef]
109. Asada, T.; Subramanian, T.; Simon, C.Z.; Singh, N.; Hirase, T.; Araghi, K.; Lu, A.Z.; Mai, E.; Kim, Y.E.; Tuma, O.; et al. Level-specific comparison of 3D navigated and robotic arm-guided screw placement: An accuracy assessment of 1210 pedicle screws in lumbar surgery. *Spine J.* **2024**, *24*, 1872–1880. [CrossRef] [PubMed]
110. Lefranc, M.; Peltier, J. Evaluation of the ROSA™ Spine robot for minimally invasive surgical procedures. *Expert Rev. Med. Devices* **2016**, *13*, 899–906. [CrossRef] [PubMed]
111. Pojskić, M.; Bopp, M.; Nimsky, C.; Carl, B.; Saβ, B. Initial Intraoperative Experience with Robotic-Assisted Pedicle Screw Placement with Cirq® Robotic Alignment: An Evaluation of the First 70 Screws. *J. Clin. Med.* **2021**, *10*, 5725. [CrossRef]
112. Kumar, R.; Waisberg, E.; Ong, J.; Lee, A.G. The potential power of Neuralink—How brain-machine interfaces can revolutionize medicine. *Expert Rev. Med. Devices* **2025**, *22*, 521–524. [CrossRef] [PubMed]
113. Liebmann, F.; von Atzigen, M.; Stütz, D.; Wolf, J.; Zingg, L.; Suter, D.; Cavalcanti, N.A.; Leoty, L.; Esfandiari, H.; Snedeker, J.G.; et al. Automatic registration with continuous pose updates for marker-less surgical navigation in spine surgery. *Npj Digit. Med.* **2023**, *91*, 103027. [CrossRef]
114. Ansari, T.S.; Maik, V.; Naheem, M.; Ram, K.; Lakshmanan, M.; Sivaprakasam, M. A Hybrid-Layered System for Image-Guided Navigation and Robot-Assisted Spine Surgery. *arXiv* **2024**, arXiv:2406.04644.
115. Paladugu, P.S.; Ong, J.; Nelson, N.; Kamran, S.A.; Waisberg, E.; Zaman, N.; Kumar, R.; Dias, R.D.; Lee, A.G. Generative Adversarial Networks in Medicine: Important Considerations for this Emerging Innovation in Artificial Intelligence. *Ann. Biomed. Eng.* **2023**, *51*, 2130–2142. [CrossRef]
116. Lee, R.; Ong, J.; Waisberg, E.; Ben-David, G.; Jaiswal, S.; Arogundade, E.; Lee, A.G. Applications of Artificial Intelligence in Neuro-Ophthalmology: Neuro-Ophthalmic Imaging Patterns and Implementation Challenges. *Neuro-Ophthalmol.* **2025**, *49*, 273–284. [CrossRef]
117. Alzubaidi, L.; Al-Dulaimi, K.; Salhi, A.; Alammar, Z.; Fadhel, M.A.; Albahri, A.S.; Alamoodi, A.H.; Albahri, O.S.; Hasan, A.F.; Bai, J.; et al. Comprehensive review of deep learning in orthopaedics: Applications, challenges, trustworthiness, and fusion. *Artif. Intell. Med.* **2024**, *155*, 102935. [CrossRef]
118. Baydili, İ.; Tasci, B.; Tasci, G. Artificial Intelligence in Psychiatry: A Review of Biological and Behavioral Data Analyses. *Diagnostics* **2025**, *15*, 434. [CrossRef] [PubMed]
119. Minerva, F.; Giubilini, A. Is AI the Future of Mental Healthcare? *Topoi* **2023**, *42*, 809–817. [CrossRef]
120. Bouguettaya, A.; Stuart, E.M.; Aboujaoude, E. Racial bias in AI-mediated psychiatric diagnosis and treatment: A qualitative comparison of four large language models. *npj Digit. Med.* **2025**, *8*, 332. [CrossRef]
121. Miller, D.J.; Lastella, M.; Scanlan, A.T.; Bellenger, C.; Halson, S.L.; Roach, G.D.; Sargent, C. A validation study of the WHOOP strap against polysomnography to assess sleep. *J. Sports Sci.* **2020**, *38*, 2631–2636. [CrossRef] [PubMed]
122. Wikimedia Commons. *What-Is-nlp*; Wikimedia Commons: San Francisco, CA, USA, 2024. Available online: https://commons.wikimedia.org/w/index.php?title=File:What-is-nlp.png&oldid=839312883 (accessed on 15 August 2025).
123. Grosicki, G.J.; Fielding, F.; Kim, J.; Chapman, C.J.; Olaru, M.; Hippel, V.; Holmes, K.E. Wearing WHOOP More Frequently Is Associated with Better Biometrics and Healthier Sleep and Activity Patterns. *Sensors* **2025**, *25*, 2437. [CrossRef]
124. Kumar, R.; Waisberg, E.; Ong, J.; Paladugu, P.; Amiri, D.; Nahouraii, R.; Jagadeesan, R.; Tavakkoli, A. Integration of Multi-Modal Imaging and Machine Learning Visualization Techniques to Optimize Structural Neuroimaging. *Preprints* **2024**, *2024*, 2024111128. [CrossRef]

125. National Academies of Sciences, Engineering, and Medicine; Division of Behavioral and Social Sciences and Education; Board on Behavioral, Cognitive, and Sensory Sciences; Committee on Future Directions for Applying Behavioral Economics to Policy. Beatty, A., Moffitt, R., Buttenheim, A., Eds.; *Behavioral Economics: Policy Impact and Future Directions*; National Academies Press (US): Washington, DC, USA, 2023. Available online: https://www.ncbi.nlm.nih.gov/books/NBK593518/ (accessed on 6 September 2025).
126. Fayers, P.; Bottomley, A.; EORTC Quality of Life Group. Quality of life research within the EORTC-the EORTC QLQ-C30. *Eur. J. Cancer* **2002**, *38* (Suppl. S4), S125–S133. [CrossRef]
127. Bushnell, D.M.; Atkinson, T.M.; McCarrier, K.P.; Liepa, A.M.; DeBusk, K.P.; Coons, S.J. Patient-Reported Outcome Consortium's NSCLC Working Group Non-Small Cell Lung Cancer Symptom Assessment Questionnaire: Psychometric Performance and Regulatory Qualification of a Novel Patient-Reported Symptom Measure. *Curr. Ther. Res.* **2021**, *95*, 100642. [CrossRef]
128. Kumar, R.; Sporn, K.; Khanna, A.; Paladugu, P.; Gowda, C.; Ngo, A.; Jagadeesan, R.; Zaman, N.; Tavakkoli, A. Integrating Radiogenomics and Machine Learning in Musculoskeletal Oncology Care. *Diagnostics* **2025**, *15*, 1377. [CrossRef]
129. Lee, Y.S.; Cho, D.C.; Kim, K.T. Navigation-Guided/Robot-Assisted Spinal Surgery: A Review Article with cost-effectiveness emphasis. *Neurospine* **2024**, *21*, 8. [CrossRef]
130. Tkachenko, A.A.; Changalidis, A.I.; Maksiutenko, E.M.; Nasykhova, Y.A.; Barbitoff, Y.A.; Glotov, A.S. Replication of Known and Identification of Novel Associations in Biobank-Scale Datasets: A Survey Using UK Biobank and FinnGen. *Genes* **2024**, *15*, 931. [CrossRef] [PubMed]
131. Kurki, M.I.; Karjalainen, J.; Palta, P.; Sipilä, T.P.; Kristiansson, K.; Donner, K.M.; Reeve, M.P.; Laivuori, H.; Aavikko, M.; Kaunisto, M.A.; et al. FinnGen provides genetic insights from a well-phenotyped isolated population. *Nature* **2023**, *613*, 508–518. [CrossRef] [PubMed]
132. Theodore, N.; Ahmed, A.K.; Fulton, T.; Mousses, S.; Yoo, C.; Goodwin, C.R.; Danielson, J.; Sciubba, D.M.; Giers, M.B.; Kalani, M.Y.S. Genetic Predisposition to Symptomatic Lumbar Disk Herniation in Pediatric and Young Adult Patients. *Spine* **2019**, *44*, E640–E649. [CrossRef]
133. Yang, J.; Xu, W.; Chen, D.; Liu, Y.; Hu, X. Evidence from Mendelian randomization analysis combined with meta-analysis for the causal validation of the relationship between 91 inflammatory factors and lumbar disc herniation. *Medicine* **2024**, *103*, e40323. [CrossRef] [PubMed]
134. Scott, H.; Panin, V.M. The role of protein N-glycosylation in neural transmission. *Glycobiology* **2014**, *24*, 407–417. [CrossRef]
135. He, M.; Zhou, X.; Wang, X. Glycosylation: Mechanisms, biological functions and clinical implications. *Signal Transduct. Target. Ther.* **2024**, *9*, 194. [CrossRef]
136. Ayoub, A.; McHugh, J.; Hayward, J.; Rafi, I.; Qureshi, N. Polygenic risk scores: Improving the prediction of future disease or added complexity? *Br. J. Gen. Pract.* **2022**, *72*, 396–398. [CrossRef]
137. Singh, O.; Verma, M.; Dahiya, N.; Senapati, S.; Kakkar, R.; Kalra, S. Integrating Polygenic Risk Scores (PRS) for Personalized Diabetes Care: Advancing Clinical Practice with Tailored Pharmacological Approaches. *Diabetes Ther.* **2025**, *16*, 149–168. [CrossRef]
138. Sporn, K.; Kumar, R.; Paladugu, P.; Ong, J.; Sekhar, T.; Vaja, S.; Hage, T.; Waisberg, E.; Gowda, C.; Jagadeesan, R.; et al. Artificial Intelligence in Orthopedic Medical Education: A Comprehensive Review of Emerging Technologies and Their Applications. *Int. Med. Educ.* **2025**, *4*, 14. [CrossRef]
139. Krupkova, O.; Cambria, E.; Besse, L.; Besse, A.; Bowles, R.; Wuertz-Kozak, K. The potential of CRISPR/Cas9 genome editing for the study and treatment of intervertebral disc pathologies. *JOR Spine* **2018**, *1*, e1003. [CrossRef]
140. Dean, L.; Kane, M. Codeine Therapy and CYP2D6 Genotype. In *Medical Genetics Summaries*; Pratt, V.M., Scott, S.A., Pirmohamed, M., Eds.; National Center for Biotechnology Information (US): Bethesda, MD, USA, 2025. Available online: https://www.ncbi.nlm.nih.gov/books/NBK100662/ (accessed on 15 August 2025).
141. Li, B.; Sangkuhl, K.; Keat, K.; Whaley, R.M.; Woon, M.; Verma, S.; Dudek, S.; Tuteja, S.; Verma, A.; Whirl-Carrillo, M.; et al. How to Run the Pharmacogenomics Clinical Annotation Tool (PharmCAT). *Clin. Pharmacol. Ther.* **2023**, *113*, 1036–1047. [CrossRef]
142. Tippenhauer, K.; Philips, M.; Largiadèr, C.; Sariyar, M. Using the PharmCAT tool for Pharmacogenetic clinical decision support. *Brief. Bioinform.* **2024**, *25*, bbad452. [CrossRef]
143. Sadee, W.; Wang, D.; Hartmann, K.; Toland, A.E. Pharmacogenomics: Driving Personalized Medicine. *Pharmacol. Rev.* **2023**, *75*, 789–814. [CrossRef]
144. Guarneri, M.; Scola, L.; Giarratana, R.M.; Bova, M.; Carollo, C.; Vaccarino, L.; Calandra, L.; Lio, D.; Balistreri, C.R.; Cottone, S. MIF rs755622 and IL6 rs1800795 Are Implied in Genetic Susceptibility to End-Stage Renal Disease (ESRD). *Genes* **2022**, *13*, 226. [CrossRef]
145. Górczyńska-Kosiorz, S.; Tabor, E.; Niemiec, P.; Pluskiewicz, W.; Gumprecht, J. Associations between the VDR Gene rs731236 (TaqI) Polymorphism and Bone Mineral Density in Postmenopausal Women from the RAC-OST-POL. *Biomedicines* **2024**, *12*, 917. [CrossRef]

146. De La Vega, R.E.; van Griensven, M.; Zhang, W.; Coenen, M.J.; Nagelli, C.V.; Panos, J.A.; Peniche Silva, C.J.; Geiger, J.; Plank, C.; Evans, C.H.; et al. Efficient healing of large osseous segmental defects using optimized chemically modified messenger RNA encoding BMP-2. *Sci. Adv.* **2022**, *8*, eabl6242. [CrossRef] [PubMed]
147. Robinson, C.; Dalal, S.; Chitneni, A.; Patil, A.; Berger, A.A.; Mahmood, S.; Orhurhu, V.; Kaye, A.D.; Hasoon, J. A Look at Commonly Utilized Serotonin Noradrenaline Reuptake Inhibitors (SNRIs) in Chronic Pain. *Health Psychol. Res.* **2022**, *10*, 32309. [CrossRef] [PubMed]
148. Wiffen, P.J.; Derry, S.; Bell, R.F.; Rice, A.S.; Tölle, T.R.; Phillips, T.; Moore, R.A. Gabapentin for chronic neuropathic pain in adults. *Cochrane Database Syst. Rev.* **2017**, *6*, CD007938. [CrossRef] [PubMed]
149. Mukherjee, A.; Abraham, S.; Singh, A.; Balaji, S.; Mukunthan, K.S. From Data to Cure: A Comprehensive Exploration of Multi-omics Data Analysis for Targeted Therapies. *Mol. Biotechnol.* **2025**, *67*, 1269–1289. [CrossRef]
150. Assi, I.Z.; Landzberg, M.J.; Becker, K.C.; Renaud, D.; Reyes, F.B.; Leone, D.M.; Benson, M.; Michel, M.; Gerszten, R.E.; Opotowsky, A.R. Correlation between Olink and SomaScan proteomics platforms in adults with a Fontan circulation. *Int. J. Cardiol. Congenit. Heart Dis.* **2025**, *20*, 100584. [CrossRef] [PubMed]
151. Yang, L.; Liu, B.; Dong, X.; Wu, J.; Sun, C.; Xi, L.; Cheng, R.; Wu, B.; Wang, H.; Tong, S.; et al. Clinical severity prediction in children with osteogenesis imperfecta caused by COL1A1/2 defects. *Osteoporos. Int.* **2022**, *33*, 1373–1384. [CrossRef]
152. Kohn, M.S.; Sun, J.; Knoop, S.; Shabo, A.; Carmeli, B.; Sow, D.; Syed-Mahmood, T.; Rapp, W. IBM's Health Analytics and Clinical Decision Support. *Yearb. Med. Inform.* **2014**, *9*, 154–162. [CrossRef]
153. Morsbach, F.; Zhang, Y.H.; Martin, L.; Lindqvist, C.; Brismar, T. Body composition evaluation with computed tomography: Contrast media and slice thickness cause methodological errors. *Nutrition* **2019**, *59*, 50–55. [CrossRef]
154. Riem, L.; DuCharme, O.; Cousins, M.; Feng, X.; Kenney, A.; Morris, J.; Tapscott, S.J.; Tawil, R.; Statland, J.; Shaw, D.; et al. AI driven analysis of MRI to measure health and disease progression in FSHD. *Sci. Rep.* **2024**, *14*, 15462. [CrossRef]
155. Moraes da Silva, W.; Cazella, S.C.; Rech, R.S. Deep learning algorithms to assist in imaging diagnosis in individuals with disc herniation or spondylolisthesis: A scoping review. *Int. J. Med. Inform.* **2025**, *201*, 105933. [CrossRef]
156. Murto, N.; Lund, T.; Kautiainen, H.; Luoma, K.; Kerttula, L. Comparison of lumbar disc degeneration grading between deep learning model SpineNet and radiologist: A longitudinal study with a 14-year follow-up. *Eur. Spine J.* **2025**, 1–7. [CrossRef]
157. van Wulfften Palthe, O.D.R.; Tromp, I.; Ferreira, A.; Fiore, A.; Bramer, J.A.M.; van Dijk, N.C.; DeLaney, T.F.; Schwab, J.H.; Hornicek, F.J. Sacral chordoma: A clinical review of 101 cases with 30-year experience in a single institution. *Spine J.* **2019**, *19*, 869–879. [CrossRef] [PubMed]
158. O'Hanlon, C.E.; Kranz, A.M.; DeYoreo, M.; Mahmud, A.; Damberg, C.L.; Timbie, J. Access, Quality, And Financial Performance Of Rural Hospitals Following Health System Affiliation. *Health Aff.* **2019**, *38*, 2095–2104. [CrossRef]
159. Vaughan, L.; Edwards, N. The problems of smaller, rural and remote hospitals: Separating facts from fiction. *Future Healthc. J.* **2020**, *7*, 38–45. [CrossRef] [PubMed]
160. Ramedani, S.; George, D.R.; Leslie, D.L.; Kraschnewski, J. The bystander effect: Impact of rural hospital closures on the operations and financial well-being of surrounding healthcare institutions. *J. Hosp. Med.* **2022**, *17*, 901–906. [CrossRef] [PubMed]
161. Kumar, R.; Waisberg, E.; Ong, J.; Paladugu, P.; Sporn, K.; Chima, K.; Amiri, D.; Zaman, N.; Tavakkoli, A. Precision health monitoring in spaceflight with integration of lower body negative pressure and advanced large language model artificial intelligence. *Life Sci. Space Res.* **2025**, *47*, 57–60. [CrossRef]
162. Agency for Healthcare Research and Quality. *2022 National Healthcare Quality and Disparities Report*; Agency for Healthcare Research and Quality (US): Rockville, MD, USA, 2022. Available online: https://www.ncbi.nlm.nih.gov/books/NBK587178/ (accessed on 15 August 2025).
163. Gillespie, E.F.; Santos, P.M.G.; Curry, M.; Salz, T.; Chakraborty, N.; Caron, M.; Fuchs, H.E.; Vicioso, N.L.; Mathis, N.; Kumar, R.; et al. Implementation Strategies to Promote Short-Course Radiation for Bone Metastases. *JAMA Netw. Open* **2024**, *7*, e2411717. [CrossRef]
164. Allen, J.; Shepherd, C.; Heaton, T.; Behrens, N.; Dorius, A.; Grimes, J. Differences in Medicare payment and practice characteristics for orthopedic surgery subspecialties. *Proc. Bayl. University. Med. Cent.* **2024**, *38*, 175–178. [CrossRef]
165. Lee, C.; Britto, S.; Diwan, K. Evaluating the Impact of Artificial Intelligence (AI) on Clinical Documentation Efficiency and Accuracy Across Clinical Settings: A Scoping Review. *Cureus* **2024**, *16*, e73994. [CrossRef]
166. Seh, A.H.; Zarour, M.; Alenezi, M.; Sarkar, A.K.; Agrawal, A.; Kumar, R.; Khan, R.A. Healthcare Data Breaches: Insights and Implications. *Healthcare* **2020**, *8*, 133. [CrossRef] [PubMed]
167. Iglesias, L.L.; Bellón, P.S.; Del Barrio, A.P.; Fernández-Miranda, P.M.; González, D.R.; Vega, J.A.; González Mandly, A.A.; Blanco, J.A.P. A primer on deep learning and convolutional neural networks for clinicians. *Insights Into Imaging* **2021**, *12*, 117. [CrossRef] [PubMed]
168. Fernández-Miranda, P.M.; Fraguela, E.M.; de Linera-Alperi, M.Á.; Cobo, M.; Del Barrio, A.P.; González, D.R.; Vega, J.A.; Iglesias, L.L. A retrospective study of deep learning generalization across two centers and multiple models of X-ray devices using COVID-19 chest-X rays. *Sci. Rep.* **2024**, *14*, 14657. [CrossRef] [PubMed]

169. Roccetti, M.; Delnevo, G.; Casini, L.; Cappiello, G. Is bigger always better? A controversial journey to the center of machine learning design, with uses and misuses of big data for predicting water meter failures. *J. Big Data* **2019**, *6*, 70. [CrossRef]
170. Kim, T.H.; Srinivasulu, A.; Chinthaginjala, R.; Zhao, X.; Obaidur Rab, S.; Tera, S.P. Improving CNN predictive accuracy in COVID-19 health analytics. *Sci. Rep.* **2025**, *15*, 29864. [CrossRef]
171. Varoquaux, G.; Cheplygina, V. Machine learning for medical imaging: Methodological failures and recommendations for the future. *NPJ Digit. Med.* **2022**, *5*, 48. [CrossRef] [PubMed]
172. Yang, Y.; Zhang, H.; Gichoya, J.W.; Katabi, D.; Ghassemi, M. The limits of fair medical imaging AI in real-world generalization. *Nat. Med.* **2024**, *30*, 2838–2848. [CrossRef] [PubMed]
173. Collins, G.S.; Moons, K.G.M.; Dhiman, P.; Riley, R.D.; Beam, A.L.; Van Calster, B.; Ghassemi, M.; Liu, X.; Reitsma, J.B.; van Smeden, M.; et al. TRIPOD+AI statement: Updated guidance for reporting clinical prediction models that use regression or machine learning methods. *BMJ Clin. Res. Ed.* **2024**, *385*, e078378. [CrossRef]
174. Yu, A.C.; Mohajer, B.; Eng, J. External Validation of Deep Learning Algorithms for Radiologic Diagnosis: A Systematic Review. *Radiol. Artif. Intell.* **2022**, *4*, e210064. [CrossRef] [PubMed]

bioengineering

MDPI

Review

Scoping Review of Machine Learning and Patient-Reported Outcomes in Spine Surgery

Christian Quinones, Deepak Kumbhare, Bharat Guthikonda and Stanley Hoang *

Department of Neurosurgery, Louisiana State University Health Shreveport, Shreveport, LA 71103, USA
* Correspondence: stanley.hoang@lsuhs.edu

Abstract

Machine learning is an evolving branch of artificial intelligence that is being applied in neurosurgical research. In spine surgery, machine learning has been used for radiographic characterization of cranial and spinal pathology and in predicting postoperative outcomes such as complications, functional recovery, and pain relief. A relevant application is the investigation of patient-reported outcome measures (PROMs) after spine surgery. Although a multitude of PROMs have been described and validated, there is currently no consensus regarding which questionnaires should be utilized. Additionally, studies have reported varying degrees of accuracy in predicting patient outcomes based on questionnaire responses. PROMs currently lack standardization, which renders them difficult to compare across studies. The purpose of this manuscript is to identify applications of machine learning to predict PROMs after spine surgery.

Keywords: artificial intelligence; machine learning; patient-reported outcomes; spine surgery; outcome measures; literature review; health informatics

1. Introduction

Research in spine surgery has been impacted by the recent rise in artificial intelligence (AI). Machine learning (ML) is a subset of AI that functions to predict outputs based on given inputs. In medical research, input data may include any combination of the following: patient demographics, spinal pathology, imaging characteristics, surgical characteristics, comorbidities, and patient-reported outcome measures (PROMs) [1]. Examples of outputs are complications, functional outcomes, surgical success, hospitalization characteristics, readmission rates, reoperation rates, survival prediction, cost prediction, and rehabilitation needs. One outcome in which ML is particularly applicable is in predicting PROMs after spine surgery.

When being evaluated for spine surgery, an important consideration is the degree of improvement that a patient experiences after surgical intervention. This question can be answered by comparing preoperative and postoperative PROMs. The original PROMs developed for use in spine surgery are currently referred to as "legacy outcome measures" and include the Oswestry Disability Index (ODI), Neck Disability Index (NDI) [2], Visual Analog Scale (VAS), Short Form Health Survey (SF-36 or SF-12), Japanese Orthopaedic Association (JOA) score, Roland-Morris Disability Questionnaire (RMDQ), EuroQol-5D (EQ-5D), and Scoliosis Research Society (SRS) questionnaire [3]. These surveys provided the foundation for defining patient-oriented, clinically significant outcomes that assess quality of life after spine surgery [4]. To quantify a standard for expected PROM improvements, clinicians defined the Minimal Clinically Important Difference (MCID) for these PROMs [5].

Due to variations in spinal pathology, surgical interventions, patient demographics, and the intrinsic disadvantages of PROMs such as time to completion, there has been a lack of consensus on which PROMs to utilize. A 2022 literature review reported the presence of 206 unique spine-specific PROMs [6]. To address this, the National Institute of Health developed the Patient-Reported Outcomes Measurement Information System (PROMIS) in an attempt to standardize PROMs and simplify their administration [7].

The decision to proceed with spine surgery is often complex, largely because there are no definitive guidelines or universal indications for when surgery is appropriate. The use of ML to accurately predict patient outcomes grants surgeons another tool to more confidently advise patients on surgical outcomes [8]. The purpose of this manuscript is to describe the extent to which ML has been used to predict PROMs after spine surgery.

2. Materials and Methods

A scoping review of the literature per the Preferred Reporting Items for Systematic Reviews and Meta-Analyses for Scoping Reviews (PRISMA-ScR) guidelines [9] was carried out in Web of Science, PubMed, and EMBASE on October 8, 2024. A combination of MeSH terms and keywords related to patient-reported outcomes and spine surgery were used. The search criteria for PubMed were as follows: ("Machine Learning" [MeSH] OR "Artificial Intelligence") AND ("Patient Reported Outcome Measures" [MeSH] OR "Patient-reported outcomes"). The search criteria for Web of Science were as follows: ("Machine Learning" OR "Artificial Intelligence") AND ("Patient Reported Outcome Measures" OR "Patient-reported outcomes" OR "PROMs" OR "Quality of Life" OR "Health Outcomes") AND ("Spine" OR "Spinal Surgery"). The search criteria for EMBASE were as follows: ('machine learning'/exp OR 'machine learning' OR 'artificial intelligence'/exp OR 'artificial intelligence') AND ('patient reported outcome'/exp OR 'patient reported outcome' OR 'quality of life'/exp OR 'quality of life' OR 'patient-reported outcomes' OR 'proms' OR 'health outcomes'/exp OR 'health outcomes') AND ('spine'/exp OR 'spine' OR 'spinal surgery'/exp OR 'spinal surgery' OR 'spine surgery'/exp OR 'spine surgery') AND [english]/lim.

English articles published from 1994 to 2024 were selected. One researcher (C.Q.) assessed the manuscripts for eligibility under the supervision of another researcher (D.K.). In cases of disagreements or uncertainties requiring further clarification, the senior author (S.H.) was consulted and a consensus was reached during research team discussions. The inclusion criteria consisted of studies that utilized ML tools to predict postoperative PROMs for patients who underwent spine surgery. Studies that did not employ ML to predict PROMs were excluded. Data extracted included the ML method used, spine pathology, number of patients, features used for model prediction, and ML performance.

3. Results

3.1. Search Results

The initial search yielded 648 articles; 60 repeats were removed, resulting in 588 unique articles for screening. Of the 37 articles that met the initial screening criteria, twelve non-surgical studies were excluded. The remaining 25 articles were further assessed for eligibility, with 3 excluded for not predicting postoperative PROMs [10–12]. A total of 22 articles were included in the qualitative synthesis (Figure 1).

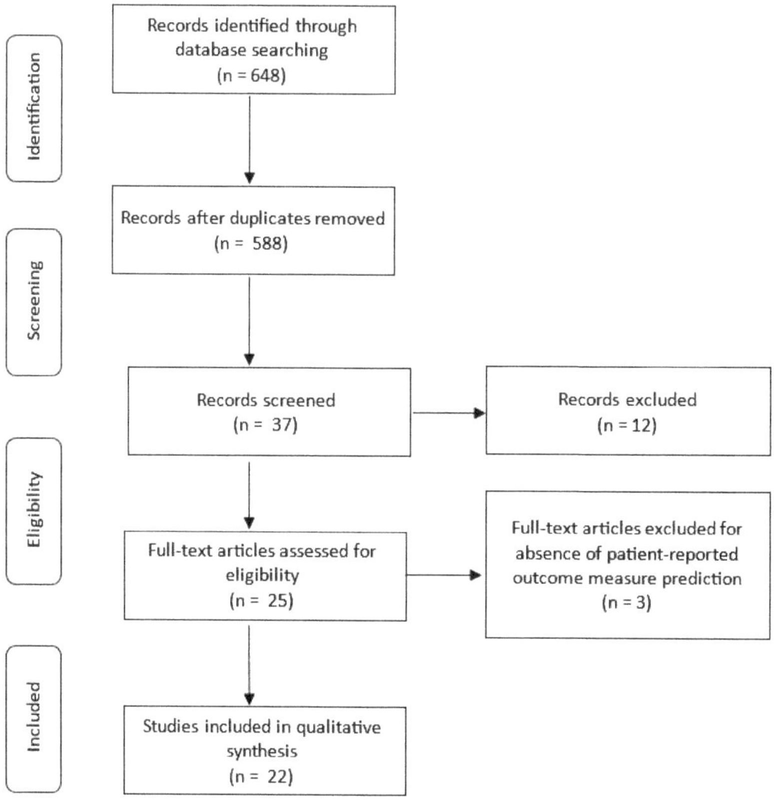

Figure 1. Literature search strategy.

3.2. Study Details

Seven articles predicted outcomes in cervical spine pathologies [13–19]. Three articles predicted outcomes for thoracolumbar pathologies [20–22]. Eleven articles predicted outcomes for lumbar spine pathology [23–33]. One study predicted outcomes for all levels of spinal pathology [34]. The postoperative timeline for PROM prediction ranged from 6 weeks to 24 months (Table 1).

A total of twenty-one PROMs were reported. Seven articles reported the ODI [19,20,23–26,31], and four articles reported the VAS [13,23,25,29], mJOA [14,15,18,19], and numeric rating scale (NRS) [20,24,30,31]. Three reported the JOA [13,25,29], NDI [13,15,17], core outcome measure index (COMI) [26,27,34], and SF-36 [15,16,26]; two articles reported the EQ-5D [13,17] and SRS [21,22]; and one article reported the EuroQol [25], Physical Component Summary (PCS) [26], PROMIS-PF [28], SF-6D [14], Mental Component Summary (MCS) [15], Mental Disability Index (MDI) [15], Disabilities of the Arm, Shoulder, and Hand (DASH) [15], North American Spine Society (NASS) [15], Japanese Orthopedic Association Back Pain Evaluation Questionnaire (JOABPEQ) [29], neck pain [17], and pain symptoms specific to quality of life, social disability, and work disability [34]. Table 2 provides a categorical breakdown and brief description of PROMs.

Table 1. Study characteristics.

Article	Pathology	# of Pts	Predicted PROMs	ML Models	Input Features	PPT (Months)	Results (AUC) *
Liew et al. [17]	Cervical	193	NDI, EQ5D, NP	Stepwise regression, LASSO, boosting, MARS	Demographics, PE, PROMs	12	Not reported
Park et al. [13]	CSM	535	VAS-NP	LR, SVM, DT, RF, extra trees, Gaussian naïve Bayes, KNN, multilayer perceptron, EGBT	Demographics, Sx chars, PROMs, spinal pathology, PE	3; 24	VAS-NP 0.773–0.762
Zhang et al. [15]	CSM	50	SF-36, PCS	SVM	Demographics, PE, PROs, imaging chars	6	SF-36 PCS 86.4, MCS 89.8
Merali et al. [14]	DCM	757	SF-6D, mJOA	RF, SVM, LR, DT, ANN models	Demographics, spinal pathology, Sx chars, comorbidities, PROMs, PE	3–24	SF-6D and mJOA0.83–0.87
Khan et al. [16]	DCM	173	SF-36 MCS, SF-36 PCS	Classification trees, SVM, partial least squares, generalized boosted models, generalized additive models, MARS, RF, LR	Demographics, PE, comorbidities, Sx Hx, spinal pathology, mJOA	12	MCS 0.77, PCS 0.78
Hoffman et al. [19]	DCM	20	ODI	MLR, SVR	Demographics, spinal pathology, Sx chars, comorbidities, PROs, PE, fine motor function	6, 12, and 24	MAA of 0.0283 with SVR
Khan et al. [18]	DCM	702	mJOA	Boosted LR, SVM, naïve Bayes, generalized boosted machines, partial least squares, LR	Demographics, Sx chars, spinal pathology, PE	12	mJOA 0.834
Grob et al. [20]	Thoraco-lumbar	1115	ODI, BP (NRS), LP (NRS)	FUSE-ML, EN regularization	MRI, PROMs, demographics, ASA, PMHx, Sx Hx	12	ODI 0.70, BP 0.72, LP 0.70
Gupta et al. [21]	AIS	6076	SRS-Pain, SRS-Self-Image	LR, gradient boosting, EGBT	PROMs, demographics, spinal pathology, Sx chars	6; 12; 24	MAE 0.47–0.55

Table 1. *Cont.*

Article	Pathology	# of Pts	Predicted PROMs	ML Models	Input Features	PPT (Months)	Results (AUC) *
Pedersen et al. [25]	LDH	1968	ODI, VAS	DL, DT, RF, BT, SVM, LR, MARS	Demographics, PROs, employment details, comorbidities, self-reported expectations to return to work	24	EQ-5D 0.82, ODI 0.75, VAS LP 0.73, VAS BP 0.81, return to work 0.84
Ve et al. [23]	LDH	422	LP (NRS), BP (NRS), ODI	DL, LR	Demographics, ASA, PROMs, Sx chars, Sx Hx, spinal pathology, social Hx	12	BP 0.90, LP 0.87, ODI 0.84
Ames et al. [22]	ASD	561	Individual SRS-22R questions	EN, gradient boosting machines, EGBT, extreme gradient boosting linear, RF, EN regularized generalized linear models	Demographics, comorbidities, Sx chars, imaging chars, hospital chars, surgeon chars	12	SRS-22R questions 0.869 with EGBT
Karhade et al. [28]	LS	906	PROMIS-PF	Stochastic gradient boosting, RF, SVM, NN, EN penalized LR	Demographics, ASA, spinal pathology, Sx chars, PROMs, Rx opioids, geographic information	12	PROMIS-PF 0.75
Yagi et al. [29]	LS	848	VAS BP, VAS LP, JOABPEQ	Generalized LR, generalized linear mixed, LR, SVM, single-layer ANN, random trees, linear-AS, tree-AS, EGBT, chi-squared automatic interaction detection classification, regression tree	Demographics, Sx chars, PROMs	10	MAE 9.3–16.5
Siccoli et al. [31]	LS	635	BP (NRS), LP (NRS), ODI	RF, EGBT, BGLM, BT, KNN, simple BGLM, ANN with a single hidden layer	Clinical data, imaging chars, PROMs, demographics, ASA, Sx Hx, spinal pathology	6 weeks; 12 months	NRS-BP 0.79, 0.92
Khor et al. [24]	LS	1965	BP (NRS), LP (NRS), ODI	Binary LR	Demographics, clinical chars, ASA, Sx Hx, PROMs, comorbidities, Sx chars, Rx opioids, hospital chars	12	ODI 0.66, BP 0.79, and LP 0.69
Berjano et al. [26]	Lumbar	1243	ODI, SF-36, PCS, COMI Back	RF	Demographics, comorbidities, spinal pathology, PROMs, past Sx Hx	6	ODI 0.808

Table 1. *Cont.*

Article	Pathology	# of Pts	Predicted PROMs	ML Models	Input Features	PPT (Months)	Results (AUC) *
Finkelstein et al. [30]	Lumbar	122	NRS	LASSO regression	Clinical and demographic variables, PROMs, patient expectations and cognitive appraisal processes	10	NRS of 0.12 MBR2
Staartjes et al. [32]	Lumbar	1115	ODI, COMI, NRS	EN regularization	Demographics, Rx opioids, Sx Hx, Sx chars, PROMs	12	ODI and COMI 0.67
Halicka et al. [27]	Lumbar	4307	COMI-BP, COMI-LP	RF, LR	Demographics, Sx chars, hospitalization chars	3–24	COMI 0.63, BP 0.72, LP 0.68
Rigoard et al. [33]	Lumbar	200	PGIC	DRFA, PCA	ODI, EQ-5D, HADS, NRS	12	PGIC 0.853
Muller et al. [34]	Cervical and lumbar	10,002	COMI	LASSO, ridge regression	Demographics, Sx chars, surgeon chars, PROMs, psychological assessment	12	MAE back patients 2.1, neck patients 1.8

* = unless otherwise specified; # = number; AIS = adolescent idiopathic scoliosis; ANN = artificial neural network; ASA = American Society of Anesthesiologist; ASD = adult spinal deformity; AUROC = area under the receiver operating characteristic curve; BGLM = Bayesian generalized linear model; BP = back pain; BT = boosted tree; CSM = cervical spondylotic myelopathy; COMI = core outcome measure index; DRFA = dimensionality reduction factor analysis; DT = decision tree; EGBT = extreme gradient boosting tree; EN = elastic net; EQ-5D = EuroQol–5 dimensions; HADS = the hospital anxiety and depression scale; Hx = history; JOABPEQ = Japanese Orthopedic Association back pain evaluation questionnaire; KNN = k-nearest neighbors; LASSO = least absolute shrinkage and selection operator; LDH = lumbar disk herniation; LP = leg pain; LR = logistic regression; MAA = mean absolute accuracy; MAE = mean absolute error; MARS = multivariate adaptive regression spline; MBR2 = mean bootstrapped R2; MCS = Mental Component Summary; MCRI = multidimensional clinical response index; mJOA = modified Japanese Orthopaedic Association; MLR = multivariate linear regression; NDI = Neck Disability Index; NP = neck pain; NRS = numeric rating scale; PE = physical exam; PCA = principal component analysis; PCS = Physical Component Summary; PGIC = Patient Global Impression of Change; PMHx = past medical history; Pts = patients; PPT = postoperative prediction timeline; PROMIS-PF = Patient-Reported Outcomes Measurement Information System-Physical Function; RF = randomforest; Rx = prescription; SF-6D = short form-6 dimensions; SF-36 = short form-36 health survey; SRS = Scoliosis Research Society; SVR = support vector regression; SVM = support vector machine; Sx = surgical; VAS = Visual Analog Scale.

Table 2. Description of common patient-reported outcome measures.

Domain	PROM	Description
Multiple Outcomes	MCRI	Modified Clinical Response Index (MCRI) evaluates pain, functional capacity, quality of life, and outcomes in spinal surgery patients with Persistent Spinal Pain syndrome
	NASS	North American Spine Society (NASS) assesses outcomes and pain related to lumbar spine disease
	EQ-5D	EuroQol-5 Dimensions (EQ-5D) measures health status across five dimensions: mobility, self-care, usual activities, pain/discomfort, anxiety/depression
	COMI	Core Outcome Measures Index (COMI) measures the impact of back and leg pain, assessing pain, function, and quality of life
	SRS	Scoliosis Research Society (SRS) assesses function, pain, self-image, mental health, and satisfaction
Physical Function	NDI	Neck Disability Index (NDI) evaluates disability related to neck pain and its impact on daily activities
	JOA	Japanese Orthopaedic Association Score (JOA) assesses neurological function in patients with cervical myelopathy
	mJOA	Modified JOA (mJOA) evaluates functional impairment in cervical spine conditions
	ODI	Oswestry Disability Index (ODI) assesses disability due to lower back pain
	PROMIS-PF	Patient-Reported Outcomes Measurement Information System (PROMIS)-Physical Function (PF) assesses physical function and the ability to perform physical activities
	PCS	Physical Component Summary (PCS) is a subscore from SF36 measuring physical health
	DASH	Disabilities of the Arm, Shoulder, and Hand (DASH) measures upper-extremity function, pain, and work and social activity participation
Mental Health	MCS	Mental Component Summary (MCS) assesses psychological well-being
	MDI	Mental Disability Index (MDI) measures mental health-related disability
	PGIC	Patient Global Impression of Change (PGIC) measures a patient's overall perception of improvement or change in condition
Quality of Life	SF-36	Short Form-36 Health Survey (SF-36) assesses overall health-related quality of life across multiple domains (physical, mental, and social)
	SF-6D	Short Form-6 Dimensions (SF-6D) is a condensed version of SF36 that measures a single index for health-related quality of life
Pain	VAS	Visual Analog Scale (VAS) measures intensity of pain using a 0–10 visual scale
	NRS	Numeric rating scale (NRS) quantifies pain on a 0–10 scale
Social	JOABPEQ	Japanese Orthopaedic Association Back Pain Evaluation Questionnaire (JOABPEQ) evaluates the impact of back pain on physical and social functioning

The features used for model prediction were demographics in all but one study [33]. Surgical characteristics were used in ten studies [13,14,18,19,21,23,27,29,32,34]. Spinal pathology characteristics were used in ten studies [13,14,16,18,19,21,23,26,28,31]. American Society of Anesthesiologist (ASA) classification was used in six studies [13,20,23,24,28,31]. Physical exam findings were used in seven studies [13–19]. Past medical history (including surgical history) was used in five studies [19,26,30,31,34]. Preoperative opioid use was used in four studies [22,24,28,32]. Hospitalization details were used in three studies [22,24,27]. Social history (including employment details) was used in two studies [23,25]. One study used geographic details [28].

Sixty unique ML models were used in the relevant studies. The most frequently used model was support vector machine (SVM), which was used in eight studies [13–16,18,25,28,29]; logistic regression (LR), which was used in seven studies [13,14,16,21,23,27,29]; and RF, which was used in six studies [14,16,22,26,27,31]. Decision tree was used in four studies [13,14,21,25], and elastic net (EN) was used in three studies [22,28,32]. Least absolute shrinkage and selection operator (LASSO) regression was used in three studies [17,30,34], and neural network was used in three studies [14,28,31]. The remaining ML models included Bayesian generalized linear models (BGLMs), boosted LR, extra trees, extreme gradient boosted trees, regression tree, Tree—AS, boosting, chi-squared, deep learning, dimensionality reduction factor analysis, EN penalized LR, EN regularization, EN, generalized additive models, generalized boosted, generalized boosted machines, generalized linear mixed model, k-nearest neighbors, linear—AS, multilayer perceptron, multivariable adaptive regression splines, multivariate linear regression, partial least squares, principal component analysis, ridge regression, simple BGLMs, single-layer artificial neural networks, stepwise regression, and stochastic gradient boosting. Model performance was most frequently reported as Area Under the Curve (AUC), which was reported in sixteen studies [13–16,18,20,22–28,31–33]. Model performance was also reported as the mean absolute error (MAE) in three studies [21,29,34]. The remaining performance measures included mean bootstrapped R2 [30], MMA [19], and coefficients [17].

3.3. Key Results

Park et al. best predicted 3- and 24-month VAS after cervical spine decompression with LR with an AUC of 0.762 and 0.773, respectively [13]. Pedersen et al. used seven ML models to predict EQ-5D, ODI, VAS leg pain (LP), VAS back pain (BP), and return to work after lumbar spine surgery with a mean AUC of 0.82, 0.75, 0.73, 0.81, and 0.84, respectively [25]. Ve et al. employed a deep learning model to predict the ODI with an AUC of 0.84 and NRS BP improvement with an AUC of 0.9 [23]. Berjano et al. predicted postoperative ODI with a combination of preoperative ODI, SF-36 Physical Component Summary (PCS), and COMI Back with an AUC of 0.808 [26]. Halicka et al. used LR to predict an AUC of 0.63, 0.72, and 0.68 for COMI, BP, and LP, respectively [27]. Karhade et al. utilized LR, neural networks, and EN penalized LR to predict PROMIS physical function, pain interference, and pain intensity, achieving AUCs of 0.75, 0.71, and 0.71, respectively, with the EN penalized LR achieving an AUC of 0.69 [28]. Merali et al. used random forest random forest (RF) to predict SF-6D and mJOA with an of AUC of 0.85, 0.83, and 0.87 at 6, 12, and 24 months, respectively [14]. Rigoard et al. found that changes in the Modified Clinical Response Index were the most accurate indicator of Patient Global Impression of Change, with an AUC of 0.853 [33]. This was higher compared to the AUC for changes in the Hospital Anxiety and Depression Scale (HADS) (0.780), ODI score (0.737), Numerical Pain Rating Scale (NPRS) (0.704), EQ-5D index (0.698), and Pain Mapping Intensity score (0.672). Grob et al. used EN regularization to predict ODI, NRS BP, and LP with an AUC of 0.70, 0.72, and 0.70, respectively [20]. Zhang et al. used SVM to predict SF-36 PCS and Mental Component Summary (MCS) with an AUC of 86.4 and 89.8, respectively [15]. Gupta et al. used gradient boosting to predict an MAE of 0.47 and 0.55 for SRS-pain prediction and SRS self-image prediction, respectively [21]. Yagi et al. used an assemblage of the top five performing algorithms to predict JOABPEQ and VAS scores following lumbar spine surgery, with MAE values ranging from 9.3 to 16.5 [29]. Muller et al. used LASSO to predict COMI subdomains for back and neck pain with an MAE of 2.1 and 1.8, respectively [34]. Khan et al. used generalized boosted models and multivariable adaptive regression models to obtain predictions with an AUC of 0.77 and 0.78 for 24-month postoperative MCS and PCS, respectively [16]. Finkelstein et al. used LASSO regression to predict NRS after lumbar surgery with a mean bootstrapped R2 of 0.12 [30]. Liew et al. was the only study evaluating cervical radiculopathy [17]. This same study used four ML models to predict the NDI and EQ-5D. In this study, stepwise regression yielded the highest accuracy for the NDI, EQ-5D, and neck pain 12 months after cervical spine surgery. Siccoli et al. employed eight ML models to predict the ODI and NRS scores for BP and LP [31]. The 6-week postoperative AUC values were as follows: ODI 0.75, NRS LP 0.79, and NRS-BP 0.92 (boosted trees model). At 12 months postoperatively, the AUC values were ODI 0.68, NRS-LP 0.72, and NRS-BP 0.79. Ames et al. used seven ML models to predict individual SRS-22R questions, achieving AUROC values for individual SRS-22R questions as high as 86.9% (extreme gradient boosting tree) [22]. Staartjes et al. used EN regularization to predict the ODI and COMI, achieving an AUC of 0.67 [32]. The model yielded an AUC of 0.72 for BP and 0.64 for LP. Khan et al. utilized a polynomial SVM model to predict an AUC of 0.834 [18]. Khor et al. applied three binary regression models to predict outcomes, achieving the following AUC values: ODI 0.66, BP 0.79, and LP 0.69 [24]. Hoffman et al. reported a mean absolute accuracy (MAA) of 0.0283 with the use of support vector regression (SVR) [19].

4. Discussion

Predicting clinically relevant outcomes after spine surgery has been increasingly performed with patient-reported outcomes [35]. These questionnaires evaluate subjective and objective measures that aid surgeons in measuring a patient's quality of life before and after surgical intervention, ultimately allowing for a better understanding of the physical and psychological burden of spinal pathology. By identifying subtle patterns in pathology, patient characteristics, and populations, ML has the potential to predict PROMs after spine surgery. There has been a significant volume of studies describing PROMs, yet the clinical relevance has yet to be determined due to the significant degree of heterogeneity [35]. To improve the consistency and completeness of prediction model studies, the Transparent Reporting of a multivariable prediction model for Individual Prognosis Or Diagnosis (TRIPOD) was devised. This TRIPOD criteria serves as a set of evidence-based guidelines designed to improve the consistency and completeness of prediction model reporting [36]. Only eleven studies [15,17,20,22,23,26,27,31,32,34] in the review claimed to adhere to the TRIPOD criteria.

PROMs often assess pain, functional status, and other relevant factors. Consistent with past literature reviews [6], the mJOA, ODI, and SRS-22 were the most frequently predicted PROMs for cervical, lumbar, and spinal deformity pathologies, respectively. This fact highlights the emphasis placed on a patient's physical function. For assessment of pain, tools like the VAS and NRS are commonly used to measure back and leg pain. Although both measure pain, some studies have found the VAS assessment to be more useful. For example, Bielewicz et al. found that VAS scores decreased to a greater degree than NRS scores three months after surgery [37], attributing the poor reproducibility of the NRS to its less detailed incremental changes [37].

The features used to predict PROMs included demographics, surgery characteristics, preoperative PROMs, spinal pathology characteristics, mental health evaluations, employment details, social history, ASA classification, comorbidities, imaging findings, fine motor function, hospital characteristics, and surgeon characteristics. Several physical exam findings have been identified as predictors of functional improvement after surgery [16]. For example, upper motor neuron signs have been associated with a decreased likelihood of recovery after lumbar spine surgery [18]. In addition to objective clinical findings, Finkelstein et al. found that cognitive factors accounted for 40% of the variance in PROMs after spine surgery [30]. This finding is consistent with a randomized control trial reporting that lumbar spine surgery patients who participated in cognitive behavioral-based physical therapy had greater improvements in pain and disability compared to those who received physical therapy-related educational training [38]. Preoperative opioid use has been identified as another factor that affects patient-reported outcomes after spine surgery. Given that unmanageable pain is often a primary reason for surgical intervention [39], this variable should be further investigated for its role in predicting PROMs.

In this report, the AUC was the most frequently reported performance metric. The AUC can be thought of as the overall performance of an ML model with values ranging from 0 to 1. Values closer to 1 indicate better performance [40]. The study reporting the highest AUC for cervical spine pathology was that by Khan et al., who used a polynomial SVM to predict mJOA with an AUC of 0.834 [18]. Siccoli et al. applied boosted trees to predict NRS-BP after lumbar spine surgery, achieving an AUC of 0.92 [31]. For adult spinal deformity, Ames et al. used extreme gradient boosting trees to predict individual SRS-22R questions, with AUC values as high as 0.869 [22]. Despite successful ML model performance, the clinical applicability of these models is limited due to the complexity of shared decision making between a patient and the provider. A review by Christodoulou et al. evaluated 71 studies investigating clinical prediction models and found no evidence of superior ML performance over LR [41].

A primary limitation of this review was the exclusion of articles not containing the term "machine learning" in the abstract or title. This may have excluded studies that employed ML to predict PROMs but did not explicitly mention "ML" in their terminology. As a result, this introduced a potential selection bias and reduced the overall comprehensiveness of the review. Another contributing limitation was the minimal volume of high-quality evidence. Due to the negligible amount of evidence and large degree of heterogeneity amongst studies, a comprehensive systematic review or meta-analysis was unable to be performed.

5. Conclusions

PROMs continue to be a valuable tool for assessing the impact of spine pathology on physical and mental health, but surgeon expertise remains pivotal when counseling patients. Providers should be aware of the evolving application of these technologies in both clinical and academic pursuits. Although ML models have the potential to accurately predict PROMs, their clinical applicability is severely limited by the variation in ML models, spinal pathology, input variables, and output variables across studies. Surgeons and researchers should collaborate to establish standardized outcome measures and evaluation metrics. This joint effort would harness the predictive potential of ML to predict postoperative PROMs.

Author Contributions: C.Q.: Contributed to Data curation, Formal analysis, Methodology, Writing—original draft, and Writing—review and editing. D.K.: Contributed to Supervision and Writing—review and editing. B.G.: Contributed to Supervision, Validation, and Writing—review and editing. S.H.: Contributed to Conceptualization, Formal analysis, Investigation, Methodology, Project administration, Supervision, Validation, Visualization, and Writing—review and editing. All authors have read and agreed to the published version of the manuscript.

Funding: This research received no external funding.

Institutional Review Board Statement: Not applicable.

Informed Consent Statement: Not applicable.

Data Availability Statement: No new data were created or analyzed in this study. Data sharing is not applicable to this article.

Conflicts of Interest: The authors declare no conflicts of interest.

References

1. Tragaris, T.; Benetos, I.S.; Vlamis, J.; Pneumaticos, S.; Tragaris, T.; Benetos, I.S.; Vlamis, J.; Pneumaticos, S.G. Machine Learning Applications in Spine Surgery. *Cureus* **2023**, *15*, e48078. [CrossRef]
2. Vernon, H.; Mior, S. The Neck Disability Index: A Study of Reliability and Validity. *J. Manip. Physiol. Ther.* **1991**, *14*, 409–415.
3. McCormick, J.D.; Werner, B.C.; Shimer, A.L. Patient-Reported Outcome Measures in Spine Surgery. *JAAOS J. Am. Acad. Orthop. Surg.* **2013**, *21*, 99. [CrossRef] [PubMed]
4. Franceschini, M.; Boffa, A.; Pignotti, E.; Andriolo, L.; Zaffagnini, S.; Filardo, G. The Minimal Clinically Important Difference Changes Greatly Based on the Different Calculation Methods. *Am. J. Sports Med.* **2023**, *51*, 1067–1073. [CrossRef]
5. Jaeschke, R.; Singer, J.; Guyatt, G.H. Measurement of Health Status. Ascertaining the Minimal Clinically Important Difference. *Control Clin. Trials* **1989**, *10*, 407–415. [CrossRef] [PubMed]
6. Beighley, A.; Zhang, A.; Huang, B.; Carr, C.; Mathkour, M.; Werner, C.; Scullen, T.; Kilgore, M.D.; Maulucci, C.M.; Dallapiazza, R.F.; et al. Patient-Reported Outcome Measures in Spine Surgery: A Systematic Review. *J. Craniovertebral Junction Spine* **2022**, *13*, 378–389. [CrossRef]
7. Intro to PROMIS. Available online: https://www.healthmeasures.net/explore-measurement-systems/promis/intro-to-promis (accessed on 17 October 2024).
8. Young, R.R. Emerging Role of Artificial Intelligence and Big Data in Spine Care. *Int. J. Spine Surg.* **2023**, *17*, S3–S10. [CrossRef] [PubMed]
9. Tricco, A.C.; Lillie, E.; Zarin, W.; O'Brien, K.K.; Colquhoun, H.; Levac, D.; Moher, D.; Peters, M.D.J.; Horsley, T.; Weeks, L.; et al. PRISMA Extension for Scoping Reviews (PRISMA-ScR): Checklist and Explanation. *Ann. Intern. Med.* **2018**, *169*, 467–473. [CrossRef] [PubMed]
10. Moustafa, I.M.; Ozsahin, D.U.; Mustapha, M.T.; Ahbouch, A.; Oakley, P.A.; Harrison, D.E. Utilizing Machine Learning to Predict Post-Treatment Outcomes in Chronic Non-Specific Neck Pain Patients Undergoing Cervical Extension Traction. *Sci. Rep.* **2024**, *14*, 11781. [CrossRef] [PubMed]
11. Janssen, E.R.; Osong, B.; van Soest, J.; Dekker, A.; van Meeteren, N.L.; Willems, P.C.; Punt, I.M. Exploring Associations of Preoperative Physical Performance With Postoperative Outcomes After Lumbar Spinal Fusion: A Machine Learning Approach. *Arch. Phys. Med. Rehabil.* **2021**, *102*, 1324–1330.e3. [CrossRef]
12. Wondra, J.P.I.; Kelly, M.P.; Greenberg, J.; Yanik, E.L.; Ames, C.P.; Pellise, F.; Vila-Casademunt, A.; Smith, J.S.; Bess, S.; Shaffrey, C.I.; et al. Validation of Adult Spinal Deformity Surgical Outcome Prediction Tools in Adult Symptomatic Lumbar Scoliosis. *Spine* **2023**, *48*, 21. [CrossRef]
13. Durand, W.M.; Lafage, R.; Hamilton, D.K.; Passias, P.G.; Kim, H.J.; Protopsaltis, T.; Lafage, V.; Smith, J.S.; Shaffrey, C.; Gupta, M.; et al. Artificial Intelligence Clustering of Adult Spinal Deformity Sagittal Plane Morphology Predicts Surgical Characteristics, Alignment, and Outcomes. *Eur. Spine J.* **2021**, *30*, 2157–2166. [CrossRef]
14. Park, C.; Mummaneni, P.V.; Gottfried, O.N.; Shaffrey, C.I.; Tang, A.J.; Bisson, E.F.; Asher, A.L.; Coric, D.; Potts, E.A.; Foley, K.T.; et al. Which Supervised Machine Learning Algorithm Can Best Predict Achievement of Minimum Clinically Important Difference in Neck Pain after Surgery in Patients with Cervical Myelopathy? A QOD Study. *Neurosurg. Focus* **2023**, *54*, E5. [CrossRef]
15. Merali, Z.G.; Witiw, C.D.; Badhiwala, J.H.; Wilson, J.R.; Fehlings, M.G. Using a Machine Learning Approach to Predict Outcome after Surgery for Degenerative Cervical Myelopathy. *PLoS ONE* **2019**, *14*, e0215133. [CrossRef] [PubMed]
16. Zhang, J.K.; Jayasekera, D.; Javeed, S.; Greenberg, J.K.; Blum, J.; Dibble, C.F.; Sun, P.; Song, S.-K.; Ray, W.Z. Diffusion Basis Spectrum Imaging Predicts Long-Term Clinical Outcomes Following Surgery in Cervical Spondylotic Myelopathy. *Spine J.* **2023**, *23*, 504–512. [CrossRef]
17. Khan, O.; Badhiwala, J.H.; Witiw, C.D.; Wilson, J.R.; Fehlings, M.G. Machine Learning Algorithms for Prediction of Health-Related Quality-of-Life after Surgery for Mild Degenerative Cervical Myelopathy. *Spine J.* **2021**, *21*, 1659–1669. [CrossRef] [PubMed]
18. Liew, B.X.W.; Peolsson, A.; Rugamer, D.; Wibault, J.; Löfgren, H.; Dedering, A.; Zsigmond, P.; Falla, D. Clinical Predictive Modelling of Post-Surgical Recovery in Individuals with Cervical Radiculopathy: A Machine Learning Approach. *Sci. Rep.* **2020**, *10*, 16782. [CrossRef]
19. Khan, O.; Badhiwala, J.H.; Akbar, M.A.; Fehlings, M.G. Prediction of Worse Functional Status After Surgery for Degenerative Cervical Myelopathy: A Machine Learning Approach. *Neurosurgery* **2021**, *88*, 584. [CrossRef]
20. Hoffman, H.; Lee, S.I.; Garst, J.H.; Lu, D.S.; Li, C.H.; Nagasawa, D.T.; Ghalehsari, N.; Jahanforouz, N.; Razaghy, M.; Espinal, M.; et al. Use of Multivariate Linear Regression and Support Vector Regression to Predict Functional Outcome after Surgery for Cervical Spondylotic Myelopathy. *J. Clin. Neurosci.* **2015**, *22*, 1444–1449. [CrossRef]
21. Grob, A.; Rohr, J.; Stumpo, V.; Vieli, M.; Ciobanu-Caraus, O.; Ricciardi, L.; Maldaner, N.; Raco, A.; Miscusi, M.; Perna, A.; et al. Multicenter External Validation of Prediction Models for Clinical Outcomes after Spinal Fusion for Lumbar Degenerative Disease. *Eur. Spine J.* **2024**, *33*, 3534–3544. [CrossRef] [PubMed]
22. Gupta, A.; Oh, I.Y.; Kim, S.; Marks, M.C.; Payne, P.R.O.; Ames, C.P.; Pellise, F.; Pahys, J.M.; Fletcher, N.D.; Newton, P.O.; et al. Machine Learning for Benchmarking Adolescent Idiopathic Scoliosis Surgery Outcomes. *Spine* **2023**, *48*, 1138. [CrossRef]

23. Ames, C.P.; Smith, J.S.; Pellisé, F.; Kelly, M.; Gum, J.L.; Alanay, A.; Acaroğlu, E.; Pérez-Grueso, F.J.S.; Kleinstück, F.S.; Obeid, I.; et al. Development of Predictive Models for All Individual Questions of SRS-22R after Adult Spinal Deformity Surgery: A Step toward Individualized Medicine. *Eur. Spine J.* **2019**, *28*, 1998–2011. [CrossRef] [PubMed]
24. Staartjes, V.E.; de Wispelaere, M.P.; Vandertop, W.P.; Schröder, M.L. Deep Learning-Based Preoperative Predictive Analytics for Patient-Reported Outcomes Following Lumbar Discectomy: Feasibility of Center-Specific Modeling. *Spine J. Off. J. N. Am. Spine Soc.* **2019**, *19*, 853–861. [CrossRef] [PubMed]
25. Khor, S.; Lavallee, D.; Cizik, A.M.; Bellabarba, C.; Chapman, J.R.; Howe, C.R.; Lu, D.; Mohit, A.A.; Oskouian, R.J.; Roh, J.R.; et al. Development and Validation of a Prediction Model for Pain and Functional Outcomes After Lumbar Spine Surgery. *JAMA Surg.* **2018**, *153*, 634–642. [CrossRef]
26. Pedersen, C.F.; Andersen, M.Ø.; Carreon, L.Y.; Eiskjær, S. Applied Machine Learning for Spine Surgeons: Predicting Outcome for Patients Undergoing Treatment for Lumbar Disc Herniation Using PRO Data. *Glob. Spine J.* **2022**, *12*, 866–876. [CrossRef] [PubMed]
27. Berjano, P.; Langella, F.; Ventriglia, L.; Compagnone, D.; Barletta, P.; Huber, D.; Mangili, F.; Licandro, G.; Galbusera, F.; Cina, A.; et al. The Influence of Baseline Clinical Status and Surgical Strategy on Early Good to Excellent Result in Spinal Lumbar Arthrodesis: A Machine Learning Approach. *J. Pers. Med.* **2021**, *11*, 1377. [CrossRef] [PubMed]
28. Halicka, M.; Wilby, M.; Duarte, R.; Brown, C. Predicting Patient-Reported Outcomes Following Lumbar Spine Surgery: Development and External Validation of Multivariable Prediction Models. *BMC Musculoskelet. Disord.* **2023**, *24*, 333. [CrossRef] [PubMed]
29. Karhade, A.; Fogel, H.A.; Cha, T.D.; Hershman, S.H.; Doorly, T.P.; Kang, J.D.; Bono, C.M.; Harris, M.B.; Schwab, J.H.; Tobert, D.G. Development of Prediction Models for Clinically Meaningful Improvement in PROMIS Scores after Lumbar Decompression. *Spine J.* **2021**, *21*, 397–404. [CrossRef] [PubMed]
30. Yagi, M.; Michikawa, T.; Yamamoto, T.; Iga, T.; Ogura, Y.; Tachibana, A.; Miyamoto, A.; Suzuki, S.; Nori, S.; Takahashi, Y.; et al. Development and Validation of Machine Learning-Based Predictive Model for Clinical Outcome of Decompression Surgery for Lumbar Spinal Canal Stenosis. *Spine J.* **2022**, *22*, 1768–1777. [CrossRef] [PubMed]
31. Finkelstein, J.A.; Stark, R.B.; Lee, J.; Schwartz, C.E. Patient Factors That Matter in Predicting Spine Surgery Outcomes: A Machine Learning Approach. *J. Neurosurg. Spine* **2021**, *35*, 127–136. [CrossRef]
32. Siccoli, A.; de Wispelaere, M.P.; Schröder, M.L.; Staartjes, V.E. Machine Learning–Based Preoperative Predictive Analytics for Lumbar Spinal Stenosis. *Neurosurg. Focus* **2019**, *46*, E5. [CrossRef] [PubMed]
33. Staartjes, V.E.; Stumpo, V.; Ricciardi, L.; Maldaner, N.; Eversdijk, H.A.J.; Vieli, M.; Ciobanu-Caraus, O.; Raco, A.; Miscusi, M.; Perna, A.; et al. FUSE-ML: Development and External Validation of a Clinical Prediction Model for Mid-Term Outcomes after Lumbar Spinal Fusion for Degenerative Disease. *Eur. Spine J.* **2022**, *31*, 2629–2638. [CrossRef] [PubMed]
34. Müller, D.; Haschtmann, D.; Fekete, T.F.; Kleinstück, F.; Reitmeir, R.; Loibl, M.; O'Riordan, D.; Porchet, F.; Jeszenszky, D.; Mannion, A.F. Development of a Machine-Learning Based Model for Predicting Multidimensional Outcome after Surgery for Degenerative Disorders of the Spine. *Eur. Spine J.* **2022**, *31*, 2125–2136. [CrossRef] [PubMed]
35. Rigoard, P.; Ounajim, A.; Goudman, L.; Louis, P.Y.; Slaoui, Y.; Roulaud, M.; Naiditch, N.; Bouche, B.; Page, P.; Lorgeoux, B.; et al. A Novel Multi-Dimensional Clinical Response Index Dedicated to Improving Global Assessment of Pain in Patients with Persistent Spinal Pain Syndrome after Spinal Surgery, Based on a Real-Life Prospective Multicentric Study (PREDIBACK) and Machine Learning Techniques. *J. Clin. Med.* **2021**, *10*, 4910. [CrossRef] [PubMed]
36. Cooper, M.E.; Torre-Healy, L.A.; Alentado, V.J.; Cho, S.; Steinmetz, M.P.; Benzel, E.C.; Mroz, T.E. Heterogeneity of Reporting Outcomes in the Spine Surgery Literature. *Clin. Spine Surg.* **2018**, *31*, E221–E229. [CrossRef]
37. Collins, G.S.; Moons, K.G.M.; Dhiman, P.; Riley, R.D.; Beam, A.L.; Calster, B.V.; Ghassemi, M.; Liu, X.; Reitsma, J.B.; van Smeden, M.; et al. TRIPOD+AI Statement: Updated Guidance for Reporting Clinical Prediction Models That Use Regression or Machine Learning Methods. *BMJ* **2024**, *385*, e078378. [CrossRef]
38. Bielewicz, J.; Daniluk, B.; Kamieniak, P. VAS and NRS, Same or Different? Are Visual Analog Scale Values and Numerical Rating Scale Equally Viable Tools for Assessing Patients after Microdiscectomy? *Pain Res. Manag.* **2022**, *2022*, 5337483. [CrossRef]
39. Archer, K.R.; Devin, C.J.; Vanston, S.W.; Koyama, T.; Phillips, S.E.; Mathis, S.L.; George, S.Z.; McGirt, M.J.; Spengler, D.M.; Aaronson, O.S.; et al. Cognitive-Behavioral-Based Physical Therapy for Patients With Chronic Pain Undergoing Lumbar Spine Surgery: A Randomized Controlled Trial. *J. Pain* **2016**, *17*, 76–89. [CrossRef]

40. Khan, A.S.R.; Mattei, T.A.; Mercier, P.J.; Cloney, M.; Dahdaleh, N.S.; Koski, T.R.; El Tecle, N.E. Outcome Reporting in Spine Surgery: A Review of Historical and Emerging Trends. *World Neurosurg.* **2023**, *179*, 88–98. [CrossRef]
41. Christodoulou, E.; Ma, J.; Collins, G.S.; Steyerberg, E.W.; Verbakel, J.Y.; Van Calster, B. A Systematic Review Shows No Performance Benefit of Machine Learning over Logistic Regression for Clinical Prediction Models. *J. Clin. Epidemiol.* **2019**, *110*, 12–22. [CrossRef] [PubMed]

bioengineering

MDPI

Review

Applications of Artificial Intelligence and Machine Learning in Spine MRI

Aric Lee [1,*,†], Wilson Ong [1,†], Andrew Makmur [1,2], Yong Han Ting [1,2], Wei Chuan Tan [1], Shi Wei Desmond Lim [1], Xi Zhen Low [1,2], Jonathan Jiong Hao Tan [3], Naresh Kumar [3] and James T. P. D. Hallinan [1,2]

1 Department of Diagnostic Imaging, National University Hospital, 5 Lower Kent Ridge Rd, Singapore 119074, Singapore; wilson.ong@mohh.com.sg (W.O.); andrew_makmur@nuhs.edu.sg (A.M.); yonghan_ting@nuhs.edu.sg (Y.H.T.); weichuan.tan@mohh.com.sg (W.C.T.); desmond.lim@mohh.com.sg (S.W.D.L.); xi_zhen_low@nuhs.edu.sg (X.Z.L.); james_hallinan@nuhs.edu.sg (J.T.P.D.H.)

2 Department of Diagnostic Radiology, Yong Loo Lin School of Medicine, National University of Singapore, 10 Medical Drive, Singapore 117597, Singapore

3 National University Spine Institute, Department of Orthopaedic Surgery, National University Health System, 1E Lower Kent Ridge Road, Singapore 119228, Singapore; jonathan_jh_tan@nuhs.edu.sg (J.J.H.T.); dosksn@nus.edu.sg (N.K.)

* Correspondence: aricleewz@gmail.com; Tel.: +65-67725207

† These authors contributed equally to this work.

Abstract: Diagnostic imaging, particularly MRI, plays a key role in the evaluation of many spine pathologies. Recent progress in artificial intelligence and its subset, machine learning, has led to many applications within spine MRI, which we sought to examine in this review. A literature search of the major databases (PubMed, MEDLINE, Web of Science, ClinicalTrials.gov) was conducted according to the Preferred Reporting Items for Systematic Reviews and Meta-Analyses (PRISMA) guidelines. The search yielded 1226 results, of which 50 studies were selected for inclusion. Key data from these studies were extracted. Studies were categorized thematically into the following: Image Acquisition and Processing, Segmentation, Diagnosis and Treatment Planning, and Patient Selection and Prognostication. Gaps in the literature and the proposed areas of future research are discussed. Current research demonstrates the ability of artificial intelligence to improve various aspects of this field, from image acquisition to analysis and clinical care. We also acknowledge the limitations of current technology. Future work will require collaborative efforts in order to fully exploit new technologies while addressing the practical challenges of generalizability and implementation. In particular, the use of foundation models and large-language models in spine MRI is a promising area, warranting further research. Studies assessing model performance in real-world clinical settings will also help uncover unintended consequences and maximize the benefits for patient care.

Keywords: artificial intelligence; machine learning; spine; spinal cord; magnetic resonance imaging

1. Introduction

The spine is an important site of pathology and can be affected by a variety of conditions, including degenerative, neoplastic, infectious, traumatic and inflammatory demyelinating diseases. Diagnostic imaging often plays a key role in the diagnosis of spinal diseases. In addition, imaging is also vital for planning treatments such as surgery and minimally invasive procedures as it allows for the localization and quantification of underlying pathologies [1].

Various imaging modalities can be used in spine imaging. Radiographs often provide initial assessment of symptoms that may be attributed to a spinal pathology, such as neck or back pain, radiculopathy, or myelopathy. They are a cost-efficient and widely available diagnostic tool that can provide rapid assessment of spinal alignment, fractures, and degenerative changes. Erosive changes can also be detected and may suggest the presence of neoplasms or underlying infection, albeit with a relatively low sensitivity. Radiographs also offer a relatively low-cost method for the dynamic assessment of spinal instability [1,2]. Computed tomography (CT) provides a superior delineation of complex spinal anatomy, which can be challenging to accurately assess using radiographs. In the setting of trauma, CT is the modality of choice for evaluating fractures and dislocations in the cervical spine as it allows for the rapid imaging of patients who may have significant traumatic injuries and be in an unstable clinical condition. It also allows for a good visualization of the cortical bone [3]. CT scans can also be used for pre-operative planning as certain pathologies, such as ossification of the posterior longitudinal ligament (OPLL), are readily visualized [4].

While radiographs and CT remain significant imaging tools, magnetic resonance imaging (MRI) has surpassed both in the range of pathologies that it is able to image. MRI scans have the advantage of being able to evaluate bone marrow signal thus allowing for an accurate detection of pathologies that alter the normal bone marrow, such as fractures or contusions, neoplastic disease or infection. In addition, MRI scans provide superior evaluation of soft tissue structures, such as the intervertebral disc, spinal ligaments, as well as the spinal cord and surrounding dural and epidural spaces [5–7]. Thus, MRIs have become widely recognized as the preferred modality to evaluate many spinal pathologies. CT myelography is an alternative modality used to assess the spinal cord and neural foramina. However, it requires the injection of contrast material into the spinal canal via lumbar puncture, making it more invasive and less widely used [8]. It is typically reserved for cases with MRI contraindications, such as patients with incompatible pacemakers.

Despite its many advantages, an important limitation of MRI is its relatively long acquisition times. To accommodate a growing number of scans, more time-efficient MRI pulse sequences have been developed. However, there is often a trade-off between diagnostic quality and time savings, resulting in faster sequences with lower resolution or tissue contrast [9]. More recent developments such as parallel imaging and compressed sensing have partially mitigated this [10,11], but scan time remains a pertinent issue. In addition, interpreting these MRIs can be a tedious and time-consuming process for the reporting radiologist. Each spinal level must be carefully examined for evidence of pathology. Additionally, there is significant interobserver variability in evaluating the severity of observed pathology [12]. The lack of standardized grading systems, particularly in the cervical and thoracic spine, further complicates this process. Finally, certain spinal pathologies present diagnostic challenges due to overlapping imaging characteristics. Differentiating between various types of spinal neoplasms or infections can be particularly difficult, especially for inexperienced radiologists, potentially impacting subsequent treatment decisions.

Artificial intelligence (AI) has been increasingly explored as a solution to many of these challenges, with widespread applications across medicine. Machine learning (ML) is a subset of AI that utilizes a combination of algorithms and statistical models to make predictions on new data [13–15]. Deep learning (DL) is a further subset of ML which has garnered significant interest in recent years. Compared to other types of ML, DL algorithms are generally more complex, requiring larger amounts of data and computational power. Such algorithms have been developed with the promise of impacting various areas of radiology. Most algorithms in radiology are 'supervised' via labeled datasets. Using labels provided by human readers, the DL model learns to identify patterns in a dataset, and its performance is studied using a separate test/validation dataset [14,15]. The number of applications for AI in radiology, including its subset ML, has increased significantly over time, now spanning areas such as image interpretation, protocolling scans, and optimizing workflows. Additionally, many of the challenges in spine imaging are not unique. Various AI techniques have been successfully applied across a broad spectrum of tasks in radiology and medicine, including endoscopic image analysis and image feature fusion and enhancement [16–18]. Many of these advancements have helped inform the innovations in spine imaging AI.

While several studies have examined the use of AI in specific aspects of spine imaging, our goal is to provide a comprehensive overview of the full spectrum of use cases in spine MRI by examining the available literature on a wide variety of applications. Additionally, we aim to identify gaps in the existing literature and propose areas for future research in the field.

2. Materials and Methods

Given the anticipated large number of studies that would be extracted, a scoping review was performed to adequately represent the breadth and depth of the current literature.

2.1. Literature Search Strategy

We performed a literature search of the major databases (PubMed, MEDLINE, Web of Science, ClinicalTrials.gov) on 8 February 2024, according to the Preferred Reporting Items for Systematic Reviews and Meta-Analyses (PRISMA) guidelines. The following medical subject headings (MeSH) and keywords were utilized: ("artificial intelligence" OR "AI" OR "machine learning" OR "ML" OR "deep learning" OR "DL") AND ("spine" OR "spinal cord" OR "cord" OR "vertebra" OR "vertebral column" OR "spinal column" OR "intervertebral disc" OR "intervertebral disk) AND ("MRI" OR "MR" OR "magnetic resonance imaging"). Limits were applied to include only English language studies from the past eight years.

2.2. Study Screening and Selection Criteria

A two-stage screening process was used. Studies were first screened independently by two authors (A.L. and W.O.) by title and abstract. A full text review was then performed for any potentially eligible studies. Any controversies at either stage were reviewed by a third author (J.T.P.D.H.).

The inclusion criteria were as follows: studies on the use of AI or ML on MRI images focusing on spine-related applications, English studies, and studies performed on human subjects. The exclusion criteria were as follows: non-original research (for example, review articles, editorial correspondence), unpublished work, conference abstracts, and case reports. Studies that primarily focused on other imaging modalities (for example, radiographs, CT, or nuclear medicine imaging) or other body regions were excluded.

2.3. Data Extraction and Reporting

The selected studies were extracted and compiled onto a spreadsheet using Microsoft Excel Version 16.81 (Microsoft Corporation, Washington DC, USA). The following data was extracted:

1. Study details: authorship, year of publication and journal name;
2. Application and primary outcome measure;
3. Study details: sample size, spine region studied, MRI sequences used;
4. Artificial intelligence technique used;
5. Key results and conclusion.

3. Results

3.1. Search Results

Our initial literature search identified 1226 studies, which were screened according to the specified criteria. Subsequently, 149 studies which did not meet the date range, 44 with an incorrect article type and 2 non-English language studies were initially excluded. This led to 1031 studies selected for full text screening, and the inclusion of 50 studies in the present review (see Figure 1 for a detailed flowchart). The studies are summarized in Table 1. Given the heterogeneity of the included studies, a formal meta-analysis could not be meaningfully performed.

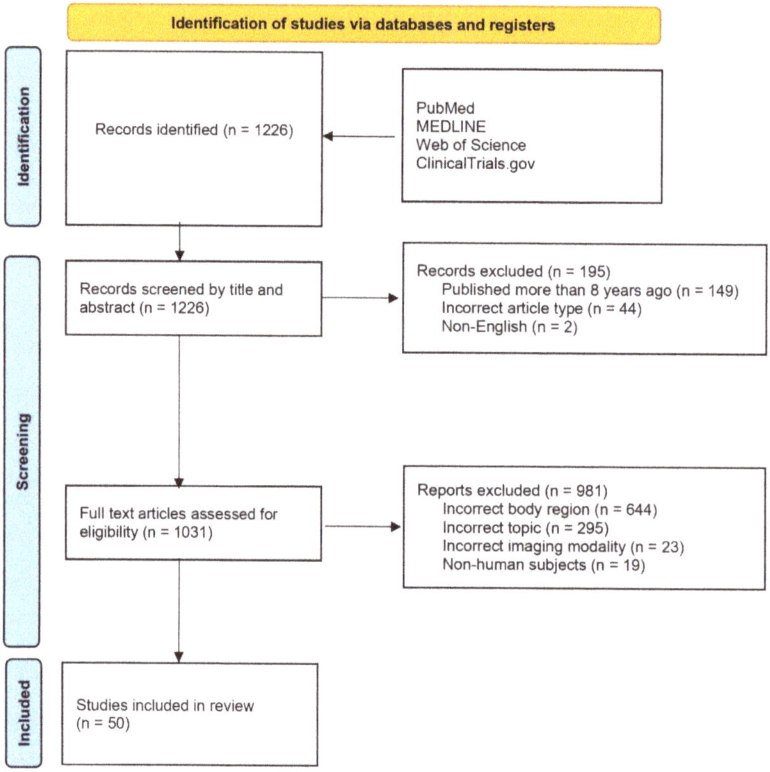

Figure 1. PRISMA flowchart showing the two-step study screening process. Adapted from PRISMA Group, 2020.

Table 1. Summary of Selected Studies.

No	Study Title	Authorship	Year of Publication	Journal Name	Application and Primary Outcome Measure	Sample Size *	Spine Region Studied	MRI Sequences Used	Artificial Intelligence Technique Used	Key Results and Conclusion
1	A quantitative evaluation of the deep learning model of segmentation and measurement of cervical spine MRI in healthy adults	Y Zhu et al. [19]	2024	J Appl Clin Med Phys	Segmentation of cervical spine structures (subarachnoid space area/diameter, spinal cord area/diameter, anterior and posterior extra-spinal space)	160	Cervical	Sagittal T1w, T2w, axial T2w	3D U-net	No comparative statistics
2	MRI radiomics-based decision support tool for a personalized classification of cervical disc degeneration: a two-center study	J Xie et al. [20]	2024	Front Physiol	Classification of cervical disc degeneration (Pfirrmann grading)	435	Cervical	Sagittal T1w, T2w	MedSAM	Disc segmentation Dice 0.93. Random forest overall performance AUC 0.95, accuracy 90%, precision 87%
3	A deep-learning model for diagnosing fresh vertebral fractures on magnetic resonance images	Y Wang et al. [21]	2024	World Neurosurg	Detection of fresh vertebral fractures	716	Whole spine	Midsagittal STIR	YoloV7, Resnet 50	Accuracy 98%, sensitivity 98%, specificity 97%. External dataset accuracy 92%
4	Diagnostic evaluation of deep learning accelerated lumbar spine MRI	KM Awan et al. [22]	2024	Neuroradiol J	Comparison of deep learning accelerated protocol to conventional protocol for neural stenosis and facet arthropathy	36	Lumbar	Sagittal T1w, T2w, STIR, axial T2w	CNN	Non-inferior in all aspects however reduced signal-to-noise ratio and increased artifact perception. Interobserver variability $\kappa = 0.50–0.76$
5	A deep neural network for MRI spinal inflammation in axial spondyloarthritis	Y Lin et al. [23]	2024	Eur Spine J	Detection of inflammatory lesions on STIR sequence for patients with axial spondyloarthritis	330	Whole spine	Sagittal STIR	U-net	AUC 0.87, sensitivity 80%, specificity 88%, comparable to a radiologist. True positive lesion Dice 0.55.

Table 1. *Cont.*

No	Study Title	Authorship	Year of Publication	Journal Name	Application and Primary Outcome Measure	Sample Size *	Spine Region Studied	MRI Sequences Used	Artificial Intelligence Technique Used	Key Results and Conclusion
6	Semi-automatic assessment of facet tropism from lumbar spine MRI using deep learning: a Northern Finland birth cohort study	N Kowlagi et al. [24]	2023	Spine (Phila Pa 1976)	Measurement of facet joint angles	490	Lumbar (L3/4 to L5/S1)	Axial T2w	U-net	Dice 0.93, IOU 0.87
7	A convolutional neural network for automated detection of cervical ossification of the posterior longitudinal ligament using magnetic resonance imaging	Z Qu et al. [25]	2023	Clin Spine Surg	Detection of ossification of posterior longitudinal ligament	684	Cervical	Sagittal MRI	ResNet	Accuracy 93–98%, AUC 0.91–0.97. ResNet50 and ResNet101 had higher accuracy and specificity than all human readers
8	Deep learning-based k-space-to-image reconstruction and super resolution for diffusion-weighted imaging in whole-spine MRI	DK Kim et al. [26]	2024	Magn Reson Imaging	K-space-to-image reconstruction for whole spine DWI in patients with hematologic and oncologic diseases	67	Whole spine	Axial single-shot echo-planar DWI	CNN	Higher diagnostic confidence scores and overall image quality
9	Automatic detection and classification of Modic changes in MRI images using deep learning: intelligent assisted diagnosis system	Gang L et al. [27]	2024	Orthop Surg	Detection and classification of Modic endplate changes	168	Lumbar	Median sagittal T1w and T2w	Single shot multibox detector, ResNet18	Internal dataset: accuracy 86%, recall 88%, precision 85%, F1-score 86%, interobserver κ = 0.79 (95%CI 0.66–0.85). External dataset: accuracy 75%, recall 77%, precision 78%, F1-score 75%, interobserver κ = 0.68 (95%CI 0.51–0.68)
10	Deep learning system for automated detection of posterior ligamentous complex injury in patients with thoracolumbar fracture on MRI	SW Jo et al. [28]	2023	Sci Rep	Detection of posterior ligamentous complex injury in patients with acute thoracolumbar fractures	500	Thoracic and lumbar	Midline sagittal T2w	Attention U-net and Inception-ResNetv2	AUC 0.92–0.93 (vs. 0.83–0.93 for radiologists)

Table 1. *Cont.*

No	Study Title	Authorship	Year of Publication	Journal Name	Application and Primary Outcome Measure	Sample Size *	Spine Region Studied	MRI Sequences Used	Artificial Intelligence Technique Used	Key Results and Conclusion
11	Cross-sectional area and fat infiltration of the lumbar spine muscles in patients with back disorders: a deep learning-based big data analysis	J Vitale et al. [29]	2023	Eur Spine J	Segmentation of lumbar paravertebral muscles and correlation with age	4434	Lumbar	Axial T2w	U-net	Higher cross-sectional area in males ($p < 0.001$). Positive correlation between age and total fat infiltration (r = 0.73, $p < 0.001$), negligible negative correlation between cross-sectional area and age (r = −0.24, $p < 0.001$)
12	MRI feature-based radiomics models to predict treatment outcome after stereotactic body radiotherapy for spinal metastases	Y Chen et al. [30]	2023	Insights Imaging	Prediction of treatment outcome after stereotactic body radiotherapy for spine metastasis	194	Whole spine	Sagittal T1w, T2w, STIR, axial T2w	Multiple (including AdaBoost, XGBoost, RF, SVM)	Combined model AUC 0.83, clinical model AUC 0.73
13	Clinical and radiomics feature-based outcome analysis in lumbar disc herniation surgery	B Saravi et al. [31]	2023	BMC Musculoskelet Disord	Combination of radiomics features and clinical features to predict lumbar disc herniation surgery outcomes	172	Lumbar	Sagittal T2w	Multiple (including XGBoost, Lagrangian SVM, RF radial basis function neural network)	Accuracy 88–93% (vs. 88–91% for clinical features alone)
14	Differentiating spinal pathologies by deep learning approach	O Haim et al. [32]	2024	Spine J	Differentiation of spinal lesions into infection, carcinoma, meningioma and schwannoma	231	Whole spine	Variable (T2w, T1w post-contrast)	Fast.ai	Accuracy 78% (validation), 93% (test)
15	Deep learning-based detection and classification of lumbar disc herniation on magnetic resonance images	W Zhang et al. [33]	2023	JOR Spine	Detection and classification of lumbar disc herniation according to the Michigan State University classification	1115	Lumbar	Axial T2w	Faster R-CNN, ResNeXt101	Internal dataset: detection IOU 0.82, classification accuracy 88%, AUC 0.97, interclass correlation 0.87. External dataset: detection IOU 0.70, classification accuracy 74%, AUC 0.92, interclass correlation 0.79

Table 1. *Cont.*

No	Study Title	Authorship	Year of Publication	Journal Name	Application and Primary Outcome Measure	Sample Size *	Spine Region Studied	MRI Sequences Used	Artificial Intelligence Technique Used	Key Results and Conclusion
16	ASNET: a novel AI framework for accurate ankylosing spondylitis diagnosis from MRI	NP Tas et al. [34]	2023	Biomedicines	Prediction of ankylosing spondylitis diagnosis on MRI	2036	Sacroiliac joints	Axial, coronal STIR, coronal T1w post-contrast	DenseNet201, ResNet50, ShuffleNet	Accuracy 100%, recall 100%, precision 100%, F1-score 100%
17	Attention-gated U-Net networks for simultaneous axial/sagittal planes segmentation of injured spinal cords	N Masse-Gignac et al. [35]	2023	J Appl Clin Med Phys	Segmentation of the spinal cord in patients with traumatic injuries	94	All (mainly cervical)	Sagittal T2w	U-Net	Dice 0.95
18	A spine segmentation method based on scene aware fusion network	EE Yilizati-Yilihamu et al. [36]	2023	BMC Neurosci	Segmentation of lumbar spine MRI into individual vertebrae and discs by level	172	Lumbar	Sagittal MRI	Scene-Aware Fusion Network (SAFNet)	Dice 0.79–0.81 (average 0.80)
19	MRI radiomics-based evaluation of Tuberculous and Brucella spondylitis	W Wang et al. [37]	2023	J Int Med Res	Differentiation of Tuberculous spondylitis from Brucella spondylitis, and culture positive from culture negative Tuberculous spondylitis	190	Whole spine	Sagittal T1w, T2w, fat suppressed	RF, SVM	SVM AUC 0.90–0.94, RF AUC 0.95
20	Deep phenotyping the cervical spine: automatic characterization of cervical degenerative phenotypes based on T2-weighted MRI	F Niemeyer et al. [38]	2023	Eur Spine J	Classification of cervical spine into degenerative phenotypes based on disc and osteophyte configuration	873	Cervical	Sagittal MRI	3D CNN	Disc $\kappa = 0.55–0.68$, disc displacement $\kappa = 0.58–0.74$, disc space narrowing $\kappa = 0.65–0.72$, osseous abnormalities $\kappa = 0.18–0.49$
21	MRI-based radiomics assessment of the imminent new vertebral fracture after vertebral augmentation	J Cai et al. [39]	2023	Eur Spine J	Evaluation of risk of new vertebral fracture after vertebral augmentation	168	Lumbar	T2w	Multiple (logistic regression, RF, SVM, XGBoost)	AUC 0.90–0.93, superior to clinical features alone ($p < 0.05$)

Table 1. *Cont.*

No	Study Title	Authorship	Year of Publication	Journal Name	Application and Primary Outcome Measure	Sample Size *	Spine Region Studied	MRI Sequences Used	Artificial Intelligence Technique Used	Key Results and Conclusion
22	Associations between vertebral localized contrast changes and adjacent annular fissures in patients with low back pain: a radiomics approach	C Waldenberg et al. [40]	2023	J Clin Med	Detection of adjacent level annular fissure based on vertebral changes on MRI	61	Lumbar	Sagittal T1w, T2w, discography, CT	Multilayer perceptron, RF, K-nearest neighbor	Accuracy 83%, sensitivity 97%, specificity 28%, AUC 0.76
23	Imaging evaluation of a proposed 3D generative model for MRI to CT translation in the lumbar spine	M Roberts et al. [41]	2023	Spine J	Generation of 3D CT from sagittal MRI data	420	Lumbar	Sagittal T1w	3D cycle-GAN	Measurements in sagittal plane <10% relative error, axial plane up to 34% relative error
24	Deep learning-generated synthetic MR imaging STIR spine images are superior in image quality and diagnostically equivalent to conventional STIR: a multicenter, multireader trial	LN Tanenbaum et al. [42]	2023	AJNR	Validation of synthetically created STIR images created from T1w and T2w	93	Whole spine	Sagittal T1w, T2w, STIR	CNN	No significant difference between synthetic and acquired STIR, higher image quality for synthetic STIR ($p < 0.0001$)
25	Prediction of osteoporosis using MRI and CT scans with unimodal and multimodal deep-learning models	Y Kucukciloglu et al. [43]	2024	Diagn Interv Radiol	Prediction of osteoporosis on lumbar spine MRI and CT against DEXA scans	120	Lumbar	Sagittal T1w, CT, DEXA	CNN	Accuracy 96–99%
26	Machine learning assisting the prediction of clinical outcomes following nucleoplasty for lumbar degenerative disc disease	PF Chiu et al. [44]	2023	Diagnostics (Basel)	Prediction of pain improvement after lumbar nucleoplasty for degenerative disc disease	181	Lumbar	Axial T2w	Multiple (SVM, light gradient boosting machine, XGBoost, XGBRF, CatBoost, iRF)	Improved RF: accuracy 76%, sensitivity 69%, specificity 83%, F1-score 0.73, AUC 0.77

Table 1. *Cont.*

No	Study Title	Authorship	Year of Publication	Journal Name	Application and Primary Outcome Measure	Sample Size *	Spine Region Studied	MRI Sequences Used	Artificial Intelligence Technique Used	Key Results and Conclusion
27	NAMSTCD: A novel augmented model for spinal cord segmentation and tumor classification using deep nets	R Mohanty et al. [45]	2023	Diagnostics (Basel)	Segmentation of spinal cord regions and tumour types	5000 images	Whole spine	Not mentioned	Multiple (Multiple Mask Regional CNN (MRCNNs), VGGNet 19, YoLo V2, ResNet 101, GoogleNet	Classification accuracy 99% (versus 81–96% for other models)
28	Benign vs. malignant vertebral compression fractures with MRI: a comparison between automatic deep learning network and radiologist's assessment	B Liu et al. [46]	2023	Eur Radiol	Differentiation of benign and malignant vertebral compression fractures	209	Whole spine	Median sagittal T1w, T2w fat suppressed	Two stream compare and contrast network (TSCCN)	AUC 92–99%, accuracy 90–96% (higher than radiologists), specificity 94–99% (higher than radiologists)
29	Automatic detection, classification, and grading of lumbar intervertebral disc degeneration using an artificial neural network model	W Liawrungrueang et al. [47]	2023	Diagnostics (Basel)	Classification of lumbar disc degeneration (Pfirrmann grading)	515	Lumbar	Sagittal T2w	Yolov5	Accuracy > 95%, F1-score 0.98
30	Differentiating magnetic resonance images of pyogenic spondylitis and spinal Modic change using a convolutional neural network	T Mukaihata et al. [48]	2023	Spine (Phila Pa 1976)	Differentiation of Modic changes from pyogenic spondylitis on MRI	100	Whole spine	Sagittal T1w, T2w, STIR	CNN	AUC 0.94–0.95, higher accuracy than clinicians ($p < 0.05$)
31	Automated classification of intramedullary spinal cord tumors and inflammatory demyelinating lesions using deep learning	Z Zhuo et al. [49]	2022	Radiol Artif Intell	Differentiation of cord tumors from demyelinating lesions	647	Whole spine	Sagittal T2w	MultiResU-net, DenseNet121	Test cohort Dice 0.50–0.80, accuracy 79–96%, AUC 0.85–0.99

Table 1. *Cont.*

No	Study Title	Authorship	Year of Publication	Journal Name	Application and Primary Outcome Measure	Sample Size *	Spine Region Studied	MRI Sequences Used	Artificial Intelligence Technique Used	Key Results and Conclusion
32	Ultrafast cervical spine MRI protocol using deep learning-based reconstruction: diagnostic equivalence to a conventional protocol	N Kashiwagi et al. [50]	2022	Eur J Radiol	Validation of an ultrafast cervical spine MRI protocol	50	Cervical	Sagittal T1w, T2w, STIR, axial T2*w	CNN	κ = 0.60–0.98, individual equivalence index 95% CI < 5%
33	Differentiation between spinal multiple myeloma and metastases originated from lung using multi-view attention-guided network	K Chen et al. [51]	2022	Front Oncol	Differentiation of multiple myeloma lesions from metastasis on MRI	217	Whole spine	T2w, T1w post-contrast (3 planes)	Multi-view attention guided (MAGN), ResNet50, Class Activation Mapping	Accuracy 79–81%, AUC 0.77–0.78, F1-score 0.67–0.71
34	Development of lumbar spine MRI referrals vetting models using machine learning and deep learning algorithms: Comparison models vs. healthcare professionals	AH Alanazi et al. [52]	2022	Radiography (Lond)	Vetting of MRI lumbar spine referrals for valid indications	1020	Lumbar	Nil	SVM, logistic regression, RF, CNN, bi-directional long-short term memory (Bi-LSTM)	RF AUC 0.99, CNN AUC 0.98 (outperforming radiographers)
35	Improved productivity using deep learning-assisted reporting for lumbar spine MRI	DSW Lim et al. [53]	2022	Radiology	Evaluation of time savings and accuracy for AI-assisted MRI lumbar spine reporting	25	Lumbar	Sagittal T1w, axial T2w	CNN, ResNet101	Reduced interpretation time ($p < 0.001$), improved or equivalent interobserver agreement with DL assistance
36	Deep learning model for classifying metastatic epidural spinal cord compression on MRI	J Hallinan et al. [54]	2022	Front Oncol	Classification of metastatic vertebral and epidural disease (Bilsky classification)	247	Thoracic	Axial T2w	ResNet50	Internal dataset: κ = 0.92–0.98, external dataset: κ = 0.94–0.95

Table 1. *Cont.*

No	Study Title	Authorship	Year of Publication	Journal Name	Application and Primary Outcome Measure	Sample Size *	Spine Region Studied	MRI Sequences Used	Artificial Intelligence Technique Used	Key Results and Conclusion
37	Vertebral deformity measurements at MRI, CT, and radiography using deep learning	A Suri et al. [55]	2021	Radiol Artif Intell	Measurement of vertebral deformity on MRI, CT and radiographs	1744	Whole spine	Sagittal T1w, T2w, CT, radiographs	Neural network	Vertebral measurement mean height percentage error 1.5–1.9% ± 0.2–0.4, lumbar lordosis angle mean absolute error 2.3–3.6°
38	Predicting postoperative recovery in cervical spondylotic myelopathy: construction and interpretation of T2*-weighted radiomic-based extra trees models	MZ Zhang et al. [56]	2022	Eur Radiol	Prediction of recovery rate after cervical spondylotic myelopathy surgery based on MRI and clinical features	151	Cervical	T2w, T2*w	Threshold selection, collinearity removal, tree-based feature selection	AUC 0.71–0.81 (vs. conventional clinical and radiologic models AUC 0.40–0.55)
39	Fully automated segmentation of lumbar bone marrow in sagittal, high-resolution T1-weighted magnetic resonance images using 2D U-NET	EJ Hwang et al. [57]	2022	Comput Biol Med	Segmentation of normal and pathological bone marrow on MRI lumbar spine	100	Lumbar	Sagittal T1w	U-net3D, Grow-cut	Healthy subjects Dice 0.91–0.96, diseased subjects Dice 0.83–0.95
40	A comparison of natural language processing methods for the classification of lumbar spine imaging findings related to lower back pain	C Jujjavarapu et al. [58]	2022	Acad Radiol	Classification of spine MRI and radiograph reports into 26 findings	871	Lumbar	MRI, radiographs	Elastic-net logistic regression	AUC 0.96 for all findings (n-grams), AUC 0.95 for potentially clinically important findings
41	Virtual magnetic resonance lumbar spine images generated from computed tomography images using conditional generative adversarial networks	M Gotoh et al. [59]	2022	Radiography (Lond)	Generation of virtual MRI images from CT	22	Lumbar	MRI	Conditional GAN	No significant difference between virtual and conventional MRI, except in visualization of spinal canal structure. Peak signal-to-noise ratio 18.4 dB

Table 1. *Cont.*

No	Study Title	Authorship	Year of Publication	Journal Name	Application and Primary Outcome Measure	Sample Size *	Spine Region Studied	MRI Sequences Used	Artificial Intelligence Technique Used	Key Results and Conclusion
42	Deep learning for adjacent segment disease at preoperative MRI for cervical radiculopathy	CMW Goedmakers et al. [60]	2021	Radiology	Prediction of adjacent segment disease after anterior cervical discectomy and fusion surgery on pre-operative MRI	344	Cervical	Sagittal T2w	CNN	Accuracy 95% (vs. 58% for clinicians), sensitivity 80% (vs. 60%), specificity 97% (vs. 58%)
43	Automatic multiclass intramedullary spinal cord tumor segmentation on MRI with deep learning	A Lemay et al. [61]	2021	Neuroimage Clin	Segmentation of three common spinal cord tumors	343	Whole spine	Sagittal T2w, T1w post-contrast	U-net	Dice 0.77 (all abnormal signal), 0.62 (tumour alone), true positive detection > 87% (all abnormal signal)
44	A preliminary study using spinal MRI-based radiomics to predict high-risk cytogenetic abnormalities in multiple myeloma	J Liu et al. [62]	2021	Radiol Med	Prediction of high-risk cytogenic abnormalities in multiple myeloma based on MRI	248 lesions	Whole spine	Sagittal T1w, T2w, T2w fat suppressed	Logistic regression	AUC 0.86–0.87, sensitivity 79%, specificity 79%, PPV 75%, NPV 82%, accuracy 79%
45	A deep learning model for detection of cervical spinal cord compression in MRI scans	Z Merali et al. [63]	2021	Sci Rep	Dichotomous spinal cord compression for cervical spine	289	Cervical	Axial T2w	CNN	AUC 0.94, sensitivity 88%, specificity 89%, F1-score 0.82
46	Deep learning model for automated detection and classification of central canal, lateral recess, and neural foraminal stenosis at lumbar spine MRI	J Hallinan et al. [64]	2021	Radiology	Grading of lumbar spinal canal, lateral recess and neural foraminal stenosis	446	Lumbar	Sagittal T1w, axial T2w	CNN	Recall 85–100%, dichotomous classification κ-range = 0.89–0.96 (vs. 0.92–0.98 for radiologists)
47	A deep convolutional neural network with performance comparable to radiologists for differentiating between spinal schwannoma and meningioma	S Maki et al. [65]	2020	Spine (Phila Pa 1976)	Differentiation of meningioma from schwannoma	84	Whole spine	Sagittal T2w, T1w post-contrast	CNN	AUC 0.87–0.88, sensitivity 78–85% (vs. 95–100% for radiologists), specificity 75–82% (vs. 26–58%), accuracy 80–81% (vs. 69–82%)

Table 1. *Cont.*

No	Study Title	Authorship	Year of Publication	Journal Name	Application and Primary Outcome Measure	Sample Size *	Spine Region Studied	MRI Sequences Used	Artificial Intelligence Technique Used	Key Results and Conclusion
48	Quantitative analysis of neural foramina in the lumbar spine: an imaging informatics and machine learning study	B Gaonkar et al. [66]	2019	Radiol Artif Intell	Segmentation and statistical modelling of lumbar neural foraminal area	1156	Lumbar	Sagittal T2w	SVM, U-net	Dice 0.63–0.68 (neural foramen), 0.84–0.91 (disc)
49	Performance of the deep convolutional neural network based magnetic resonance image scoring algorithm for differentiating between Tuberculous and pyogenic spondylitis	K Kim et al. [67]	2018	Sci Rep	Differentiation of pyogenic from Tuberculous spondylitis	161	Whole spine	Axial T2w	Deep CNN	AUC 0.80 (vs. 0.73 for radiologists, $p = 0.079$)
50	SpineNet: automated classification and evidence visualization in spinal MRIs	A Jamaludin et al. [68]	2017	Med Image Anal	Detection and classification of multiple abnormalities (Pfirrmann grading, disc narrowing, endplate defects, marrow changes, spondylolisthesis, central canal stenosis)	2009	Lumbar spine	T2w sagittal	CNN	Pfirmann inter-rater $\kappa = 0.69$–0.81, overall accuracy 74%

Artificial intelligence (AI), magnetic resonance imaging (MRI), T1-weighted (T1w), T2-weighted (T2w), T2*-weighted (T2*w), area under the curve (AUC), segment anything model (SAM), convolutional neural network (CNN), short-tau inversion recovery (STIR), intersection over union (IOU), diffusion-weighted imaging (DWI), random forest (RF), support vector machine (SVM), computed tomography (CT), generative adversarial network (GAN), dual-energy X-ray absorptiometry (DEXA). * numbers are patients unless stated otherwise.

We classified the included studies based on the following themes: Image Acquisition and Processing (6/50, 12%), Segmentation (8/50, 16%), Diagnosis (27/50, 54%), Treatment Planning, Patient Selection and Prognosis (6/50, 12%) and Others (3, 6%) (Figure 2). We further sub-divided the Diagnosis theme into Degenerative (13/50, 26%), Neoplastic Diseases (7/50, 14%), Infection (3/50, 6%), Trauma (2/50, 4%), and Spondyloarthropathy (2/50, 4%).

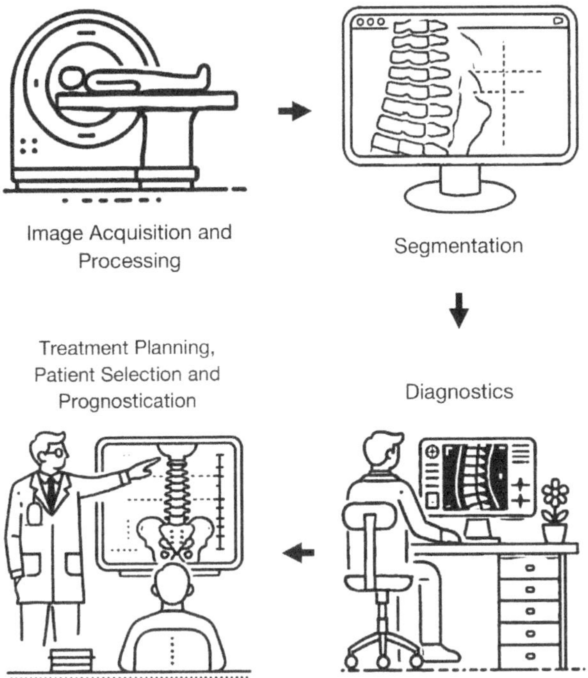

Figure 2. Key themes identified through the literature search representing potential areas where advances in artificial intelligence and machine learning can improve the field of spine MRI.

3.2. Image Acquisition and Processing

AI has demonstrated promise in the area of image acquisition and processing, with multiple studies demonstrating the ability of deep learning (DL)-assisted acquisition and reconstruction techniques to reduce image acquisition times while maintaining similar image quality to conventional protocols. Kashiwagi et al. (2022) studied an ultrafast cervical spine MRI protocol (sagittal T1-, T2-weighted, short-tau inversion recovery (STIR), and axial T2*-weighted sequences) using a convolutional neural network (CNN)-based reconstruction which reduces the matrix size, oversampling rate, and number of excitations by applying a noise reduction algorithm. Scan quality was rated by three neuroradiologists, who graded various degenerative changes including central canal stenosis, foraminal stenosis and disc degeneration. Compared with a conventional MRI protocol, the DL-based reconstruction technique reduced scan time from 12 min 54 s to 2 min 57 s (achieving a time reduction of 9 min 57 s, 77% faster), with high levels of agreement (κ = 0.60–0.98) between the protocols [50]. In another study by Awan et al. (2024), the authors evaluated a lumbar spine MRI DL-accelerated protocol (sagittal T1-, T2-weighted, STIR, axial T2-weighted sequences) that was 57% faster compared to a conventional protocol (287 s versus 654 s). This protocol employs an unrolled variational network and neural networks to reduce the number of signal averages needed while preserving high image fidelity. The DL-accelerated protocol demonstrated non-inferiority for the assessment of foraminal and spinal canal stenosis, nerve compression, and facet arthropathy. However, there was increased artifact perception in the DL group. The authors proposed that further work could focus on other pathologies, such as spinal cord evaluation, to ensure the broad applicability of such protocols across various clinical scenarios [22]. Such protocols promise to generate significant time- and cost-savings for radiology departments. In addition, reducing examination time would potentially improve patient comfort, especially for those who may not be able to fully cooperate with long examination times due to pre-existing medical conditions or claustrophobia.

AI can also be applied to generate synthetic MRI sequences. In a multi-center trial, Tanenbaum et al. (2023) used existing sagittal T1- and T2-weighted MRI images to generate STIR images, which is the preferred MRI sequence to assess certain pathologies such as vertebral fractures and infection. The authors demonstrated that both acquired and synthetic STIR sequences were diagnostically equivalent; five radiologists (four subspecialists and one general radiologist) had similar interobserver agreements for both the conventional and AI-generated sequences for the detection of three findings (prevertebral fluid collections, fracture-related bone edema, and posterior soft tissue/ligamentous injury) against the reference standard. Additionally, synthetic images had a higher mean image quality score. Nonetheless, the authors acknowledged that artifacts in the input images could potentially affect synthetic image quality [42]. Thus, while synthetic MRI sequences could also help reduce scan times, further work is necessary to better understand the effects of MRI artifacts, such as metal or susceptibility artifacts on such algorithms.

Furthermore, certain DL models such as generative adversarial networks (GANs) have been successfully deployed to generate MRI-like images from CT data, and vice versa [41,59]. Gotoh et al. (2022) utilized a conditional GAN (pix2pix) to generate synthetic T2-weighted MRI images from lumbar spine CTs. They achieved a modest peak signal-to-noise ratio of 18.4 dB, although, on qualitative evaluation by two radiologists, there was no significant difference in the image quality with conventional MRI images [59]. These models can be potentially useful for patients who have contraindications to MRI, such as non-MRI compatible implants.

3.3. Segmentation

Segmentation comprised the second highest proportion of studies reviewed. Notably, many early studies concentrated on segmentation. Various regions of the spine, including the vertebrae, intervertebral discs, and spinal cord, have been studied for this application. Recently, more sophisticated and complex models have been employed to achieve higher levels of accuracy across a broader range of tasks. Mohanty et al. (2023) demonstrated the use of a novel segmentation technique that initially segments the spinal cord into different regions. A combination of multiple mask regional CNNs (MRCNNs) is then used for each spinal cord segment, which provides a higher overall accuracy of 99% compared to accuracies of 81–96% for the other models (a CNN, deep neural network, and statistical parametric mapping) [45]. Newer models are also able to segment a larger number of structures, improving granularity. Yilizati-Yilihamu et al. (2023) employed a SAFNet-based model to segment 17 unique spinal structures, overcoming issues posed by intra- and inter-class differences across a range of spinal levels. This method extracted low-, mid- and high-level features on MRI images which were then processed separately before being concatenated. The model achieved an overall mean Dice score of 80% against a radiologist, surpassing other models whose Dice scores ranged from 75–79%, with 3D UNet performing the worst. However, SAFNet exhibited relatively poor segmentation for certain structures, such as the L5 vertebra and sacrum. While SAFNet had high Dice scores on most vertebrae, it struggled with accurately depicting the borders of L5 and the sacral intervertebral discs [36]. The sacrum's unique shape and poorly formed intervertebral discs may have contributed to these difficulties. In contrast, models like 3D DeepLabv3 and ResUNet, which employ superior boundary detection techniques, were more successful in achieving accurate segmentation in these challenging areas. Despite these challenges,

SAFNet demonstrated better generalization and overall performance, making it a robust choice for segmentation tasks.

Interpreting MRIs with spinal abnormalities presents a significant challenge for accurate segmentation due to distorted anatomy and altered relationships between normal structures. To address this, several models have been developed for segmentation in specific clinical scenarios, such as spinal cord trauma. Specifically, Masse-Gignac et al. (2023) employed an attention-gated U-net to segment injured spinal cords. The attention gating mechanism helped the architecture focus on the most relevant features while reducing the number of feature maps, leading to a considerable Dice score of 0.95, even in the presence of distorted segmentation boundaries [35].

Additionally, segmentation has been expanded beyond normal anatomical structures to include pathology itself. For instance, Lemay et al. (2021) trained a cascaded neural network for segmentation of intramedullary tumors across different spinal regions. The study included 343 patients with various tumors (namely, astrocytomas, ependymomas and hemangioblastomas) and utilized T2-weighted and T1-weighted post-contrast images. A Dice score of 62% was achieved for segmentation of the tumor itself compared to radiologists' segmentation, with a higher Dice score of 77% when the tumor cavity and edema were also included. Compared to a single model architecture (a 3D U-net), the cascaded architecture demonstrated increased Dice scores of 30% for edema, and 5% for tumor and tumor cavity [61]. The segmentation of pathology is potentially useful in clinical practice to allow more accurate quantification and post-treatment follow-up.

3.4. *Diagnostics*

There has been considerable interest in using AI for diagnostic applications in spine MRI, and this represented the largest proportion of studies in our review. To provide more focus, we have further categorized the studies based on the type of disease examined.

3.4.1. Degenerative Disease

Degenerative disease along the spine is found in a sizeable proportion of all MRIs performed. Multiple studies have investigated the use of AI models in the detection and classification of degenerative pathologies. These mainly focused on the cervical [20,38,63] and lumbar [33,47,64,68] spine, given the relatively higher incidence in these regions compared to the semi-rigid thoracic spine [1]. Models have also been utilized to allow for the detection of specific pathologies on MRI, such as OPLL [25], which is typically assessed on CT.

A number of studies have focused on identifying the sites of spinal cord or nerve compression. Merali et al. (2021) trained a CNN (ResNet50) to classify cervical spine MRIs for the presence or absence of cord compression on axial T2-weighted images, achieving a high AUC of 0.94. While this model could be used to quickly classify patients with high accuracy, the authors noted that a more precise model that stratifies the severity of spinal cord compression (for example, partial versus circumferential compression, with the latter being more severe) would offer greater clinical utility [63].

In a study by Hallinan et al. (2021), the authors examined the ability of a CNN-based model to perform automated grading of lumbar spinal stenosis at different regions of interest. The model was trained on axial T2-weighted and sagittal T1-weighted sequences and achieved high levels of agreement compared with the reference standard (an expert radiologist with 31 years of experience). Its performance was comparable to that of subspecialist radiologists for dichotomous grading at the central canal (κ = 0.96 versus 0.98 for radiologists) and lateral recesses (κ = 0.92 versus 0.92–0.95 for radiologists) but slightly lower at the neural foramina (κ = 0.89 versus 0.94–0.95 for radiologists) [64]. In a follow-up study, Lim et al. (2022) assessed whether this model could enhance radiologist performance. The authors evaluated the performance of eight radiologists (comprising subspecialists, general radiologists, and in-training radiologists) with and without DL model assistance. They found that DL model assistance generated significant time savings (reduced interpretation time by 76–203 s, $p < 0.001$), with the greatest benefit for in-training radiologists. DL-assisted readers had improved or similar performance compared to the baseline [53]. Such studies that assess the real-world impact of DL models are useful in identifying the areas of greatest benefit and potential problems. In this context, using AI alongside radiologists during image interpretation has the potential to enhance both the efficiency and consistency of reporting by reducing variability in their assessments.

Other studies have focused on specific degenerative pathologies, such as intervertebral disc degeneration. Liawrungrueang et al. (2023) trained a CNN (YOLOv5) to classify lumbar discs on sagittal T2-weighted images using the Pfirrmann classification system [69], a widely used system for communicating the severity of disc degeneration and destruction. Compared to a musculoskeletal radiologist, the model achieved accuracies of more than 95% [47]. Recent work by Xie et al. (2024) employed a combined model using MedSAM followed by radiomics analysis to perform Pfirrmann grading for degenerate cervical discs. The model was trained on sagittal T1- and T2-weighted images and achieved an AUC of 0.95 on a test set, compared against an orthopedic radiologist. It demonstrated the highest accuracy of 90% when using T1- and T2-weighted images in combination (versus 81–86% when trained on either sequence alone) [20]. The ability to classify degenerative pathologies using standardized grading systems can allow for the rapid identification of cases with more severe disease. The use of established criteria would also help facilitate communication among different specialists.

3.4.2. Neoplastic Diseases

Neoplastic disease can affect different structures along the spine including the vertebral column and epidural space with risk of spinal cord compression, potentially leading to significant disability. Bone neoplasms include metastases, myeloma, and primary neoplastic lesions [70]. Additionally, neoplasms can involve the thecal sac/dura and spinal cord. Several models have been utilized to address diagnostic challenges in spine oncology [32,49,51,65], facilitating the distinction between different pathologies with overlapping imaging characteristics. For example, Zhuo et al. (2022) employed the MultiResUNet and DenseNet121-based models to differentiate demyelinating disease from neoplasms (namely ependymoma and astrocytoma) on sagittal T2-weighted MRI alone, without contrast-enhanced sequences. Scans were evaluated by seven neuroradiologists, with the model achieving high accuracies of 79–96% (AUC 0.85–0.99), which was similar or superior to the performance of the neuroradiologists (accuracies of 67–97%). Accuracy for differentiating between the types of demyelinating diseases (multiple sclerosis versus neuromyelitis optica spectrum disorders) was the lowest. This pipeline could potentially be useful for cases where intravenous gadolinium contrast is contraindicated, for example, in patients with renal impairment. However, the authors also performed lesion segmentation and noted relatively poor Dice scores of 0.50–0.58 for the segmentation of demyelinating lesions (versus Dice scores of 0.77–0.80 for neoplasms), suggesting that further work in this area is necessary before AI-based quantification can be applied to clinical practice [49].

Other models have been applied to evaluate complications resulting from neoplastic diseases. For instance, Liu et al. (2023) used a Two-Stream Compare and Contrast Network (TSCCN) model to differentiate between benign and malignant vertebral compression fractures on sagittal T1-weighted and T2-weighted fat-saturated images, a common diagnostic dilemma. In clinical practice, malignant fractures (usually due to metastases) may require surgical management, and the primary malignancy must also be sought. In their study, all cases of malignant fractures were confirmed histologically (total of 14 cancer types). The model achieved higher accuracies of 90–96% (highest accuracy using both MRI sequences in combination) relative to clinical radiologists (accuracies of 81–90%). The TSCCN model does not require the manual segmentation of fractures and allows for the rapid identification of malignant fractures. The authors, however, acknowledge that the generalizability of the model may be limited for other cancer types not included in the study [46].

Additionally, in routine practice, radiologists also evaluate the extent of spinal cord compression resulting from neoplastic disease as it helps guide management and identify patients at risk of neurologic compromise. To this end, Hallinan et al. (2022) used a CNN to grade the severity of metastatic epidural spinal cord compression (MESCC) using the Bilsky classification on axial T2-weighted images. Compared against an experienced musculoskeletal radiologist as the reference standard, the model achieved an almost-perfect agreement for dichotomous grading on internal validation ($\kappa = 0.92$) and external testing ($\kappa = 0.94$). It was also compared to three clinicians who had similar performance (κ-range = 0.94–0.98). This could be used to identify patients with severe cord compression for prompt specialist review [54]. In a separate study, the authors also demonstrated the feasibility of automated MESCC grading (normal/low/high-grade) on a matched set of contrast-enhanced CT images that had corresponding MRIs. The CT model had a high agreement (κ = 0.87–91) with the expert and was superior to two radiologists (κ = 0.73–0.82). This would potentially allow for even earlier diagnosis on staging CT scans which are routinely performed for patients with cancer [71–73].

3.4.3. Infection

MRI is the modality of choice for evaluating spondylodiscitis, allowing for an accurate diagnosis, characterization of the extent of infection, and assessment of complications. However, infections can present a diagnostic challenge as degenerative or inflammatory lesions may exhibit similar MRI findings.

Mukaihata et al. (2023) developed an algorithm to differentiate pyogenic spondylitis from Modic endplate changes, a common diagnostic dilemma. Using a CNN backbone, the authors assessed the model's performance on sagittal T1-, T2-weighted, and STIR images against a radiologist and specialist orthopedic and spine surgeons. The model demonstrated comparable performance to the clinicians and had a high AUC (0.94–0.95) [48]. Additionally, MRI can be useful in suggesting the likely causative organism for spine infections, helping guide treatment and follow-up. Several studies have applied AI to this effect [37,69]. Wang et al. (2023) evaluated a combined model to predict whether Brucella or Tuberculous spondylitis was more likely using sagittal T1-, T2-, T2-weighted fat-saturated, and axial T2-weighted sequences. Various AI models were used to assess images against the reference standard (defined by clinical and microbiological diagnostic criteria). A random forest model achieved the highest AUC of 0.95, higher than a support vector machine (AUC 0.90–0.94) [37]. Such models are potentially useful as the choice of microbiological therapy and management strategy differs significantly between these conditions.

3.4.4. Trauma

MRI is often used in the assessment of traumatic injuries, providing a detailed visualization of soft tissues including the spinal cord and vertebrae, aiding in the detection of subtle injuries and fractures crucial for accurate diagnosis and treatment planning. Wang et al. (2024) demonstrated that CNNs (YoloV7 and ResNet50) may be used to evaluate for acute vertebral fractures. In their study, sagittal STIR images were used, with the model demonstrating a high accuracy of 98% (sensitivity of 98%, specificity of 97%) against assessments by spine surgeons. While the performance on an external dataset was slightly poorer, this was still relatively high at 92% (sensitivity of 93%, specificity of 92%) [21].

In another application, Jo et al. (2023) developed a two-step algorithm (Attention U-net and Inception-ResNet-V2) for the diagnosis and localization of posterior ligamentous complex injury in patients with thoracolumbar fractures on midsagittal T2-weighted fat-saturated images, which can be particularly difficult for inexperienced readers. Assessment by two experienced musculoskeletal radiologists was used as the reference standard. The algorithm demonstrated comparable performance (AUC 0.93 on internal testing, 0.92 on external testing) to a musculoskeletal radiologist (AUC 0.93), and higher performance than a radiology trainee (AUC 0.83). In addition, they showed that the performance of the radiology trainee was significantly improved when aided by the model (improved from AUC 0.83 to AUC 0.92) [28]. Such models can be used to improve diagnostic confidence for junior readers.

3.4.5. Spondyloarthropathy

MRIs play an important role in the diagnosis and monitoring of spondyloarthropathies, such as ankylosing spondylitis, given its increased sensitivity over conventional techniques like radiographs and CT. It can identify lesions in the pre-clinical stage of the disease and guide the decision on the use of disease-modifying drugs. Tas et al. (2023) demonstrated the use of a multi-stage CNN-based model (termed "ASNet") in the diagnosis of ankylosing spondylitis with high accuracy (96–100%) on both non-contrast (axial and coronal STIR) and contrast-enhanced T1-weighted MRI sequences. All the included ankylosing spondylitis patients had a clinico-radiological diagnosis and were on follow-up with a rheumatologist. The authors achieved higher accuracies compared to previous similar studies which used ResNet and U-net models (accuracies of 88–92%). Of note, the authors demonstrated the highest accuracy with non-contrast images (99% on coronal and 100% on axial images), which may obviate the need for intravenous contrast in the future [34]. This could improve diagnosis for patients with contraindications such as contrast medium allergy or impaired renal function. In another sample of 330 patients with axial spondyloarthritis, Lin et al. (2024) employed a UNet-based model to detect inflammatory lesions on sagittal STIR images, using combined assessment by an experienced radiologist and rheumatologist as the ground truth. The DL model demonstrated similar results (sensitivity 80%, specificity 88%, on a per-image basis) to a radiologist of four years' experience (sensitivity 82%, specificity 87%) [23].

3.5. Treatment Planning, Patient Selection, and Prognostication

Another growing application of AI is its use in patients who are being evaluated for specific treatments. Models have been developed to predict outcomes for patients undergoing various spinal procedures or surgeries, such as lumbar disc surgery [31], lumbar nucleoplasty [44], and cervical spine surgery [56,60]. Of note, Goedmakers et al. (2021) employed three CNNs (VGGNet19, ResNet19, and ResNet50) to predict which patients would develop adjacent segment disease (on clinical and radiologic follow-up) after undergoing cervical radiculopathy surgery (anterior discectomy and fusion). Conventionally, the prediction of this relatively common complication relies on subjective clinical assessment. The authors used sagittal T2-weighted images and demonstrated a higher accuracy of 95% (using ResNet50) compared to 58% by the clinicians (a neurosurgeon and neuroradiologist). This model offers to provide useful prognostic information and can guide decisions on patient selection, although future work could also account for other variables such as patient demographics and surgical technique [60].

Apart from surgery, other treatments can also be analyzed using predictive algorithms. Chen et al. (2023) investigated an ML-based radiomics algorithm to evaluate sagittal T1-, T2-weighted, STIR, and axial T2-weighted MRIs for radiotherapy prognostication. Follow-up data on tumor progression were classified into "progressive disease" and "non-progressive disease" groups based on established tumor response criteria. The clinical model achieved an AUC of 0.73 (based on features such as multiplicity of tumors, Bilsky score, symptoms) whereas a combined clinical–radiomics model had an improved AUC of 0.83. Although this study was relatively small, with only 52 lesions in the progressive disease group, and benefits over the conventional model were relatively modest, it shows the potential applicability of radiomics models to assist radiation oncologists in treatment selection for difficult cases [30].

3.6. Others

A variety of other applications exist. These include various non-interpretative tasks such as vetting MRI requests. Alanazi et al. (2022) compared the performance of experienced radiographers to various AI models in determining whether a lumbar spine MRI request was indicated or not. A random forest model was found to achieve the highest area under the curve of 0.99 [52]. Further models have also been applied to tasks such as processing radiology reports. For instance, Jujjavarapu et al. applied various natural language processing methods to analyze lumbar spine radiograph and MRI reports. High accuracy was achieved (AUC 0.96 with n-grams) for the identification of 26 radiologic findings. The authors also showed reliable extraction of potentially clinically important findings (AUC 0.95 with document embeddings). Such models could be employed to facilitate early clinical review for patients with time-critical pathology [58].

3.7. AI and ML Techniques

The reviewed studies employed various AI and ML techniques, with CNNs being the most frequently used, both appearing in studies from the earlier years to the most recent. CNNs are versatile and have been applied across a wide range of tasks, including segmentation, detection, and classification. In more recent years, advanced CNN architectures (such as ResNet, DenseNet, YOLO) have been developed. These architectures incorporate new mechanisms to overcome several limitations of conventional models (including the vanishing gradient problem and overfitting), allowing for deeper networks and better performance [21,25,27,28,33,34,45].

U-nets are another common technique, being particularly favored in image segmentation tasks for their precision and efficiency. In later studies, U-net variants (such as 3D U-net, Attention U-net, and MultiRes U-net) were employed to further enhance their capabilities [19,28,49,57]. For instance, 3D U-nets enable the segmentation of volumetric data like MRI scans, preserving spatial information across slices and leading to greater accuracy.

Some studies also implemented ensemble models, where outputs from multiple individual models are aggregated to produce superior results than each model alone. Common ensemble models in this review include Random Forest and boosting models (XGBoost, AdaBoost), which were used to improve the performance for advanced classification tasks such as predicting outcomes after spinal surgery or stereotactic radiotherapy [30,31,39,44].

Overall, there was a noticeable transition from simple, single-model approaches to more sophisticated models over time. Hybrid and ensemble models became increasingly common, reflecting the need for more robust models capable of effectively handling complex tasks.

4. Discussion

AI and ML in spine MRI have the potential to address several shortcomings of conventional technology and assessment. However, there remain important gaps and limitations that need to be addressed and studied.

As previously alluded to, one of the major challenges that modern radiology departments face is the significant time required to perform MRIs, despite ongoing advances in MRI technology, acceleration techniques, and pulse sequences. The ability of DL reconstructions to significantly reduce imaging time has the potential to improve scanner utilization and patient comfort [74]. These are pertinent issues, given the increasing demand for advanced imaging such as MRI and the longer examination times compared to other imaging modalities. Many DL reconstruction algorithms promise minimal to no degradation of image quality, ensuring high diagnostic accuracy, and some are already commercially available. In particular, the synthetic MRI sequences generated from CT images could allow clinicians to leverage the speed of the CT with the superior soft tissue resolution of MRI, facilitating more accurate diagnoses for patients who cannot undergo MRI (e.g., patients with MRI-incompatible implants or claustrophobia) [59]. Conversely, synthetic MRI-generated CT sequences can eliminate radiation exposure. However, there are limitations to the current DL technology. Reconstruction algorithms, especially those used for denoising, can exaggerate artifacts and may cause instability in output images, potentially leading to small lesions being overlooked [74,75].

Advances in spine segmentation have served as an important foundation on which more complex applications can be built. Most recently, models developed to segment pathology have given rise to new clinical applications [61]. The segmentation of other diseases such as neoplasms could also lead to more objective and accurate monitoring for treatment response. Further work in this area is necessary to determine the impact on patient outcomes.

With advances in diagnostics, interpretative tasks conventionally performed by trained radiologists can be augmented by AI. An important area of potential impact is increased efficiency and productivity leading to time savings. Given the ever-increasing radiology workloads, AI could potentially be used to reduce interpretation times and reader fatigue, allowing radiologists to focus on more complex cases and patient care [76]. Additionally, AI tools may supplement radiologists by improving their diagnostic accuracy. AI augmentation has been shown to improve radiologists' performance, particularly those with less experience [28,53]. Another area of particular interest is the synergy between radiomics and deep learning. This field involves quantitative image analysis, offering more precise and accurate lesion characterization or classification than what is possible by human readers alone [20,77]. Additionally, AI models, such as those applied to spondyloarthropathy [34], have the potential to reduce the need for intravenous gadolinium contrast, which is commonly used to enhance diagnostic quality in MRI scans. This reduction could lead to significant cost savings and minimize the potential risks of gadolinium toxicity.

In the field of treatment planning, patient selection, and prognostication, predictive algorithms have shown promise in allowing for the better anticipation of patient outcomes and complications. Spinal surgery and interventions carry significant risks and should be offered to patients who are likely to benefit the most. While existing clinical decision support and predictive tests are available, these often lack consensus and can have conflicting evidence [78,79]. AI systems that accurately predict outcomes can improve patient care and resource optimization.

However, despite widespread optimism about the purported benefits of these AI technologies, there are important limitations and potential areas for further study, which we will address in the next sections.

4.1. Generalizability

Generalizability refers to the ability of an AI model to perform its intended function on a new set of data that was not part of the model development process [80]. While models may exhibit high levels of accuracy on test sets, developing a generalizable model presents unique challenges. Ethical, legislative, and practical concerns often lead to the development of models based on patient data from a single healthcare institution or country. Variability in institutional imaging protocols, MRI equipment, and pulse sequences introduces significant challenges to consistent AI model performance. In addition, variations in treatment approaches further complicate the development of generalizable models. These factors collectively limit the performance of AI models when applied in different settings [81,82].

Several strategies can be employed to improve generalizability. Firstly, ensuring the availability of data from varied populations is crucial. For instance, Xu et al. (2023) used a large training dataset to develop an AI model for thyroid nodule classification on ultrasound. They utilized data from 10,023 patients across 208 hospitals and 12 equipment vendors, achieving a high AUC of 0.90. The use of scans from a heterogeneous patient population was cited as an important factor for the model's strong performance [83]. Large medical image datasets, including RadImageNet, MedPix, CheXpert, have been made available in recent years. Additionally, the Radiological Society of North America (RSNA) and the American Society of Neuroradiology (ASNR) recently launched a publicly available dataset of cases annotated by 50 expert radiologists across eight institutions, with the goal of encouraging the development of AI tools for degenerative lumbar spine MRIs [84].

Improving the availability of diverse, high-quality data can potentially overcome some of the challenges posed by limited diversity in training datasets, potentially resulting in more robust models.

Secondly, techniques such as transfer learning can be employed. Transfer learning, which includes domain adaptation, involves making modifications to a model in order to improve its performance on previously unseen tasks [85]. Xuan et al. (2023) employed transfer learning on CNNs (YOLOv3, YOLOv5, PP-YOLOv2) that were pre-trained on general image datasets. Transfer learning was applied by using these models to train a CNN, together with sagittal T2-weighted MRI images labeled by experienced spinal surgeons for evaluation of various features (including disc bulges and spondylolisthesis). The model had a higher accuracy (98%) compared to three spine doctors (accuracies ranging from 70 to 88%) [86]. Similar approaches could be applied to other spine AI models, ensuring their validity when applied to varied settings.

Thirdly, "stress testing" involves evaluating an AI model under varied or extreme conditions to identify potential weak points [81]. In radiology, this may include modifying the input image by rotating, cropping, or adjusting the brightness. Such tests help simulate clinical variability. Santomartino et al. (2024) recently evaluated a bone age prediction algorithm on external images before and after applying transformations to simulate real-world variations (for example, rotating or flipping the image, altering brightness and contrast). The algorithm performed well on the external dataset with a mean absolute difference of 6.9 months and 16.2% clinically significant errors (CSEs) when compared to radiologists. However, its performance significantly worsened when tested on the altered images; when the image resolution was altered, the mean absolute difference increased to 118.3 months. This process helped demonstrate the important pitfalls of the model [87]. Stress testing allows for the simulation of real-world variations in image quality that can significantly impact model performance.

As more AI models become commercially available, it is crucial that they are rigorously validated before they can be applied to new healthcare settings, ensuring their accuracy and safety for patient use.

4.2. Implementation

Implementing AI in clinical practice involves overcoming several hurdles. Most recently, a multi-society statement was released by several radiological organizations (ACR, CAR, ESR, RANZCR, RSNA) that provided guidance on the application of AI tools, from development to implementation and use [88]. The statement highlighted the need for rigorous evaluation to ensure patient safety and supported the integration of AI into existing healthcare information technology (IT) infrastructure. Other authors have emphasized the importance of using vendor-neutral platforms, which can streamline algorithms from multiple developers and facilitate end-user access to AI-generated results [89]. Addressing these concerns will ensure that AI algorithms are reliable and effective.

A key challenge in healthcare is maintaining patient confidentiality while leveraging large volumes of medical data for AI training and deployment. Privacy concerns arise due to the sensitive nature of medical data, and the risk of data breaches or misuse could compromise patient trust and legal compliance. Designing AI systems that protect patient identities through techniques like data anonymization and encryption is essential [90].

The use of AI in healthcare settings such as radiology also raises ethical concerns. Patient well-being, equity, privacy, and dignity should be prioritized. Responsible use of AI includes ensuring that patient data are properly regulated and kept secure. AI models may also exaggerate pre-existing biases in healthcare, particularly the effects of selection bias. Such bias is inadvertently introduced when algorithms are applied to patient data that differ from the data on which they were trained, where the incidence of various pathologies may differ. For example, an AI model trained primarily on data from urban hospitals may underperform when used in rural settings, where the prevalence of certain conditions and patient demographics differ significantly. Even within a single health system, AI systems may inadvertently introduce bias against minority populations due to unrepresentative training data. This can potentially lead to less accurate predictions for certain groups and increase healthcare disparity. Minimizing bias is crucial to ensuring fairness and accuracy [88,90–94].

Trust is another key factor in the successful implementation of AI models into clinical care. Radiologists' trust in AI has been identified as one of the most common barriers to its adoption [95]. Many commonly used algorithms operate as "black box" solutions, making it difficult to fully understand how conclusions are derived. Building patient trust in AI is also important for its role to be widely accepted in patient care. Clear communication about how AI works and its benefits can foster this trust. Involving end-users and patients in the AI development process and addressing their concerns is also vital [96]. For example, saliency maps (heat maps) can be used to improve model explainability. These are visual representations that highlight parts of the image that are most relevant to a DL model's predictions. Brima and Atemkeng (2024) used various saliency methods (GradCAM, Score-CAM, XRAI) on datasets comprising MRI scans depicting brain tumors and COVID-19 chest radiographs. Employing both qualitative visual assessment and quantitative (Accuracy and Softmax Information Curves) metrics, they showed that saliency maps can offer accurate representations of a model's decision-making process [97].

Ongoing research and close collaboration between researchers, healthcare providers, and regulatory bodies is necessary to ensure the smooth implementation of AI in routine practice. Establishing robust regulatory frameworks and continuously monitoring AI systems will be essential to addressing any emerging issues and maintaining high standards of patient care.

4.3. Study Limitations

While this review provides a comprehensive analysis of the current applications of AI and ML in spine MRI, several limitations should be acknowledged. Firstly, the heterogeneity of the included studies and lack of inferential statistics limit the robustness and ability to draw generalized conclusions. Differences in study designs, patient populations, MRI protocols, and models make it difficult to directly compare outcomes between studies. Nonetheless, we sought to provide a comprehensive overview across the range of applications that have been studied in this field, with the aim of highlighting current trends and identifying key gaps in the literature which could serve as targets for further research. Secondly, a majority of the studies reviewed were retrospective in nature, which limits the ability to assess the real-world applicability of these AI tools in prospective clinical settings. Another notable limitation is the lack of standardized evaluation metrics across studies, making it challenging to objectively compare the performance of different AI models. Finally, the review did not consider the potential biases that could be introduced by AI models, such as those related to patient demographics, which could impact the fairness and equity of AI-driven healthcare solutions.

4.4. Proposed Areas of Future Research

Firstly, the exploration of foundation AI models in healthcare presents an exciting opportunity. These models are trained on varied and much more extensive datasets than the conventional models, making them adaptable for a wide range of tasks. Furthermore, they have the potential to integrate multiple data types to provide comprehensive insights. However, there are several limitations, including the increased complexity in training and validating these generalist models [98,99]. Thus, further work is necessary to evaluate potential applications in spine MRI.

One such application is the development of comprehensive models for image interpretation. Such models have already been developed and validated for applications like interpreting chest radiographs, where the detection of multiple pathologies is possible [100–102]. However, in this application, many existing models focus on detecting a single pathology or differentiating between a small number of pathologies. Currently, many of these models still require radiologist input for image interpretation. Comprehensive AI models that can detect and classify a wide range of pathologies—including degenerative disease, fractures and vertebral malalignment, marrow signal abnormality, spinal cord abnormalities and incidental extra-spinal findings—will significantly enhance the diagnostic process. These advanced models could also integrate information from the patient's electronic medical records. Multidisciplinary collaboration among computer scientists, radiologists, and clinicians is necessary to identify areas where clinically relevant models can provide the greatest benefit for patients [103].

Another area where foundation models can improve patient care is through large language models (LLMs). Privacy-protecting LLMs (PP-LLMs), which can manage large volumes of healthcare data while ensuring patient privacy and security, are particularly promising. In radiology, LLMs have already been employed for a range of tasks. For example, they have been used to determine the most appropriate imaging protocol for different types of scans [104], generate radiology reports, and summarize reports [105,106]. Spine MRI reports are a suitable area for LLM assistance as they are typically structured by spinal level, which can make the reporting process tedious and time-consuming. LLMs could automate much of this work, generating consistent and accurate reports more efficiently than manual methods. In addition, LLMs have the potential to enhance the understanding of radiological findings by both referring clinicians and patients. LLMs can help translate complicated medical jargon into language that is accessible to patients, helping them to better understand their diagnosis [107,108]. As the performance of LLMs continues to improve, their range of applications in healthcare is likely to expand. Future advancements could include more varied diagnostic tasks. In particular, recent multimodal LLMs which can interpret both text and images are particularly useful in radiology, with the potential to aid in tasks such as identifying errors in radiology reports [109]. Such algorithms could be developed for spine imaging thus ensuring patient safety.

A final key area of future research is the evaluation of real-world applications of AI, particularly its impact on diagnostic accuracy, productivity, and patient outcomes. Studies like those by Lim et al. (2022), where the radiologist's performance in interpreting the lumbar spine MRI was assessed with and without a DL model, provide valuable insight. The largest improvements in time and accuracy were seen for in-training and general radiologists, with subspeciality radiologists achieving the least productivity gains [53]. Studies on the application of AI systems for other diseases have helped demonstrate unexpected or unintended consequences. A recent study by Yu et al. (2024) examined the impact of AI assistance on 140 radiologists who were tasked with interpreting chest radiographs. The authors found that the impact of AI assistance on radiologist performance was variable, and that AI errors significantly impacted treatment outcomes [110]. Similar studies will be useful in evaluating other interpretative tasks, such as spine imaging, to understand the influence of AI more holistically.

5. Conclusions

Our review has highlighted the significant potential that AI and ML have in revolutionizing spine MRI by addressing important challenges in image acquisition, diagnostic accuracy, and treatment planning. We have examined key advancements in AI including the development of DL reconstruction algorithms that allow for faster image acquisition, and models that allow for improved diagnostic performance. We also acknowledge the limitations of current AI technology. Future work will require collaborative efforts to fully exploit new technologies and address practical challenges related to generalizability and implementation.

Author Contributions: Conceptualization, methodology, validation, data curation, writing—review and editing, A.L., W.O., A.M., Y.H.T., W.C.T., S.W.D.L., X.Z.L. and J.T.P.D.H.; software, resources, A.L., W.C.T., S.W.D.L., J.J.H.T., N.K. and J.T.P.D.H.; writing—original draft preparation, A.L., W.O. and W.C.T.; project administration, A.L., W.O., Y.H.T., A.M. and J.J.H.T.; supervision, funding acquisition, J.T.P.D.H. All authors have read and agreed to the published version of the manuscript.

Funding: This research was directly funded by the Ministry of Health/National Medical Research Council, Singapore under the NMRC Clinician Innovator Award (CIA). The grant was awarded for the project titled "Deep learning pipeline for augmented reporting of MRI whole spine" (Grant ID: CIAINV23jan-0001, MOH-001405, J.T.P.D.H.).

Institutional Review Board Statement: Not applicable.

Informed Consent Statement: Not applicable.

Data Availability Statement: Not applicable.

Conflicts of Interest: The authors declare no conflicts of interest.

References

1. Kim, G.-U.; Chang, M.C.; Kim, T.U.; Lee, G.W. Diagnostic Modality in Spine Disease: A Review. *Asian Spine J.* **2020**, *14*, 910–920. [CrossRef] [PubMed]
2. Leone, A.; Guglielmi, G.; Cassar-Pullicino, V.N.; Bonomo, L. Lumbar Intervertebral Instability: A Review. *Radiology* **2007**, *245*, 62–77. [CrossRef] [PubMed]
3. Blackmore, C.C.; Mann, F.A.; Wilson, A.J. Helical CT in the Primary Trauma Evaluation of the Cervical Spine: An Evidence-Based Approach. *Skelet. Radiol.* **2000**, *29*, 632–639. [CrossRef]
4. Selopranoto, U.S.; Soo, M.Y.; Fearnside, M.R.; Cummine, J.L. Ossification of the Posterior Longitudinal Ligament of the Cervical Spine. *J. Clin. Neurosci.* **1997**, *4*, 209–217. [CrossRef]
5. Hartley, K.G.; Damon, B.M.; Patterson, G.T.; Long, J.H.; Holt, G.E. MRI Techniques: A Review and Update for the Orthopaedic Surgeon. *J. Am. Acad. Orthop. Surg.* **2012**, *20*, 775–787. [CrossRef]
6. Alyas, F.; Saifuddin, A.; Connell, D. MR Imaging Evaluation of the Bone Marrow and Marrow Infiltrative Disorders of the Lumbar Spine. *Magn. Reson. Imaging Clin. N. Am.* **2007**, *15*, 199–219. [CrossRef] [PubMed]
7. Henninger, B.; Kaser, V.; Ostermann, S.; Spicher, A.; Zegg, M.; Schmid, R.; Kremser, C.; Krappinger, D. Cervical Disc and Ligamentous Injury in Hyperextension Trauma: MRI and Intraoperative Correlation. *J. Neuroimaging* **2020**, *30*, 104–109. [CrossRef]
8. Landman, J.A.; Hoffman, J.C., Jr.; Braun, I.F.; Barrow, D.L. Value of Computed Tomographic Myelography in the Recognition of Cervical Herniated Disk. *AJNR Am. J. Neuroradiol.* **1984**, *5*, 391–394.
9. Runge, V.M.; Richter, J.K.; Heverhagen, J.T. Speed in Clinical Magnetic Resonance. *Investig. Radiol.* **2017**, *52*, 1–17. [CrossRef]
10. Nölte, I.; Gerigk, L.; Brockmann, M.A.; Kemmling, A.; Groden, C. MRI of Degenerative Lumbar Spine Disease: Comparison of Non-Accelerated and Parallel Imaging. *Neuroradiology* **2008**, *50*, 403–409. [CrossRef]
11. Gao, T.; Lu, Z.; Wang, F.; Zhao, H.; Wang, J.; Pan, S. Using the Compressed Sensing Technique for Lumbar Vertebrae Imaging: Comparison with Conventional Parallel Imaging. *Curr. Med. Imaging Rev.* **2021**, *17*, 1010–1017. [CrossRef] [PubMed]
12. Hajiahmadi, S.; Shayganfar, A.; Askari, M.; Ebrahimian, S. Interobserver and Intraobserver Variability in Magnetic Resonance Imaging Evaluation of Patients with Suspected Disc Herniation. *Heliyon* **2020**, *6*, e05201. [CrossRef]
13. SITNFlash. The History of Artificial Intelligence. Science in the News. Available online: https://sitn.hms.harvard.edu/flash/2017/history-artificial-intelligence/ (accessed on 16 June 2024).
14. European Society of Radiology (ESR). What the Radiologist Should Know about Artificial Intelligence—An ESR White Paper. *Insights Imaging* **2019**, *10*, 44. [CrossRef] [PubMed]
15. Noguerol, M.; Paulano-Godino, T.; Martín-Valdivia, F.; Menias, M.T.; Luna, C.O. Strengths, Weaknesses, Opportunities, and Threats Analysis of Artificial Intelligence and Machine Learning Applications in Radiology. *J. Am. Coll. Radiol.* **2019**, *16 Pt B*, 1239–1247. [CrossRef]
16. Khan, S.A.; Hussain, S.; Yang, S. Contrast Enhancement of Low-Contrast Medical Images Using Modified Contrast Limited Adaptive Histogram Equalization. *J. Med. Imaging Health Inform.* **2020**, *10*, 1795–1803. [CrossRef]
17. Khan, S.A.; Khan, M.A.; Song, O.-Y.; Nazir, M. Medical Imaging Fusion Techniques: A Survey Benchmark Analysis, Open Challenges and Recommendations. *J. Med. Imaging Health Inform.* **2020**, *10*, 2523–2531. [CrossRef]
18. Nouman Noor, M.; Nazir, M.; Khan, S.A.; Song, O.-Y.; Ashraf, I. Efficient Gastrointestinal Disease Classification Using Pretrained Deep Convolutional Neural Network. *Electronics* **2023**, *12*, 1557. [CrossRef]
19. Zhu, Y.; Li, Y.; Wang, K.; Li, J.; Zhang, X.; Zhang, Y.; Li, J.; Wang, X. A Quantitative Evaluation of the Deep Learning Model of Segmentation and Measurement of Cervical Spine MRI in Healthy Adults. *J. Appl. Clin. Med. Phys.* **2024**, *25*, e14282. [CrossRef] [PubMed]
20. Xie, J.; Yang, Y.; Jiang, Z.; Zhang, K.; Zhang, X.; Lin, Y.; Shen, Y.; Jia, X.; Liu, H.; Yang, S.; et al. MRI Radiomics-Based Decision Support Tool for a Personalized Classification of Cervical Disc Degeneration: A Two-Center Study. *Front. Physiol.* **2023**, *14*, 1281506. [CrossRef] [PubMed]
21. Wang, Y.-N.; Liu, G.; Wang, L.; Chen, C.; Wang, Z.; Zhu, S.; Wan, W.-T.; Weng, Y.-Z.; Lu, W.W.; Li, Z.-Y.; et al. A Deep-Learning Model for Diagnosing Fresh Vertebral Fractures on Magnetic Resonance Images. *World Neurosurg.* **2024**, *183*, e818–e824. [CrossRef]
22. Awan, K.M.; Goncalves Filho, A.L.M.; Tabari, A.; Applewhite, B.P.; Lang, M.; Lo, W.-C.; Sellers, R.; Kollasch, P.; Clifford, B.; Nickel, D.; et al. Diagnostic Evaluation of Deep Learning Accelerated Lumbar Spine MRI. *Neuroradiol. J.* **2024**, *37*, 323–331. [CrossRef]

23. Lin, Y.; Chan, S.C.W.; Chung, H.Y.; Lee, K.H.; Cao, P. A Deep Neural Network for MRI Spinal Inflammation in Axial Spondyloarthritis. *Eur. Spine J.* 2024, *ahead of print*. [CrossRef]
24. Kowlagi, N.; Kemppainen, A.; Panfilov, E.; McSweeney, T.; Saarakkala, S.; Nevalainen, M.; Niinimäki, J.; Karppinen, J.; Tiulpin, A. Semiautomatic Assessment of Facet Tropism from Lumbar Spine MRI Using Deep Learning: A Northern Finland Birth Cohort Study. *Spine* **2024**, *49*, 630–639. [CrossRef] [PubMed]
25. Qu, Z.; Deng, B.; Sun, W.; Yang, R.; Feng, H. A Convolutional Neural Network for Automated Detection of Cervical Ossification of the Posterior Longitudinal Ligament Using Magnetic Resonance Imaging. *Clin. Spine Surg.* **2024**, *37*, E106–E112. [CrossRef]
26. Kim, D.K.; Lee, S.-Y.; Lee, J.; Huh, Y.J.; Lee, S.; Lee, S.; Jung, J.-Y.; Lee, H.-S.; Benkert, T.; Park, S.-H. Deep Learning-Based k-Space-to-Image Reconstruction and Super Resolution for Diffusion-Weighted Imaging in Whole-Spine MRI. *Magn. Reson. Imaging* **2024**, *105*, 82–91. [CrossRef] [PubMed]
27. Liu, G.; Wang, L.; You, S.-N.; Wang, Z.; Zhu, S.; Chen, C.; Ma, X.-L.; Yang, L.; Zhang, S.; Yang, Q. Automatic Detection and Classification of Modic Changes in MRI Images Using Deep Learning: Intelligent Assisted Diagnosis System. *Orthop. Surg.* **2024**, *16*, 196–206. [CrossRef] [PubMed]
28. Jo, S.W.; Khil, E.K.; Lee, K.Y.; Choi, I.; Yoon, Y.S.; Cha, J.G.; Lee, J.H.; Kim, H.; Lee, S.Y. Deep Learning System for Automated Detection of Posterior Ligamentous Complex Injury in Patients with Thoracolumbar Fracture on MRI. *Sci. Rep.* **2023**, *13*, 19017. [CrossRef] [PubMed]
29. Vitale, J.; Sconfienza, L.M.; Galbusera, F. Cross-Sectional Area and Fat Infiltration of the Lumbar Spine Muscles in Patients with Back Disorders: A Deep Learning-Based Big Data Analysis. *Eur. Spine J.* **2024**, *33*, 1–10. [CrossRef]
30. Chen, Y.; Qin, S.; Zhao, W.; Wang, Q.; Liu, K.; Xin, P.; Yuan, H.; Zhuang, H.; Lang, N. MRI Feature-Based Radiomics Models to Predict Treatment Outcome after Stereotactic Body Radiotherapy for Spinal Metastases. *Insights Imaging* **2023**, *14*, 169. [CrossRef]
31. Saravi, B.; Zink, A.; Ülkümen, S.; Couillard-Despres, S.; Wollborn, J.; Lang, G.; Hassel, F. Clinical and Radiomics Feature-Based Outcome Analysis in Lumbar Disc Herniation Surgery. *BMC Musculoskelet. Disord.* **2023**, *24*, 791. [CrossRef]
32. Haim, O.; Agur, A.; Gabay, S.; Azolai, L.; Shutan, I.; Chitayat, M.; Katirai, M.; Sadon, S.; Artzi, M.; Lidar, Z. Differentiating Spinal Pathologies by Deep Learning Approach. *Spine J.* **2024**, *24*, 297–303. [CrossRef] [PubMed]
33. Zhang, W.; Chen, Z.; Su, Z.; Wang, Z.; Hai, J.; Huang, C.; Wang, Y.; Yan, B.; Lu, H. Deep Learning-Based Detection and Classification of Lumbar Disc Herniation on Magnetic Resonance Images. *JOR Spine* **2023**, *6*, e1276. [CrossRef] [PubMed]
34. Tas, N.P.; Kaya, O.; Macin, G.; Tasci, B.; Dogan, S.; Tuncer, T. ASNET: A Novel AI Framework for Accurate Ankylosing Spondylitis Diagnosis from MRI. *Biomedicines* **2023**, *11*, 2441. [CrossRef]
35. Masse-Gignac, N.; Flórez-Jiménez, S.; Mac-Thiong, J.-M.; Duong, L. Attention-Gated U-Net Networks for Simultaneous Axial/Sagittal Planes Segmentation of Injured Spinal Cords. *J. Appl. Clin. Med. Phys.* **2023**, *24*, e14123. [CrossRef] [PubMed]
36. Yilizati-Yilihamu, E.E.; Yang, J.; Yang, Z.; Rong, F.; Feng, S. A Spine Segmentation Method Based on Scene Aware Fusion Network. *BMC Neurosci.* **2023**, *24*, 49. [CrossRef]
37. Wang, W.; Fan, Z.; Zhen, J. MRI Radiomics-Based Evaluation of Tuberculous and Brucella Spondylitis. *J. Int. Med. Res.* **2023**, *51*, 3000605231195156. [CrossRef]
38. Niemeyer, F.; Galbusera, F.; Tao, Y.; Phillips, F.M.; An, H.S.; Louie, P.K.; Samartzis, D.; Wilke, H.-J. Deep Phenotyping the Cervical Spine: Automatic Characterization of Cervical Degenerative Phenotypes Based on T2-Weighted MRI. *Eur. Spine J.* **2023**, *32*, 3846–3856. [CrossRef]
39. Cai, J.; Shen, C.; Yang, T.; Jiang, Y.; Ye, H.; Ruan, Y.; Zhu, X.; Liu, Z.; Liu, Q. MRI-Based Radiomics Assessment of the Imminent New Vertebral Fracture after Vertebral Augmentation. *Eur. Spine J.* **2023**, *32*, 3892–3905. [CrossRef]
40. Waldenberg, C.; Brisby, H.; Hebelka, H.; Lagerstrand, K.M. Associations between Vertebral Localized Contrast Changes and Adjacent Annular Fissures in Patients with Low Back Pain: A Radiomics Approach. *J. Clin. Med.* **2023**, *12*, 4891. [CrossRef]
41. Roberts, M.; Hinton, G.; Wells, A.J.; Van Der Veken, J.; Bajger, M.; Lee, G.; Liu, Y.; Chong, C.; Poonnoose, S.; Agzarian, M.; et al. Imaging Evaluation of a Proposed 3D Generative Model for MRI to CT Translation in the Lumbar Spine. *Spine J.* **2023**, *23*, 1602–1612. [CrossRef]
42. Tanenbaum, L.N.; Bash, S.C.; Zaharchuk, G.; Shankaranarayanan, A.; Chamberlain, R.; Wintermark, M.; Beaulieu, C.; Novick, M.; Wang, L. Deep Learning-Generated Synthetic MR Imaging STIR Spine Images Are Superior in Image Quality and Diagnostically Equivalent to Conventional STIR: A Multicenter, Multireader Trial. *AJNR Am. J. Neuroradiol.* **2023**, *44*, 987–993. [CrossRef] [PubMed]
43. Küçükçiloğlu, Y.; Şekeroğlu, B.; Adalı, T.; Şentürk, N. Prediction of Osteoporosis Using MRI and CT Scans with Unimodal and Multimodal Deep-Learning Models. *Diagn. Interv. Radiol.* **2024**, *30*, 9–20. [CrossRef]
44. Chiu, P.-F.; Chang, R.C.-H.; Lai, Y.-C.; Wu, K.-C.; Wang, K.-P.; Chiu, Y.-P.; Ji, H.-R.; Kao, C.-H.; Chiu, C.-D. Machine Learning Assisting the Prediction of Clinical Outcomes Following Nucleoplasty for Lumbar Degenerative Disc Disease. *Diagnostics* **2023**, *13*, 1863. [CrossRef]
45. Mohanty, R.; Allabun, S.; Solanki, S.S.; Pani, S.K.; Alqahtani, M.S.; Abbas, M.; Soufiene, B.O. NAMSTCD: A Novel Augmented Model for Spinal Cord Segmentation and Tumor Classification Using Deep Nets. *Diagnostics* **2023**, *13*, 1417. [CrossRef] [PubMed]
46. Liu, B.; Jin, Y.; Feng, S.; Yu, H.; Zhang, Y.; Li, Y. Benign vs Malignant Vertebral Compression Fractures with MRI: A Comparison between Automatic Deep Learning Network and Radiologist's Assessment. *Eur. Radiol.* **2023**, *33*, 5060–5068. [CrossRef] [PubMed]
47. Liawrungrueang, W.; Kim, P.; Kotheeranurak, V.; Jitpakdee, K.; Sarasombath, P. Automatic Detection, Classification, and Grading of Lumbar Intervertebral Disc Degeneration Using an Artificial Neural Network Model. *Diagnostics* **2023**, *13*, 663. [CrossRef]

48. Mukaihata, T.; Maki, S.; Eguchi, Y.; Geundong, K.; Shoda, J.; Yokota, H.; Orita, S.; Shiga, Y.; Inage, K.; Furuya, T.; et al. Differentiating Magnetic Resonance Images of Pyogenic Spondylitis and Spinal Modic Change Using a Convolutional Neural Network. *Spine* **2023**, *48*, 288–294. [CrossRef] [PubMed]
49. Zhuo, Z.; Zhang, J.; Duan, Y.; Qu, L.; Feng, C.; Huang, X.; Cheng, D.; Xu, X.; Sun, T.; Li, Z.; et al. Automated Classification of Intramedullary Spinal Cord Tumors and Inflammatory Demyelinating Lesions Using Deep Learning. *Radiol. Artif. Intell.* **2022**, *4*, e210292. [CrossRef] [PubMed]
50. Kashiwagi, N.; Sakai, M.; Tsukabe, A.; Yamashita, Y.; Fujiwara, M.; Yamagata, K.; Nakamoto, A.; Nakanishi, K.; Tomiyama, N. Ultrafast Cervical Spine MRI Protocol Using Deep Learning-Based Reconstruction: Diagnostic Equivalence to a Conventional Protocol. *Eur. J. Radiol.* **2022**, *156*, 110531. [CrossRef]
51. Chen, K.; Cao, J.; Zhang, X.; Wang, X.; Zhao, X.; Li, Q.; Chen, S.; Wang, P.; Liu, T.; Du, J.; et al. Differentiation between Spinal Multiple Myeloma and Metastases Originated from Lung Using Multi-View Attention-Guided Network. *Front. Oncol.* **2022**, *12*, 981769. [CrossRef]
52. Alanazi, A.H.; Cradock, A.; Rainford, L. Development of Lumbar Spine MRI Referrals Vetting Models Using Machine Learning and Deep Learning Algorithms: Comparison Models vs. Healthcare Professionals. *Radiography* **2022**, *28*, 674–683. [CrossRef] [PubMed]
53. Lim, D.S.W.; Makmur, A.; Zhu, L.; Zhang, W.; Cheng, A.J.L.; Sia, D.S.Y.; Eide, S.E.; Ong, H.Y.; Jagmohan, P.; Tan, W.C.; et al. Improved Productivity Using Deep Learning-Assisted Reporting for Lumbar Spine MRI. *Radiology* **2022**, *305*, 160–166. [CrossRef] [PubMed]
54. Hallinan, J.T.P.D.; Zhu, L.; Zhang, W.; Lim, D.S.W.; Baskar, S.; Low, X.Z.; Yeong, K.Y.; Teo, E.C.; Kumarakulasinghe, N.B.; Yap, Q.V.; et al. Deep Learning Model for Classifying Metastatic Epidural Spinal Cord Compression on MRI. *Front. Oncol.* **2022**, *12*, 849447. [CrossRef] [PubMed]
55. Suri, A.; Jones, B.C.; Ng, G.; Anabaraonye, N.; Beyrer, P.; Domi, A.; Choi, G.; Tang, S.; Terry, A.; Leichner, T.; et al. Vertebral Deformity Measurements at MRI, CT, and Radiography Using Deep Learning. *Radiol. Artif. Intell.* **2022**, *4*, e210015. [CrossRef]
56. Zhang, M.-Z.; Ou-Yang, H.-Q.; Liu, J.-F.; Jin, D.; Wang, C.-J.; Ni, M.; Liu, X.-G.; Lang, N.; Jiang, L.; Yuan, H.-S. Predicting Postoperative Recovery in Cervical Spondylotic Myelopathy: Construction and Interpretation of T2*-Weighted Radiomic-Based Extra Trees Models. *Eur. Radiol.* **2022**, *32*, 3565–3575. [CrossRef] [PubMed]
57. Hwang, E.-J.; Kim, S.; Jung, J.-Y. Fully Automated Segmentation of Lumbar Bone Marrow in Sagittal, High-Resolution T1-Weighted Magnetic Resonance Images Using 2D U-NET. Comput. *Biol. Med.* **2022**, *140*, 105105. [CrossRef] [PubMed]
58. Jujjavarapu, C.; Pejaver, V.; Cohen, T.A.; Mooney, S.D.; Heagerty, P.J.; Jarvik, J.G. A Comparison of Natural Language Processing Methods for the Classification of Lumbar Spine Imaging Findings Related to Lower Back Pain. *Acad. Radiol.* **2022**, *29* (Suppl. S3), S188–S200. [CrossRef]
59. Gotoh, M.; Nakaura, T.; Funama, Y.; Morita, K.; Sakabe, D.; Uetani, H.; Nagayama, Y.; Kidoh, M.; Hatemura, M.; Masuda, T.; et al. Virtual Magnetic Resonance Lumbar Spine Images Generated from Computed Tomography Images Using Conditional Generative Adversarial Networks. *Radiography* **2022**, *28*, 447–453. [CrossRef]
60. Goedmakers, C.M.W.; Lak, A.M.; Duey, A.H.; Senko, A.W.; Arnaout, O.; Groff, M.W.; Smith, T.R.; Vleggeert-Lankamp, C.L.A.; Zaidi, H.A.; Rana, A.; et al. Deep Learning for Adjacent Segment Disease at Preoperative MRI for Cervical Radiculopathy. *Radiology* **2021**, *301*, E446. [CrossRef]
61. Lemay, A.; Gros, C.; Zhuo, Z.; Zhang, J.; Duan, Y.; Cohen-Adad, J.; Liu, Y. Automatic Multiclass Intramedullary Spinal Cord Tumor Segmentation on MRI with Deep Learning. *NeuroImage Clin.* **2021**, *31*, 102766. [CrossRef]
62. Liu, J.; Wang, C.; Guo, W.; Zeng, P.; Liu, Y.; Lang, N.; Yuan, H. A Preliminary Study Using Spinal MRI-Based Radiomics to Predict High-Risk Cytogenetic Abnormalities in Multiple Myeloma. *Radiol. Med.* **2021**, *126*, 1226–1235. [CrossRef] [PubMed]
63. Merali, Z.; Wang, J.Z.; Badhiwala, J.H.; Witiw, C.D.; Wilson, J.R.; Fehlings, M.G. A Deep Learning Model for Detection of Cervical Spinal Cord Compression in MRI Scans. *Sci. Rep.* **2021**, *11*, 10473. [CrossRef] [PubMed]
64. Hallinan, J.T.P.D.; Zhu, L.; Yang, K.; Makmur, A.; Algazwi, D.A.R.; Thian, Y.L.; Lau, S.; Choo, Y.S.; Eide, S.E.; Yap, Q.V.; et al. Deep Learning Model for Automated Detection and Classification of Central Canal, Lateral Recess, and Neural Foraminal Stenosis at Lumbar Spine MRI. *Radiology* **2021**, *300*, 130–138. [CrossRef] [PubMed]
65. Maki, S.; Furuya, T.; Horikoshi, T.; Yokota, H.; Mori, Y.; Ota, J.; Kawasaki, Y.; Miyamoto, T.; Norimoto, M.; Okimatsu, S.; et al. A Deep Convolutional Neural Network with Performance Comparable to Radiologists for Differentiating between Spinal Schwannoma and Meningioma. *Spine* **2020**, *45*, 694–700. [CrossRef]
66. Gaonkar, B.; Beckett, J.; Villaroman, D.; Ahn, C.; Edwards, M.; Moran, S.; Attiah, M.; Babayan, D.; Ames, C.; Villablanca, J.P.; et al. Quantitative Analysis of Neural Foramina in the Lumbar Spine: An Imaging Informatics and Machine Learning Study. *Radiol. Artif. Intell.* **2019**, *1*, 180037. [CrossRef] [PubMed]
67. Kim, K.; Kim, S.; Lee, Y.H.; Lee, S.H.; Lee, H.S.; Kim, S. Performance of the Deep Convolutional Neural Network Based Magnetic Resonance Image Scoring Algorithm for Differentiating between Tuberculous and Pyogenic Spondylitis. *Sci. Rep.* **2018**, *8*, 13124. [CrossRef] [PubMed]
68. Jamaludin, A.; Kadir, T.; Zisserman, A. SpineNet: Automated Classification and Evidence Visualization in Spinal MRIs. *Med. Image Anal.* **2017**, *41*, 63–73. [CrossRef]
69. Pfirrmann, C.W.; Metzdorf, A.; Zanetti, M.; Hodler, J.; Boos, N. Magnetic Resonance Classification of Lumbar Intervertebral Disc Degeneration. *Spine* **2001**, *26*, 1873–1878. [CrossRef]

70. Kumar, N.; Tan, W.L.B.; Wei, W.; Vellayappan, B.A. An Overview of the Tumors Affecting the Spine-inside to Out. *Neuro-Oncol. Pract.* **2020**, *7* (Suppl. S1), i10–i17. [CrossRef]
71. Hallinan, J.T.P.D.; Zhu, L.; Zhang, W.; Kuah, T.; Lim, D.S.W.; Low, X.Z.; Cheng, A.J.L.; Eide, S.E.; Ong, H.Y.; Muhamat Nor, F.E.; et al. Deep Learning Model for Grading Metastatic Epidural Spinal Cord Compression on Staging CT. *Cancers* **2022**, *14*, 3219. [CrossRef]
72. Hallinan, J.T.P.D.; Zhu, L.; Zhang, W.; Ge, S.; Muhamat Nor, F.E.; Ong, H.Y.; Eide, S.E.; Cheng, A.J.L.; Kuah, T.; Lim, D.S.W.; et al. Deep Learning Assessment Compared to Radiologist Reporting for Metastatic Spinal Cord Compression on CT. *Front. Oncol.* **2023**, *13*, 1151073. [CrossRef] [PubMed]
73. Hallinan, J.T.P.D.; Zhu, L.; Tan, H.W.N.; Hui, S.J.; Lim, X.; Ong, B.W.L.; Ong, H.Y.; Eide, S.E.; Cheng, A.J.L.; Ge, S.; et al. A Deep Learning-Based Technique for the Diagnosis of Epidural Spinal Cord Compression on Thoracolumbar CT. *Eur. Spine J.* **2023**, *32*, 3815–3824. [CrossRef]
74. Kiryu, S.; Akai, H.; Yasaka, K.; Tajima, T.; Kunimatsu, A.; Yoshioka, N.; Akahane, M.; Abe, O.; Ohtomo, K. Clinical Impact of Deep Learning Reconstruction in MRI. *Radiographics* **2023**, *43*, e220133. [CrossRef]
75. Antun, V.; Renna, F.; Poon, C.; Adcock, B.; Hansen, A.C. On Instabilities of Deep Learning in Image Reconstruction and the Potential Costs of AI. *Proc. Natl. Acad. Sci. USA* **2020**, *117*, 30088–30095. [CrossRef] [PubMed]
76. Hsu, W.; Hoyt, A.C. Using Time as a Measure of Impact for AI Systems: Implications in Breast Screening. *Radiol. Artif. Intell.* **2019**, *1*, e190107. [CrossRef] [PubMed]
77. Avanzo, M.; Wei, L.; Stancanello, J.; Vallières, M.; Rao, A.; Morin, O.; Mattonen, S.A.; El Naqa, I. Machine and Deep Learning Methods for Radiomics. *Med. Phys.* **2020**, *47*, e185–e202. [CrossRef]
78. Willems, P.; de Bie, R.; Öner, C.; Castelein, R.; de Kleuver, M. Clinical Decision Making in Spinal Fusion for Chronic Low Back Pain. Results of a Nationwide Survey among Spine Surgeons. *BMJ Open* **2011**, *1*, e000391. [CrossRef]
79. Fairbank, J.; Frost, H.; Wilson-MacDonald, J.; Yu, L.-M.; Barker, K.; Collins, R.; Spine Stabilisation Trial Group. Randomised Controlled Trial to Compare Surgical Stabilisation of the Lumbar Spine with an Intensive Rehabilitation Programme for Patients with Chronic Low Back Pain: The MRC Spine Stabilisation Trial. *BMJ* **2005**, *330*, 1233. [CrossRef]
80. Azad, T.D.; Zhang, Y.; Weiss, H.; Alamin, T.; Cheng, I.; Huang, B.; Veeravagu, A.; Ratliff, J.; Malhotra, N.R. Fostering Reproducibility and Generalizability in Machine Learning for Clinical Prediction Modeling in Spine Surgery. *Spine J.* **2021**, *21*, 1610–1616. [CrossRef] [PubMed]
81. Eche, T.; Schwartz, L.H.; Mokrane, F.-Z.; Dercle, L. Toward Generalizability in the Deployment of Artificial Intelligence in Radiology: Role of Computation Stress Testing to Overcome Underspecification. *Radiol. Artif. Intell.* **2021**, *3*, e210097. [CrossRef]
82. Huisman, M.; Hannink, G. The AI Generalization Gap: One Size Does Not Fit All. *Radiol. Artif. Intell.* **2023**, *5*, e230246. [CrossRef] [PubMed]
83. Xu, W.; Jia, X.; Mei, Z.; Gu, X.; Lu, Y.; Fu, C.-C.; Zhang, R.; Gu, Y.; Chen, X.; Luo, X.; et al. Chinese Artificial Intelligence Alliance for Thyroid and Breast Ultrasound. Generalizability and Diagnostic Performance of AI Models for Thyroid US. *Radiology* **2023**, *307*, e221157. [CrossRef]
84. RSNA Lumbar Spine Degenerative Classification AI Challenge. 2024. Rsna.org. Available online: https://www.rsna.org/rsnai/ai-image-challenge/lumbar-spine-degenerative-classification-ai-challenge (accessed on 12 July 2024).
85. Kim, H.E.; Cosa-Linan, A.; Santhanam, N.; Jannesari, M.; Maros, M.E.; Ganslandt, T. Transfer Learning for Medical Image Classification: A Literature Review. *BMC Med. Imaging* **2022**, *22*, 69. [CrossRef]
86. Xuan, J.; Ke, B.; Ma, W.; Liang, Y.; Hu, W. Spinal Disease Diagnosis Assistant Based on MRI Images Using Deep Transfer Learning Methods. *Front. Public Health* **2023**, *11*, 1044525. [CrossRef] [PubMed]
87. Santomartino, S.M.; Putman, K.; Beheshtian, E.; Parekh, V.S.; Yi, P.H. Evaluating the Robustness of a Deep Learning Bone Age Algorithm to Clinical Image Variation Using Computational Stress Testing. *Radiol. Artif. Intell.* **2024**, *6*, e230240. [CrossRef] [PubMed]
88. Brady, A.P.; Allen, B.; Chong, J.; Kotter, E.; Kottler, N.; Mongan, J.; Oakden-Rayner, L.; Pinto Dos Santos, D.; Tang, A.; Wald, C.; et al. Developing, Purchasing, Implementing and Monitoring AI Tools in Radiology: Practical Considerations. A Multi-Society Statement from the ACR, CAR, ESR, RANZCR and RSNA. *J. Am. Coll. Radiol.* **2021**, *18*, 710–717. [CrossRef] [PubMed]
89. Kim, B.; Romeijn, S.; van Buchem, M.; Mehrizi, M.H.R.; Grootjans, W. A Holistic Approach to Implementing Artificial Intelligence in Radiology. *Insights Imaging* **2024**, *15*, 22. [CrossRef]
90. Suran, M.; Hswen, Y. How to Navigate the Pitfalls of AI Hype in Health Care. *JAMA* **2024**, *331*, 273–276. [CrossRef] [PubMed]
91. Geis, J.R.; Brady, A.; Wu, C.C.; Spencer, J.; Ranschaert, E.; Jaremko, J.L.; Langer, S.G.; Kitts, A.B.; Birch, J.; Shields, W.F.; et al. Ethics of Artificial Intelligence in Radiology: Summary of the Joint European and North American Multisociety Statement. *Insights Imaging* **2019**, *10*, 101. [CrossRef]
92. Jaremko, J.L.; Azar, M.; Bromwich, R.; Lum, A.; Alicia Cheong, L.H.; Gilbert, M.; Laviolette, F.; Gray, B.; Reinhold, C.; Cicero, M.; et al. Canadian Association of Radiologists White Paper on Ethical and Legal Issues Related to Artificial Intelligence in Radiology. *Can. Assoc. Radiol. J.* **2019**, *70*, 107–118. [CrossRef]
93. Plackett, B. The Rural Areas Missing out on AI Opportunities. *Nature* **2022**, *610*, S17. [CrossRef]
94. Celi, L.A.; Cellini, J.; Charpignon, M.-L.; Dee, E.C.; Dernoncourt, F.; Eber, R.; Mitchell, W.G.; Moukheiber, L.; Schirmer, J.; Situ, J.; et al. Sources of Bias in Artificial Intelligence That Perpetuate Healthcare Disparities-A Global Review. *PLoS Digit. Health* **2022**, *1*, e0000022. [CrossRef]

95. Eltawil, F.A.; Atalla, M.; Boulos, E.; Amirabadi, A.; Tyrrell, P.N. Analyzing Barriers and Enablers for the Acceptance of Artificial Intelligence Innovations into Radiology Practice: A Scoping Review. *Tomography* **2023**, *9*, 1443–1455. [CrossRef]
96. Borondy Kitts, A. Patient Perspectives on Artificial Intelligence in Radiology. *J. Am. Coll. Radiol.* **2023**, *20*, 243–250. [CrossRef]
97. Brima, Y.; Atemkeng, M. Saliency-Driven Explainable Deep Learning in Medical Imaging: Bridging Visual Explainability and Statistical Quantitative Analysis. *BioData Min.* **2024**, *17*, 18. [CrossRef] [PubMed]
98. Moor, M.; Banerjee, O.; Abad, Z.S.H.; Krumholz, H.M.; Leskovec, J.; Topol, E.J.; Rajpurkar, P. Foundation Models for Generalist Medical Artificial Intelligence. *Nature* **2023**, *616*, 259–265. [CrossRef] [PubMed]
99. Hafezi-Nejad, N.; Trivedi, P. Foundation AI Models and Data Extraction from Unlabeled Radiology Reports: Navigating Uncharted Territory. *Radiology* **2023**, *308*, e232308. [CrossRef] [PubMed]
100. Seah, J.; Tang, C.; Buchlak, Q.D.; Holt, X.G.; Wardman, J.B.; Aimoldin, A. Effect of a Comprehensive Deep-Learning Model on the Accuracy of Chest X-ray Interpretation by Radiologists: A Retrospective, Multireader Multicase Study. *Lancet Digit. Health* **2021**, *3*, e496–e506. [CrossRef]
101. van Beek, E.J.R.; Ahn, J.S.; Kim, M.J.; Murchison, J.T. Validation Study of Machine-Learning Chest Radiograph Software in Primary and Emergency Medicine. *Clin. Radiol.* **2023**, *78*, 1–7. [CrossRef]
102. Niehoff, J.H.; Kalaitzidis, J.; Kroeger, J.R.; Schoenbeck, D.; Borggrefe, J.; Michael, A.E. Evaluation of the Clinical Performance of an AI-Based Application for the Automated Analysis of Chest X-rays. *Sci. Rep.* **2023**, *13*, 3680. [CrossRef]
103. Hayashi, D. Deep Learning for Lumbar Spine MRI Reporting: A Welcome Tool for Radiologists. *Radiology* **2021**, *300*, 139–140. [CrossRef] [PubMed]
104. Gertz, R.J.; Bunck, A.C.; Lennartz, S. GPT-4 for Automated Determination of Radiological Study and Protocol Based on Radiology Request Forms: A Feasibility Study. *Radiology* **2023**, *307*, e230877. [CrossRef] [PubMed]
105. Beddiar, D.-R.; Oussalah, M.; Seppänen, T. Automatic Captioning for Medical Imaging (MIC): A Rapid Review of Literature. *Artif. Intell. Rev.* **2023**, *56*, 4019–4076. [CrossRef] [PubMed]
106. Sun, Z.; Ong, H.; Kennedy, P. Evaluating GPT4 on Impressions Generation in Radiology Reports. *Radiology* **2023**, *307*, e231259. [CrossRef]
107. Ayers, J.W.; Poliak, A.; Dredze, M. Comparing Physician and Artificial Intelligence Chatbot Responses to Patient Questions Posted to a Public Social Media Forum. *JAMA Intern. Med.* **2023**, *183*, 589–596. [CrossRef] [PubMed]
108. Kuckelman, I.J.; Yi, P.H.; Bui, M.; Onuh, I.; Anderson, J.A.; Ross, A.B. Assessing AI-Powered Patient Education: A Case Study in Radiology. *Acad. Radiol.* **2024**, *31*, 338–342. [CrossRef]
109. Wu, J.; Kim, Y.; Keller, E.C.; Chow, J.; Levine, A.P.; Pontikos, N.; Ibrahim, Z.; Taylor, P.; Williams, M.C.; Wu, H. Exploring Multimodal Large Language Models for Radiology Report Error-Checking. *arXiv* **2023**, arXiv:2312.13103.
110. Yu, F.; Moehring, A.; Banerjee, O.; Salz, T.; Agarwal, N.; Rajpurkar, P. Heterogeneity and Predictors of the Effects of AI Assistance on Radiologists. *Nat. Med.* **2024**, *30*, 837–849. [CrossRef]

bioengineering

MDPI

Article

Evaluation of Operator Variability and Validation of an AI-Assisted α-Angle Measurement System for DDH Using a Phantom Model

Yusuke Ohashi [1], Tomohiro Shimizu [1,*], Hidenori Koyano [2], Yumejiro Nakamura [1], Daisuke Takahashi [1], Katsuhisa Yamada [1] and Norimasa Iwasaki [1]

[1] Department of Orthopaedic Surgery, Faculty of Medicine and Graduate School of Medicine, Hokkaido University, Sapporo 060-8638, Japan; yuk1274go@gmail.com (Y.O.); nakamurayjiro33@gmail.com (Y.N.); rainbow-quest@pop02.odn.ne.jp (D.T.); yka2q@pop.med.hokudai.ac.jp (K.Y.); niwasaki@med.hokudai.ac.jp (N.I.)

[2] Department of Medical Physics, Graduate School of Medicine, Hokkaido University, Sapporo 060-8638, Japan; koyano@med.hokudai.ac.jp

* Correspondence: simitom@wg8.so-net.ne.jp; Tel.: +81-11-706-5936

Abstract

Ultrasound examination using the Graf method is widely applied for early detection of developmental dysplasia of the hip (DDH), but intra- and inter-operator variability remains a limitation. This study aimed to quantify operator variability in hip ultrasound assessments and to validate an AI-assisted system for automated α-angle measurement to improve reproducibility. Thirty participants of different experience levels, including trained clinicians, residents, and medical students, each performed six ultrasound scans on a standardized infant hip phantom. Examination time, iliac margin inclination, and α-angle measurements were analyzed to assess intra- and inter-operator variability. In parallel, an AI-based system was developed to automatically detect anatomical landmarks and calculate α-angles from static images and dynamic video sequences. Validation was conducted using the phantom model with a known α-angle of 70°. Clinicians achieved shorter examination times and higher reproducibility than residents and students, with manual measurements systematically underestimating the reference α-angle. Static AI produced closer estimates with greater variability, whereas dynamic AI achieved the highest accuracy (mean 69.2°) and consistency with narrower limits of agreement than manual measurements. These findings confirm substantial operator variability and demonstrate that AI-assisted dynamic ultrasound analysis can improve reproducibility and reliability in routine DDH screening.

Keywords: Developmental Dysplasia of the Hip (DDH); ultrasound imaging; Artificial Intelligence (AI); α-angle measurement; operator variability

1. Introduction

Although ultrasound examination using the Graf method is widely employed for the early detection of developmental dysplasia of the hip (DDH), concerns regarding the reliability of its measurements remain [1,2]. Both intra-operator variability—where repeated measurements by the same examiner yield inconsistent results—and inter-operator variability—differences between examiners—have been recognized as significant limitations. Contributing factors include probe angulation, applied pressure, transducer positioning, and subjective interpretation of anatomical landmarks [3–5]. Even experienced

 https://doi.org/10.3390/bioengineering12091004

examiners are susceptible to such variability, and prior studies have demonstrated that key diagnostic parameters, particularly the α- and β-angles, are highly sensitive to subtle deviations in technique [4,6]. Despite efforts to reduce these discrepancies through standardized training, a moderate degree of inconsistency persists, underscoring the inherent difficulty in achieving fully reliable and reproducible ultrasound-based assessments of the infant hip [3,7].

In response to these challenges, recent research has turned to artificial intelligence (AI) as a means to improve diagnostic consistency and reduce operator dependence in DDH ultrasound assessments [8]. Deep learning–based models have shown promising performance in automating critical components of the Graf classification, including landmark detection, standard plane identification, and α-angle measurement, with diagnostic accuracy comparable to that of expert clinicians [9–11]. These AI-assisted systems offer the potential to standardize assessments, improve reproducibility, and expand access to high-quality screening. Previous AI-assisted approaches for DDH ultrasound have primarily relied on static image analysis, often using manually selected frames to detect anatomical landmarks or estimate α-angles. While these studies demonstrated the feasibility of applying deep learning to DDH diagnosis, they did not capture operator-dependent variability or provide real-time diagnostic support. Our study builds on this body of work by introducing a dynamic, video-based AI system capable of frame-by-frame α-angle measurement during continuous scanning and validating its accuracy against a phantom with a known reference angle. This provides both real-time applicability and objective benchmarking that have been lacking in previous reports. However, before the benefits of such technologies can be accurately evaluated, it is essential to establish a quantitative understanding of the variability that exists among human examiners with different levels of training and experience.

To that end, we designed a two-part study to explore these issues. First, we conducted a phantom-based experiment (Study 1) to assess diagnostic accuracy and examination time among medical students, residents, and experienced physicians, thereby quantifying intra- and inter-operator variability under controlled conditions. Second (Study 2), we developed and validated an AI-based system capable of automatically selecting diagnostic-quality frames and calculating α-angles from both static ultrasound images and video sequences.

Previous studies have mainly addressed operator variability or AI-assisted systems in isolation, without integrating both perspectives within a unified framework. This has left two key gaps: (1) a limited quantitative understanding of how examiner experience affects measurement accuracy and reproducibility, and (2) insufficient validation of AI-assisted methods against objective reference standards under controlled conditions. Our two-part design was chosen specifically to address these gaps: Study 1 established a benchmark of human performance, and Study 2 directly evaluated an AI-assisted solution under the same conditions, enabling meaningful comparison between human and AI performance. In particular, the novelty of this work lies in extending α-angle measurement to dynamic video-based ultrasound and validating its accuracy against a phantom with a known reference angle.

2. Materials and Methods

2.1. Study 1

This study investigated the diagnostic accuracy and efficiency of Graf method ultrasound assessments across different levels of clinical experience using a standardized phantom model. Participants were divided into three groups: the trained group (T group), comprising seven individuals who had completed a specialized infant hip ultrasound seminar; the resident group (R group), consisting of seven orthopedic residents without formal ultrasound seminar training; and the student group (S group), composed of sixteen medical students without prior specialized ultrasound education.

All ultrasound examinations were performed using the same ultrasound device (Hitachi-Aloka, Mitaka, Japan) and a pediatric hip phantom model (Kyoto Kagaku Co., Ltd., Kyoto, Japan) simulating the anatomical structure of an infant hip (Figure 1). Participants conducted the examinations according to the Graf method, with the phantom positioned in the lateral decubitus position. Each participant was instructed to align the iliac outer margin vertically, identify key anatomical landmarks, and acquire an appropriate image for subsequent α-angle measurement. A total of four independent measurements were obtained per participant.

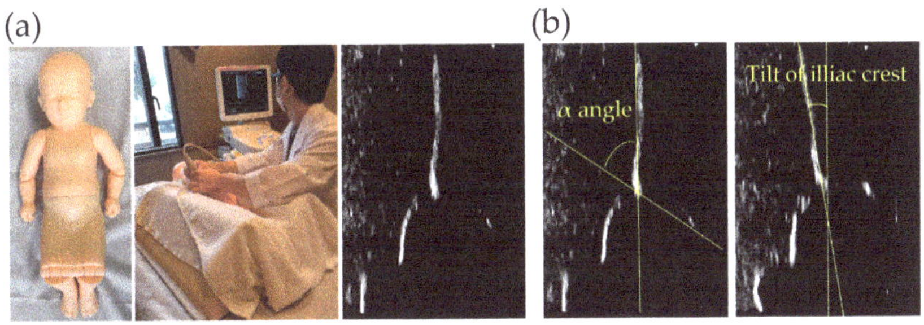

Figure 1. (**a**) Standardized infant hip phantom model (Kyoto Kagaku Co., Ltd., Kyoto, Japan) used for ultrasound examination and demonstration of the scanning procedure according to the Graf method. (**b**) Representative ultrasound images of the phantom hip. The α-angle is defined as the angle between the baseline along the iliac outer margin and a line extending to the bony acetabular rim. The tilt of the iliac crest relative to the vertical axis was also measured to evaluate probe positioning and image acquisition quality.

The evaluation focused on three key parameters: the time required to obtain a diagnostic-quality image, the inclination of the iliac outer margin relative to the vertical axis, and the measured α-angle. Examination time was recorded for each trial, and the iliac inclination angle was assessed to verify correct probe positioning. α-angles were measured from the acquired images according to the standard Graf technique [12].

This study was a phantom-based experiment designed to evaluate the effect of clinical experience on operator variability. The sample size was intentionally limited to representative participants from three experience levels within our institution (trained clinicians, residents, and medical students), which was considered sufficient to demonstrate experience-related trends rather than clinical outcomes. Participants were randomly selected from available rotating clinicians and medical students during the study period. No exclusion criteria were applied, and each participant performed five independent examinations per hip joint to allow intra-operator analysis.

2.2. *Study 2*

To address the operator-dependent variability identified in Study 1, we evaluated the performance of an automated α-angle measurement system using static ultrasound images acquired from the same standardized hip phantom. A different group of orthopedic residents, not involved in Study 1, performed four independent measurements each, following the Graf method under standardized conditions. Four static ultrasound images per participant were collected for analysis.

Manual measurements of the α-angle and iliac outer margin inclination were performed by the same physicians who acquired the ultrasound images, strictly following

Graf's method. The baseline was defined along the iliac outer margin, and a second line was extended to the bony acetabular rim. The α-angle was then calculated using the built-in angle measurement tool of the ultrasound system. Each participant repeated the measurements independently, and duplicate trials per hip joint were used to assess intra-operator consistency.

2.2.1. Static-Image-Based Diagnostic Algorithm for DDH

Subsequently, the same static ultrasound images were analyzed using an automated algorithm developed in accordance with a previously published method [13]. The images were first preprocessed to enhance quality and suppress noise, followed by automatic detection of key anatomical landmarks, including the bony acetabular rim using a convolutional neural network [14] (Figure 2a). After landmark detection, the system segmented relevant bone and cartilage regions and applied line fitting based on the Hough transform to construct a baseline along the iliac outer margin (Figure 2b). The α-angle was then calculated as the angle between this baseline and a line extending to the tip of the labrum (Figure 2c).

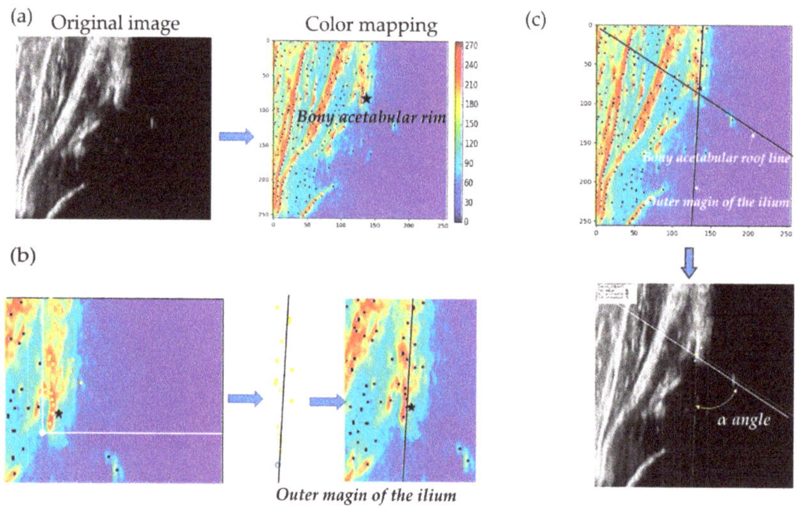

Figure 2. Schematic illustration of the AI-assisted α-angle measurement system. (**a**) Original ultrasound image of the hip joint and corresponding color-mapped image highlighting structural features, with the bony acetabular rim indicated. (**b**) Automatic extraction of anatomical landmarks: detection of the outer margin of the ilium and localization of the bony acetabular rim. (**c**) Determination of the baseline along the iliac outer margin and the bony acetabular roof line, followed by automated calculation of the α-angle on the reconstructed ultrasound image.

All automated measurements were generated without human intervention. For validation, manual measurements were obtained independently by the same physicians who acquired the ultrasound images, strictly following Graf's method. Both manual and automated measurements were performed in a blinded manner, and agreement and consistency between the two approaches were subsequently evaluated.

2.2.2. Dynamic-Image-Based Diagnostic Algorithm for DDH

To extend the capabilities of static image analysis to real-time ultrasound video sequences, we developed a novel diagnostic system capable of automatically extracting diagnostic-quality frames and calculating key angular measurements during continuous scanning. This system was built upon an enhanced image-processing pipeline based on our previous work [13], with critical modifications for real-time application.

First, a deep learning model based on YOLO v3 was employed to perform bounding box inference on each frame [15]. The model simultaneously detected key anatomical features, specifically the bony acetabular rim (osseous acetabular beak) and the lower limb of the ilium. By using bounding box predictions instead of traditional point detection methods, the computational burden was significantly reduced, enabling near real-time analysis (Figure 3a). Subsequent processing steps included: (1) extraction of local maxima from grayscale ultrasound images to identify high-intensity bone surfaces; (2) application of intensity-based filtering to eliminate minor peaks and improve landmark reliability; (3) linear approximation using screened local maxima to construct the iliac outer wall line; and (4) establishment of a baseline parallel to the iliac outer margin that passes through the detected acetabular rim (Figure 3b).

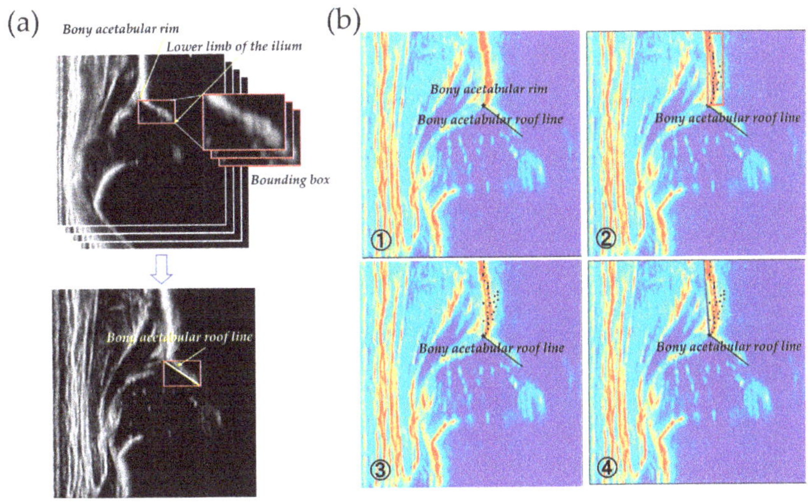

Figure 3. AI-assisted α angle measurement process. (**a**) A deep learning model based on YOLO v3 was employed to perform bounding box inference on each frame, simultaneously detecting key anatomical features including the bony acetabular rim (osseous acetabular beak) and the lower limb of the ilium. (**b**) Subsequent image processing steps: (**1**) extraction of local maxima from grayscale ultrasound images to identify high-intensity bone surfaces; (**2**) screening of local maxima through intensity-based filtering to remove minor peaks and improve landmark reliability; (**3**) linear approximation using screened local maxima to construct the iliac outer wall line; and (**4**) establishment of a baseline parallel to the iliac outer margin passing through the detected acetabular rim.

The α-angle was calculated in each extracted diagnostic-quality frame by measuring the angle between the constructed baseline and the identified acetabular rim line. This bounding box–based approach, combined with optimized peak screening, reduced processing time by approximately 100 to 200 milliseconds per frame compared to previous methods. These enhancements allowed for near real-time guidance during ultrasound examinations, assisting operators in identifying appropriate frames for diagnosis and enabling continuous automated assessment of hip morphology. All calculations were performed automatically without human intervention, and the results were compared with manual measurements under blinded conditions to ensure consistency.

2.3. Statistical Analysis

Statistical analyses were performed using JMP Pro version 17.0 (SAS Institute, Cary, NC, USA). For Study 1, group differences were assessed by one-way ANOVA. In addition to p-values, the observed effect size (η^2 and Cohen's f) and post hoc statistical power were calculated to evaluate the adequacy of the sample size. For reliability analyses, intra- and inter-operator consistency was assessed using intraclass correlation coefficients (ICCs), and 95% confidence intervals were reported together with point estimates. For Study 2, agreement with the phantom reference (70°) was evaluated by comparing mean α-angle values and the variability of measurements across methods, with bias and variability reported as the most relevant metrics. A p-value < 0.05 was considered statistically significant.

3. Results

3.1. Study 1

Manual Ultrasound Measurements Across Different Experience Levels in Study 1, 30 participants (7 trained clinicians, 7 residents, and 16 medical students) each performed six independent ultrasound measurements on a standardized phantom model with a known reference α-angle of 70°. The mean examination time was significantly shorter in the trained group compared to the resident and student groups (T group: 5.1 ± 2.3 s; R group: 11.4 ± 5.5 s; S group: 21.6 ± 15.0 s; $p < 0.001$), with a large effect size ($\eta^2 = 0.291$; Cohen's f = 0.64) and adequate post hoc power (0.85). The inclination of the iliac outer margin relative to the vertical axis was closest in the trained group, with greater deviations observed in the resident and student groups ($p < 0.01$). Intra-operator variability, assessed by intraclass correlation coefficients (ICCs), was highest in the trained group (ICC = 0.92 (95% CI: 0.89–0.95)), followed by the resident group (ICC = 0.85 (95% CI: 0.79–0.91)) and the student group (ICC = 0.78 (95% CI: 0.69–0.87)). Inter-operator reproducibility followed a similar trend (T group ICC = 0.89 (95% CI: 0.83–0.95); R group ICC = 0.81 (95% CI: 0.74–0.87); S group ICC = 0.74 (95% CI: 0.69–0.79)).

3.2. Study 2: Comparison of Manual and Automated α-Angle Measurements

3.2.1. Manual Measurements

The mean α-angle measured manually was 64.0° (SD = 4.7°), substantially underestimating the reference value of 70°. Bland–Altman analysis indicated a mean bias of −6.0°, with 95% limits of agreement ranging from −15.2° to +3.2°, confirming systematic underestimation by manual measurement.

3.2.2. Static-Image-Based Automated Measurements

The static-image-based diagnostic algorithm yielded a mean α-angle of 69.3° (SD = 10.4°). Although the mean value closely approximated the reference, Bland–Altman analysis against the phantom reference (70°) showed a small mean bias of −0.7°, but with wide 95% limits of agreement (−21.1° to +19.7°), indicating considerable variability despite acceptable mean accuracy. Error distribution plots confirmed the wide dispersion of static-image measurements around the reference, reflecting limited reproducibility.

3.2.3. Dynamic-Image-Based Automated Measurements

The dynamic-image-based diagnostic system analyzed continuous ultrasound video sequences. The mean α-angle measured from automatically extracted diagnostic-quality frames was 69.2° (SD = 2.4°), demonstrating both high accuracy and low variability. Bland–Altman analysis against the phantom reference (70°) showed a mean bias of −0.8°, with narrow 95% limits of agreement (−5.5° to +3.9°), indicating excellent agreement and reproducibility. Compared to static-image analysis, the dynamic system achieved greater consistency and precision. The diagnostic success rate was 100% (40/40 frames correctly assessed), with a mean absolute error of 0.8° relative to the reference value. The processing time per frame was reduced by approximately 100–200 milliseconds, enabling near real-time assessment. Error distribution plots confirmed that dynamic AI measurements were tightly clustered around the true value with minimal variance, whereas manual measurements systematically underestimated and static-AI assessments exhibited wide variability (Figure 4).

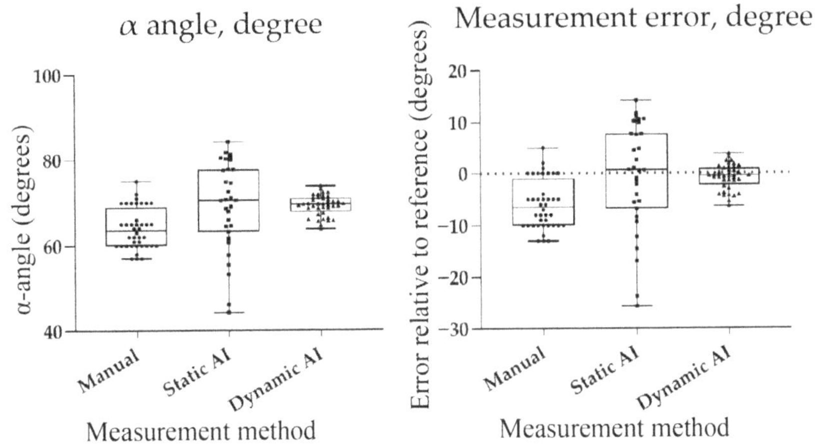

Figure 4. Comparison of manual, static AI, and dynamic AI measurements of the α-angle using a phantom model. (**Left**): Distribution of α-angle measurements. The dashed horizontal line indicates the true reference value (70°). Manual measurements underestimated the reference, static AI approximated the reference but with large variability, and dynamic AI clustered tightly around the true value. (**Right**): Distribution of measurement errors relative to the reference value (70°). Dynamic AI demonstrated the lowest median error and smallest variability, highlighting its superior accuracy and reproducibility compared with manual and static AI.

4. Discussion

Early and accurate diagnosis of DDH is critical for preventing long-term sequelae and reducing the need for invasive interventions [16]. Although ultrasound examination using the Graf method has become the standard for infant hip screening 16, its reliability remains significantly influenced by examiner technique. Recent systematic reviews and studies have emphasized persistent intra- and inter-operator variability in α- and β-angle measurements, even among trained practitioners [17–19]. Minor deviations in probe angulation, pressure, and landmark identification can significantly impact diagnostic outcomes, highlighting the inherent difficulty of achieving fully reproducible manual assessments.

Our first study confirmed that operator variability persists across different levels of clinical experience. Trained clinicians demonstrated significantly shorter examination times, better iliac margin alignment, and more consistent α-angle measurements compared to residents and medical students. These findings align with previous reports showing that even novice operators can achieve high reproducibility after brief, structured training programs, typically consisting of 1.5–2 h of instruction and supervised practice [3,7,20]. Intraclass correlation coefficients exceeding 0.9 have been reported after such interventions [3,7]. However, our results also suggest that a major source of measurement variability may lie not only in the angle measurement itself, but in the ability to acquire an appropriate standard plane for evaluation. Since α-angle accuracy is inherently dependent on the quality of the acquired image, especially the alignment of the iliac margin and identification of key landmarks, acquiring the correct standard plane appears to be a particularly critical and experience-sensitive skill. Supporting operators in obtaining such images may therefore be essential to improving reproducibility in DDH screening.

To address these limitations, several strategies have been proposed. Immediate feedback during scanning, continuous quality assurance programs, and refresher training are essential to sustain diagnostic accuracy and minimize technical drift over time. Common error sources, such as misalignment of the iliac margin and incorrect landmark identification, continue to affect measurement reliability, particularly among less experienced operators. Adjunctive technologies, including computer-aided diagnosis (CAD) systems and three-dimensional (3D) ultrasound, have shown promise in further reducing operator-dependent variability [4,21]. These tools can provide real-time feedback, enhance standardization, and support novice examiners in acquiring diagnostic-quality images.

Building on these observations, we evaluated an AI-assisted system for automated α-angle measurement using static ultrasound images and dynamic video sequences. The system showed high accuracy: static-image results closely matched the reference, and dynamic analysis achieved even greater consistency with narrower Bland–Altman limits of agreement. These findings support the utility of AI in DDH screening, where prior studies have reported classification accuracies of 90–98% and mean absolute errors of 1.7–2.5°. Compared to earlier methods such as that by Chen et al. [22], our system focuses specifically on α-angle measurement—central to early DDH diagnosis—and enables real-time processing by combining bounding box inference with local peak detection. Phantom-based validation with a known reference angle allowed for the objective assessment of measurement error, independent of clinical variability. A principal strength of this study is the novelty of applying a dynamic, video-based AI system for α-angle measurement, moving beyond previously reported static-image approaches. This real-time capability is particularly relevant to clinical practice, as continuous frame analysis can support consistent identification of diagnostic-quality planes. Moreover, validation against a phantom with a known reference angle provides a robust and objective benchmark, reinforcing the reliability of both human and AI performance. Although clinical validation is still needed, these results suggest that AI tools may improve reproducibility and standardization in ultrasound-based DDH screening.

Several limitations of this study should be acknowledged. First, the validation of the AI-assisted system was conducted using a phantom model rather than clinical ultrasound images. Although the use of a phantom with a known reference α-angle enabled objective quantification of measurement error, the performance of the system in real-world clinical settings remains to be evaluated. Clinical images typically present greater variability due to patient movement, anatomical diversity, and differences in operator technique, which could affect the system's accuracy and robustness. Second, the number of participants involved in the manual ultrasound assessments was relatively limited. While significant differences were observed between groups with different levels of experience, larger sample sizes across diverse institutions would be necessary to generalize the findings regarding operator-dependent variability. Third, the AI algorithm focused exclusively on α-angle measurement without incorporating β-angle evaluation. Although α-angle is the primary determinant for early DDH classification, comprehensive assessment following Graf's original methodology also considers β-angle measurements, which may contribute additional diagnostic information in certain cases. Finally, this study did not directly assess the system's usability or integration within real-time clinical workflows. Future work should include prospective clinical trials to evaluate not only diagnostic accuracy but also the practical impact on workflow efficiency, examiner confidence, and training effectiveness when AI-assisted tools are deployed in routine DDH screening programs. Future work should therefore include prospective clinical trials to evaluate not only diagnostic accuracy but also the practical impact on workflow efficiency, examiner confidence, and training effectiveness when AI-assisted tools are deployed in routine DDH screening programs, as well as investigations of system performance under real-world conditions of patient motion, anatomical variability, and variable image quality. Moreover, extending the algorithm to incorporate β-angle analysis and optimizing it for seamless integration into daily practice will be important next steps to maximize clinical applicability.

5. Conclusions

This study confirmed that substantial operator variability persists in infant hip ultrasound despite structured training, with trained clinicians achieving shorter examination times and more reproducible measurements than residents and medical students. Using a phantom model with a known reference α-angle, we demonstrated that manual measurements systematically underestimated the true value, static AI achieved closer estimates with higher variability, and dynamic AI provided the highest accuracy and consistency with near real-time performance. Compared to previous frameworks, our system therefore offers improved reproducibility and real-time diagnostic support, focusing on the most clinically critical parameter. In practical terms, these findings suggest that integrating AI-assisted α-angle measurement into routine DDH screening could reduce operator dependence, improve diagnostic reproducibility, and support the training of less experienced examiners. Future clinical validation will be essential to establish its broader applicability for standardized DDH screening.

6. Patents

A Japanese patent application related to the methodology described in this manuscript has been filed by the authors.

Author Contributions: Conceptualization, T.S. and H.K.; methodology, Y.O. and Y.N.; software, H.K.; validation, K.Y. and D.T.; formal analysis, Y.O.; investigation, Y.O.; resources, Y.O.; data curation, T.S.; writing—original draft preparation, Y.O.; writing—review and editing, T.S.; visualization, T.S.; supervision, N.I.; project administration, T.S.; funding acquisition, T.S. All authors have read and agreed to the published version of the manuscript.

Funding: This research was funded by AMED under Grant number 25ym0126801.

Institutional Review Board Statement: The study was conducted in accordance with the Declaration of Helsinki, and approved by the Institutional Review Board of the Hokkaido University Hospital (019-0292).

Informed Consent Statement: Informed consent was obtained from all subjects involved in the study.

Data Availability Statement: The data presented in this study are available on request from the corresponding author.

Acknowledgments: During the preparation of this manuscript, the authors used ChatGPT (GPT-5, OpenAI) for the purpose of English language minor editing. The authors have reviewed and edited the output and take full responsibility for the content of this publication.

Conflicts of Interest: The authors declare no conflict of interest.

Abbreviations

The following abbreviations are used in this manuscript:

DDH	Developmental Dysplasia of the Hip
AI	Artificial Intelligence

ICC	Intraclass Correlation Coefficient
YOLO	You Only Look Once (deep learning model)
3D	Three-Dimensional
CAD	Computer-Aided Diagnosis

References

1. Kolb, A.; Benca, E.; Willegger, M.; Puchner, S.E.; Windhager, R.; Chiari, C. Measurement considerations on examiner-dependent factors in the ultrasound assessment of developmental dysplasia of the hip. *Int. Orthop.* **2017**, *41*, 1245–1250. [CrossRef]
2. Heisinger, S.; Chiari, C.; Willegger, M.; Windhager, R.; Kolb, A. Clinical Evaluation of an Electronic Guidance System for Optimizing the Ultrasound Screening for Developmental Hip Dysplasia in Newborns. *J. Clin. Med.* **2024**, *13*, 7656. [CrossRef] [PubMed]
3. Shirai, Y.; Wakabayashi, K.; Wada, I.; Goto, H.; Ueki, Y.; Tsuchiya, A.; Tsuboi, Y.; Ha, M.; Otsuka, T. Reproducibility of acquiring ultrasonographic infant hip images by the Graf method after an infant hip ultrasound training course. *J. Med. Ultrason.* **2018**, *45*, 583–589. [CrossRef]
4. Hu, X.; Wang, L.; Yang, X.; Zhou, X.; Xue, W.; Cao, Y.; Liu, S.; Huang, Y.; Guo, S.; Shang, N.; et al. Joint Landmark and Structure Learning for Automatic Evaluation of Developmental Dysplasia of the Hip. *IEEE J. Biomed. Health Inform.* **2022**, *26*, 345–358. [CrossRef] [PubMed]
5. Liu, R.; Liu, M.; Sheng, B.; Li, H.; Li, P.; Song, H.; Zhang, P.; Jiang, L.; Shen, D. NHBS-Net: A Feature Fusion Attention Network for Ultrasound Neonatal Hip Bone Segmentation. *IEEE Trans. Med. Imaging* **2021**, *40*, 3446–3458. [CrossRef]
6. Hareendranathan, A.R.; Mabee, M.; Punithakumar, K.; Noga, M.; Jaremko, J.L. Toward automated classification of acetabular shape in ultrasound for diagnosis of DDH: Contour alpha angle and the rounding index. *Comput. Methods Programs Biomed.* **2016**, *129*, 89–98. [CrossRef]
7. Jejurikar, N.; Moscona-Mishy, L.; Rubio, M.; Cavallaro, R.; Castañeda, P. What is the Interobserver Reliability of an Ultrasound-enhanced Physical Examination of the Hip in Infants? A Prospective Study on the Ease of Acquiring Skills to Diagnose Hip Dysplasia. *Clin. Orthop. Relat. Res.* **2021**, *479*, 1889–1896. [CrossRef]
8. Shen, Y.-T.; Chen, L.; Yue, W.-W.; Xu, H.-X. Artificial intelligence in ultrasound. *Eur. J. Radiol.* **2021**, *139*, 109717. [CrossRef]
9. Lee, S.-W.; Ye, H.-U.; Lee, K.-J.; Jang, W.-Y.; Lee, J.-H.; Hwang, S.-M.; Heo, Y.-R. Accuracy of New Deep Learning Model-Based Segmentation and Key-Point Multi-Detection Method for Ultrasonographic Developmental Dysplasia of the Hip (DDH) Screening. *Diagnostics* **2021**, *11*, 1174. [CrossRef]
10. Den, H.; Ito, J.; Kokaze, A. Diagnostic accuracy of a deep learning model using YOLOv5 for detecting developmental dysplasia of the hip on radiography images. *Sci. Rep.* **2023**, *13*, 6693. [CrossRef] [PubMed]
11. Kinugasa, M.; Inui, A.; Satsuma, S.; Kobayashi, D.; Sakata, R.; Morishita, M.; Komoto, I.; Kuroda, R. Diagnosis of Developmental Dysplasia of the Hip by Ultrasound Imaging Using Deep Learning. *J. Pediatr. Orthop.* **2023**, *43*, e538–e544. [CrossRef] [PubMed]
12. Graf, R. Fundamentals of sonographic diagnosis of infant hip dysplasia. *J. Pediatr. Orthop.* **1984**, *4*, 735–740. [CrossRef]
13. Shimizu, H.; Enda, K.; Koyano, H.; Ogawa, T.; Takahashi, D.; Tanaka, S.; Iwasaki, N.; Shimizu, T. Diagnosis on Ultrasound Images for Developmental Dysplasia of the Hip with a Deep Learning-Based Model Focusing on Signal Heterogeneity in the Bone Region. *Diagnostics* **2025**, *15*, 403. [CrossRef] [PubMed]
14. Desai, N.; Bala, P.; Richardson, R.; Raper, J.; Zimmermann, J.; Hayden, B. OpenApePose, a database of annotated ape photographs for pose estimation. *eLife* **2023**, *12*, RP86873. [CrossRef] [PubMed]
15. Zhang, X.; Yang, W.; Tang, X.; Liu, J. A Fast Learning Method for Accurate and Robust Lane Detection Using Two-Stage Feature Extraction with YOLO v3. *Sensors* **2018**, *18*, 4308. [CrossRef]
16. O'bEirne, J.G.; Chlapoutakis, K.; Alshryda, S.; Aydingoz, U.; Baumann, T.; Casini, C.; de Pellegrin, M.; Domos, G.; Dubs, B.; Hemmadi, S.; et al. International Interdisciplinary Consensus Meeting on the Evaluation of Developmental Dysplasia of the Hip. *Ultraschall Der Med.* **2019**, *40*, 454–464. [CrossRef]
17. Quader, N.; Schaeffer, E.K.; Hodgson, A.J.; Abugharbieh, R.; Mulpuri, K. A Systematic Review and Meta-analysis on the Reproducibility of Ultrasound-based Metrics for Assessing Developmental Dysplasia of the Hip. *J. Pediatr. Orthop.* **2018**, *38*, e305–e311. [CrossRef]
18. Chavoshi, M.; Mirshahvalad, S.A.; Mahdizadeh, M.; Zamani, F. Diagnostic Accuracy of Ultrasonography Method of Graf in the detection of Developmental Dysplasia of the Hip: A Meta-Analysis and Systematic Review. *Arch. Bone Jt. Surg.* **2021**, *9*, 297–305. [CrossRef]
19. Chen, M.; Cai, R.; Zhang, A.; Chi, X.; Qian, J. The diagnostic value of artificial intelligence-assisted imaging for developmental dysplasia of the hip: A systematic review and meta-analysis. *J. Orthop. Surg. Res.* **2024**, *19*, 522. [CrossRef]
20. Ulziibat, M.; Munkhuu, B.; Schmid, R.; Wyder, C.; Baumann, T.; Essig, S.; Wojcik, M. Comparison of quality and interpretation of newborn ultrasound screening examinations for developmental dysplasia of the hip by basically trained nurses and junior physicians with no previous ultrasound experience. *PLoS ONE* **2024**, *19*, e0300753. [CrossRef]

21. Mostofi, E.; Chahal, B.; Zonoobi, D.; Hareendranathan, A.; Roshandeh, K.P.; Dulai, S.K.; Jaremko, J.L. Reliability of 2D and 3D ultrasound for infant hip dysplasia in the hands of novice users. *Eur. Radiol.* **2019**, *29*, 1489–1495. [CrossRef] [PubMed]
22. Chen, T.; Zhang, Y.; Wang, B.; Wang, J.; Cui, L.; He, J.; Cong, L. Development of a Fully Automated Graf Standard Plane and Angle Evaluation Method for Infant Hip Ultrasound Scans. *Diagnostics* **2022**, *12*, 1423. [CrossRef] [PubMed]

bioengineering

MDPI

Article

Automated Risser Grade Assessment of Pelvic Bones Using Deep Learning

Jeoung Kun Kim [1], Donghwi Park [2] and Min Cheol Chang [3,*]

[1] Department of Business Administration, School of Business, Yeungnam University, Gyeongsan-si 38541, Republic of Korea; kimjk70@yu.ac.kr

[2] Seoul Spine Rehabilitation Clinic, Ulsan-si 44607, Republic of Korea; bdome@hanmail.net

[3] Department of Rehabilitation Medicine, College of Medicine, Yeungnam University, Daegu 42415, Republic of Korea

* Correspondence: wheel633@gmail.com

Abstract

(1) Background: This study aimed to develop a deep learning model using a convolutional neural network (CNN) to automate Risser grade assessment from pelvic radiographs. (2) Methods: We used 1619 pelvic radiographs from patients aged 12–18 years with scoliosis to train two CNN models—one for the right pelvis and one for the left. A multimodal approach incorporated 224 × 224-pixel regions of interest from radiographs, alongside patient age and gender. The models were optimized with Adam, weight decay, rectified linear unit (ReLU) activation, dropout, and batch normalization, while synthetic data augmentation addressed class imbalance. Performance was evaluated through accuracy, precision, recall, F1-score, and area under the receiver operating characteristic curve (ROC AUC). (3) Results: The right pelvis model achieved 83.64% accuracy; the left pelvis model reached 80.56%. Both models performed well for Risser Grades 0, 2, and 4, with the right pelvis model achieving a microaverage F1-score of 0.836 and ROC AUC of 0.895. The left pelvis model achieved a microaverage F1-score of 0.806 and ROC AUC of 0.872. Challenges arose from class imbalance in less frequent grades. (4) Conclusions: CNN models effectively automated Risser grade assessment, reducing clinician workload and variability.

Keywords: Risser grade; pelvic bone; bone age; radiograph; deep learning; artificial intelligence

1. Introduction

Bone age assessment (BAA) is a clinical approach that evaluates skeletal development stages in children [1–3]. BAA for boys and girls relies on findings from hand and elbow radiographs up to ages 15 and 13, respectively [1–3]. Beyond these ages, bone age is measured using ossification and fusion levels of iliac crest apophyses, following the Risser grading system, which includes the following stages [4,5]: Grade 0 indicates no ossification center at the level of an iliac crest apophysis; Grade 1 represents an apophysis under 25% of the iliac crest; Grade 2 corresponds to an apophysis over 25–50% of the iliac crest; Grade 3 indicates an apophysis over 50–75% of the iliac crest; Grade 4 reflects an apophysis over 75% of the iliac crest; and Grade 5 means complete ossification and fusion of the iliac crest apophysis. This classification provides a standardized method for assessing skeletal maturity in adolescents.

BAA with the Risser grading system presents several challenges that limit its efficiency and consistency in clinical practice [6]. The process is inherently time-consuming,

 https://doi.org/10.3390/bioengineering12060589

necessitating detailed visual inspection and manual grading by trained radiologists or pediatricians. Additionally, BAA has low inter- (0.46) and intra-observer variability (0.49), meaning that different practitioners—or even the same practitioner at different times—may arrive at varying conclusions based on the same radiographic images [6]. Such subjectivity introduces uncertainty in clinical decisions, particularly when treatment plans hinge on precise skeletal maturity assessment.

Recent advancements in deep learning technology have revolutionized medical image analysis [7–9]. In particular, convolutional neural networks (CNNs) have shown significant promise in enabling automated diagnoses through complex pattern recognition in medical imaging [10–12]. Recent advancements in CNNs have significantly improved image tasks and focus on enhancing model performance by combining features from different layers or modalities, including transformer-based models, efficient architecture, multiscale feature fusion, and early and late fusion [10–12].

CNN models are extensively utilized in various medical applications. For instance, SpineNet employs intervertebral disk volumes as input and is trained with disk-specific class labels to automatically interpret the radiological grades from lumbar spine magnetic resonance images [13]. Furthermore, a multimodal CNN-based regression model has been developed to automatically perform BAA by learning from hand X-ray images in conjunction with patient age and gender. The developed model demonstrates robust overall performance in BAA. Specifically, it achieves an overall mean absolute error of 0.410 years, a root mean square error of 0.637 years, and an accuracy of 91.1% [3].

Recent CNN models, such as ConvNeXt, offer significant advantages for vision tasks by automatically learning hierarchical features and leveraging inherent spatial inductive biases. They contradict traditional ML models, such as support vector machine and random forest, which necessitate manual feature engineering and often lose spatial context. When compared to transformer models, the ConvNeXt CNN model retains crucial vision-specific inductive biases that can lead to good sample efficiency, while its architectural design promotes computational efficiency, providing a strong performance-to-resource ratio through optimized convolutional operations.

Feature fusion in a CNN enhances performance by aggregating information from diverse sources, such as multimodal data or different network layers [14–16]. This allows for a more comprehensive representation of input data, capturing both fine-grained details and the global context, leading to improved performance in various tasks [14–16]. We hypothesize that a CNN-based deep learning model can achieve comparable or superior accuracy in Risser grade assessment compared to traditional expert-based evaluation while significantly reducing assessment time and observer variability. Therefore, this study developed a deep learning algorithm using CNN to automatically determine Risser grades of pelvic bones and evaluated its efficacy.

2. Materials and Methods

2.1. Subjects

This study was approved by the Institutional Review Board of Yeungnam University Hospital (2024-06-005). The requirement for informed consent was waived by the institutional review board of Yeungnam University Hospital owing to the retrospective nature of the study. The data were accessed from 14 June 2024 to 31 December 2024. The authors had access to information that could identify individual participants during data collection.

The study cohort comprised patients aged 12–18 years who were confirmed to have scoliosis in the screening conducted at Yeungnam University Hospital from January 2010 to December 2022. Posteroanterior pelvic radiographs were utilized for algorithm development. The exclusion criteria were as follows: (I) radiographs with interference from extracorporeal objects and (II) radiographs with surgical implants. The radiographs were retrieved from the institution's picture archiving and communication system, anonymized, and exported as JPEG images. A radiologist with over 20 years of clinical experience determined Risser grades from posteroanterior pelvic radiographs.

2.2. Deep Learning Model Development

This study developed two deep learning models for automated Risser grade assessment using Python 3.10.15 and TensorFlow 2.16.2 with Keras. To address the challenges posed by class imbalance and limited data, a multimodal approach incorporating both radiographic images and patient clinical data was implemented. Specifically, 224 × 224-pixel regions of interest from right and left pelvic radiographs, along with patient age and gender, were used as input. The synthetic minority oversampling technique (SMOTE) was used to address class imbalance [17], and traditional image augmentation techniques (tf.image random_flip_left_right, random_flip_up_down, and random_brightness with max_delta = 0.05) were applied to enhance data diversity.

Class imbalance, a prevalent challenge in medical research, can significantly hinder the performance of classification algorithms. SMOTE addresses this issue by augmenting the minority class through the generation of synthetic samples. Unlike simple duplication, which risks overfitting, SMOTE interpolates between existing minority instances and their k-nearest neighbors in the feature space. This process effectively expands the minority class representation, enhancing the classifier performance on imbalanced datasets and improving the prediction of rare yet clinically significant events.

The deep learning models determining Risser grades of the right and left pelvises utilized a ConvNextTiny CNN architecture [18], which was optimized with Adam with weight decay (AdamW) and rectified linear unit (ReLU) activation. Regularization was achieved through dropout and batch normalization. The system also employed a separate deep neural network (DNN) to process clinical data. Features extracted from the CNNs and DNN were fused using a concatenation layer, followed by additional dense layers culminating in an output layer generating Risser grade predictions. Furthermore, iterative hyperparameter optimization, guided by performance metrics (accuracy, precision, recall, F1-score, and area under the receiver operating characteristic curve [ROC AUC]), was conducted to refine the model performance. This integrated multimodal approach provides a comprehensive and automated pipeline for Risser grade assessment. Figure 1 provides an overview of the model development process for Risser grade determination.

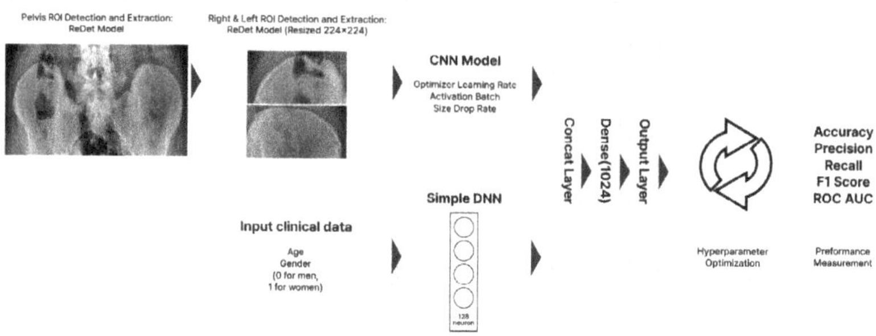

Figure 1. Summary of the model development process for assessing Risser grades.

2.3. Statistical Analyses

Statistical analyses were conducted using Python (version 3.10.15) with the Scikit-learn library (version 1.5.2) [19]. The diagnostic performance of the deep learning classification model for Risser grade assessment was evaluated by calculating accuracy, precision, recall,

F1-score, and ROC AUC. These metrics were reported separately for models determining Risser grades on the right and left pelvises.

3. Results

A total of 1619 pelvic radiographs were used for the development of the deep learning model. The mean age of the subjects was 13.13 ± 1.73 years, comprising 582 males and 1037 females. Of these images, 1295 (80%) were used for training, whereas 324 (20%) were utilized for validation. The dataset exhibited a marked class imbalance, wherein the number of data for Risser Grade 4 was the largest (right and left sides: 42.1%), and that for Risser Grade 1 was the smallest (right side: 5.4%, left side: 5.8%). The specific ratios of each Risser grade are presented in the "Sample class size and ratio" columns of Tables 1 and 2. During training, the model for determining Risser grades of the right pelvis (RT model) reached 100% accuracy while achieving a validation accuracy of 83.64%. In comparison, the model for the left side (LT model) obtained a training accuracy of 98.07% and a validation accuracy of 80.56%. Tables 1 and 2 show the details of the developed models.

Evaluation metrics derived from the validation dataset indicated generally robust performances for both the RT and LT models. Specifically, the RT model demonstrated a microaverage F1-score of 0.836, a macroaverage F1-score of 0.727, and a microaverage ROC AUC of 0.895 (Figure 2). Meanwhile, the LT model achieved a microaverage F1-score of 0.806, a macroaverage F1-score of 0.708, and a microaverage ROC AUC of 0.872 (Figure 2).

The confusion matrices for the RT and LT models (Figure 3) revealed specific patterns in Risser grade classification. The RT model showed prediction accuracies of 96%, 71%, and 93% for Risser Grades 0, 2, and 4, respectively, with lower accuracies of 47%, 66%, and 55% for Grades 1, 3, and 5, respectively. Similarly, the LT model showed accuracies of 95%, 77%, and 87% for Grades 0, 2, and 4, respectively, with lower prediction accuracies of 53%, 57%, and 53% for Grades 1, 3, and 5. These matrices highlighted the impact of class imbalance. Both models demonstrated strong performance in identifying Risser Grades 0, 2, and 4. However, both models exhibited challenges in accurately classifying Grades 1, 3, and 5, which were often misclassified as adjacent grades. In particular, the models frequently assigned lower grades than the actual values for Grades 1 and 5, which had the least training data.

Table 1. Details of the model for determining Risser grades of the right pelvis (RT model).

Sample size and ratio	- 80% for training: 1295; 20% for validation: 324; total: 1619					
Sample class size and ratio	- Class 0, 394 (24.3%); Class 1, 94 (5.8%); Class 2, 158 (9.8%); Class 3, 194 (12%); Class 4, 682 (42.1%); Class 5, 97 (6%)					
Gender ratio	- Male: 582 (35.9%); Female: 1037 (64.1%)					
Age distribution	- 9 (42, 2.59%); 10 (80, 4.94%); 11 (161, 9.94%); 12 (285, 17.6%); 13 (349, 21.56%); 14 (308, 19.02%); 15 (236, 14.58%); 16 (133, 8.21%); 17 (23, 1.42%); 18 (2, 0.12%)					
RT model	- ConvNextTiny CNN model - AdamW optimizer, ReLU activation, batch size 16 - Image input: right pelvis ROI (224 × 224) - Clinical data for input: age and gender - Dropout and batch normalization layer for regularization - Training accuracy: 100%; validation accuracy: 83.64%					
Model performance	Class	Precision	Recall	F1-score	Support	ROC AUC
	0	0.894	0.962	0.927	79	0.963
	1	0.533	0.472	0.500	17	0.724
	2	0.649	0.706	0.676	34	0.831
(Validation data)	3	0.758	0.658	0.704	38	0.815
	4	0.914	0.934	0.924	136	0.935
	5	0.733	0.550	0.629	20	0.768
	Microaverage	0.836	0.836	0.836	324	0.895
	Macroaverage	0.747	0.713	0.727	324	0.839

CNN, convolutional neural network; AdamW, Adam with weight decay; ReLU, rectified linear unit; ROI, region of interest; ROC, receiver operating characteristic; AUC, area under the curve.

Table 2. Details of the model for determining Risser grades of the left pelvis (LT model).

Sample size and ratio Sample class size and ratio	- 80% for training: 1295; 20% for validation: 324; total: 1619 - Class 0, 402 (24.8%); Class 1, 87 (5.4%); Class 2, 149 (9.2%), Class 3, 202 (12.5%); Class 4, 682 (42.1%); Class 5, 97 (6%)					
Gender ratio Age distribution	- Male: 582 (35.9%); Female: 1037 (64.1%) - 9 (42, 2.59%); 10 (80, 4.94%); 11 (161, 9.94%); 12 (285, 17.6%); 13 (349, 21.56%); 14 (308, 19.02%); 15 (236, 14.58%); 16 (133, 8.21%); 17 (23, 1.42%); 18 (2, 0.12%)					
LT model	- ConvNextTiny CNN model - AdamW optimizer, ReLU activation, batch size 32 - Image input: left pelvis ROI (224 × 224) - Clinical data for input: age and gender - Dropout and batch normalization layer for regularization - Training accuracy: 98.07%; validation accuracy: 80.56%					
Model performance	Class	Precision	Recall	F1-score	Support	ROC AUC
	0	0.906	0.951	0.928	81	0.959
	1	0.692	0.529	0.600	17	0.758
	2	0.657	0.767	0.708	30	0.863
	3	0.639	0.575	0.605	40	0.765
(Validation data)	4	0.869	0.869	0.869	137	0.886
	5	0.556	0.526	0.541	19	0.750
	Microaverage	0.806	0.806	0.806	324	0.872
	Macroaverage	0.720	0.703	0.708	324	0.830

CNN, convolutional neural network; AdamW, Adam with weight decay; ReLU, rectified linear unit; ROI, region of interest; ROC, receiver operating characteristic; AUC, area under the curve.

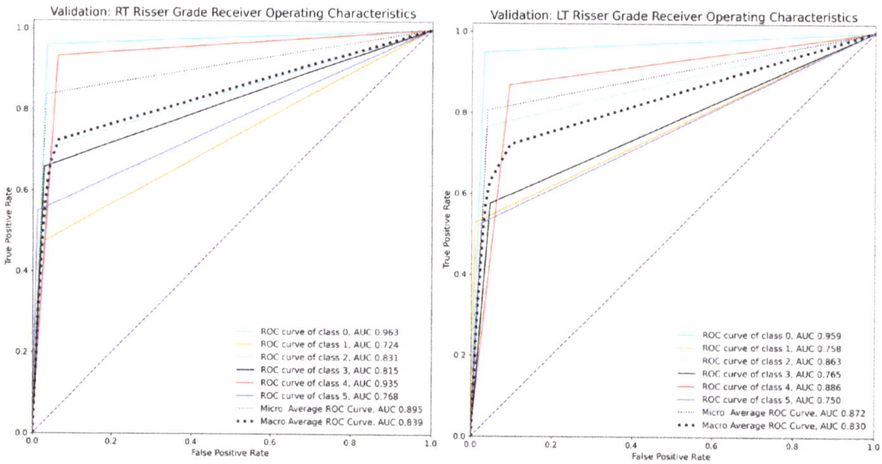

Figure 2. ROC AUC of the RT and LT models.

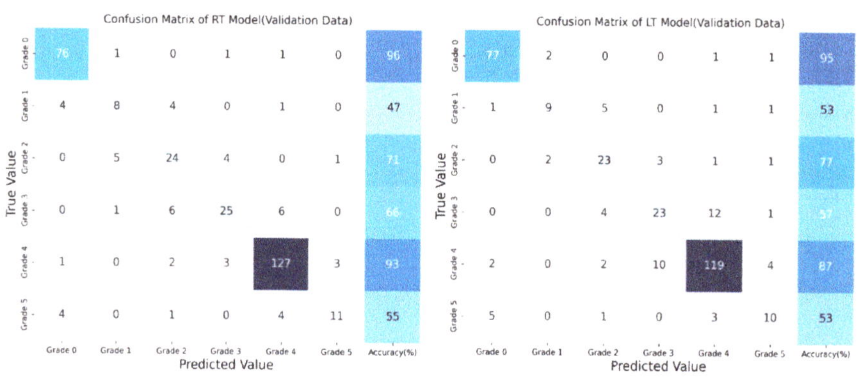

Figure 3. Confusion matrix of the RT and LT models.

Furthermore, precision–recall analysis evaluated the RT and LT models across Grades 0–5, revealing significant grade-specific performance disparities (Figure 4). Both models achieved optimal performance in early skeletal maturity detection, with Grade 0 demonstrating the highest average precision scores (RT: 0.849, LT: 0.897) and Grade 1 maintaining relatively weak performance (RT: 0.271, LT: 0.380). However, intermediate grades (2–3) showed markedly reduced performance, with Grade 4 exhibiting particularly superior results (RT: 0.891, LT: 0.820), while Grade 5 demonstrated relatively weak performance (RT: 0.493, LT: 0.315).

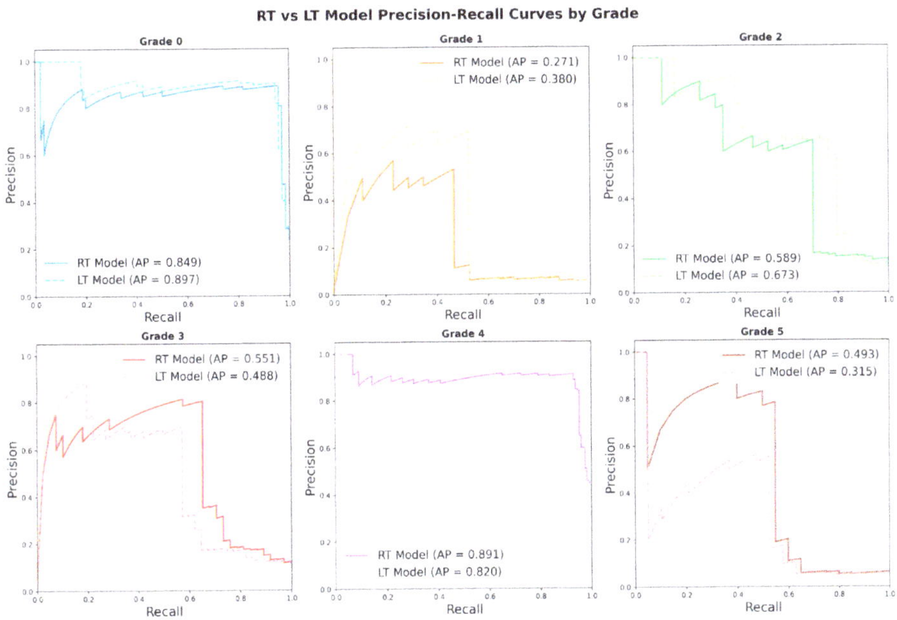

Figure 4. RT vs. LT model precision–recall curves by grade.

4. Discussion

Herein, we developed an automated deep-learning-based system for assessing Risser grades of pelvic bones using CNN to analyze radiographs and patient clinical data. The results demonstrated the potential of deep learning in assessing skeletal maturity using the Risser grading system, traditionally reliant on expert assessment. The model showed good performance in determining Risser grades, especially for the more common grades (Risser Grades 0, 2, and 4).

Regarding the performance of our deep learning model for both right and left pelvic radiographs, the RT model achieved a validation accuracy of 83.64%, whereas the LT model had a validation accuracy of 80.56%, indicating that the models can reliably predict Risser grades. Evaluation metrics such as F1-score, precision, recall, and ROC AUC revealed the models' overall good classification performance, with the RT and LT models achieving microaverage F1-scores of 0.836 and 0.806 and microaverage ROC AUC of 0.895 and 0.872, respectively, indicating good model sensitivity and specificity [20,21].

This study identified class imbalance in the dataset as a major challenge. Risser Grade 4 was the most prevalent class, representing a substantial portion of the training data (42.1% for both right and left pelvic images). Conversely, the data portion for Risser Grade 1 was low at 5.4% for the right pelvic images and 5.8% for the left pelvic images. This imbalance caused misclassification, particularly for Risser Grades 1, 3, and 5, which were frequently predicted as adjacent grades. The lower accuracies for these grades (i.e., 47%, 66%, and 55% for Risser Grades 1, 3, and 5, respectively, in the RT model and 53%, 57%, and 53% for Risser Grades 1, 3, and 5, respectively, in the LT model) seemed to be due to their lower amount of data compared to Risser Grades 0, 2, and 4. Despite the use of SMOTE to address the data imbalance by generating synthetic samples for underrepresented classes, the models still tended to classify less common grades as more prevalent ones. These findings highlight the need for a balanced dataset to enhance the model's accuracy in classifying less frequent Risser grades.

Several studies have addressed class imbalance using focal loss, cost-sensitive learning, or ensemble methods [22–24]. Additionally, Kim et al. developed a deep learning model that predicts bone age in hand radiographs [3]. They showed that a multimodal regression-based model integrating radiographic and clinical data can achieve high accuracy (91.1%), despite significant imbalance in gender distribution (2162 females vs. 812 males). We addressed the data imbalance issue using SMOTE, which generates synthetic examples for minority classes by interpolating between existing minority class samples. This approach helps balance class distribution without simply duplicating data, thereby reducing the risk of overfitting [19]. Furthermore, SMOTE is known to enhance classifier performance on underrepresented classes by providing a more diverse and informative training set [19].

The development of an automated system for Risser grade assessment has important clinical implications. As the manual measurement of Risser grading is time-consuming, highly dependent on physician experience, and prone to interobserver variability [25], automating this process using deep learning models can help reduce the workload of clinicians and provide more consistent and accurate assessments.

A limitation of this study is the residual overfitting in our models, despite employing mitigation strategies such as early stopping, regularization (dropout and batch normalization), and SMOTE-based data augmentation. The persistent discrepancy between training and validation accuracies for both the RT and LT models indicates limited generalization to unseen data. This factor warrants consideration when interpreting the study's findings.

To enhance the model's classification of Risser grades accurately, it is necessary to balance datasets by increasing representation of less frequent grades or employing advanced oversampling techniques. Although our model currently determines Risser grades, future research should focus on developing a model to assess potential height increase using longitudinal data on height change. In addition, the dataset used for model training is limited to a single institution, potentially reducing the model's generalizability to other patient populations or institutions. Additionally, a larger amount of training data can improve the model's performance. Moreover, a study comparing time saved using the developed model versus manual assessment would demonstrate the model's effectiveness.

5. Conclusions

Our study demonstrated the potential of deep learning models, particularly CNN-based architectures, for automating the assessment of Risser grades in pelvic radiographs. The right pelvis model achieved an accuracy of 83.64%, with a microaverage F1-score of 0.836 and ROC AUC of 0.895. The left pelvis model reached an accuracy of 80.56%, with a microaverage F1-score of 0.806 and ROC AUC of 0.872. Both models performed well for Risser Grades 0, 2, and 4. The model performed well in identifying common Risser grades, but addressing class imbalance is necessary to improve accuracy across all grades. Overall, the findings suggest that deep learning can effectively enhance the efficiency and consistency of BAA in clinical practice.

Author Contributions: Conceptualization, J.K.K., D.P. and M.C.C.; methodology, J.K.K., D.P. and M.C.C.; software, J.K.K., D.P. and M.C.C.; validation, J.K.K., D.P. and M.C.C.; formal analysis, J.K.K.,

D.P. and M.C.C.; investigation, J.K.K., D.P. and M.C.C.; resources, J.K.K., D.P. and M.C.C.; data curation, J.K.K., D.P. and M.C.C.; writing—original draft preparation, J.K.K., D.P. and M.C.C.; writing—review and editing, J.K.K., D.P. and M.C.C.; visualization, J.K.K., D.P. and M.C.C.; supervision, M.C.C. All authors have read and agreed to the published version of the manuscript.

Funding: This work was supported by the 2025 Yeungnam University Research Grant.

Institutional Review Board Statement: The study was conducted in accordance with the Declaration of Helsinki and approved by the Institutional Review Board of Yeungnam University Hospital (protocol code 2024-06-005, date of approval: 14 June 2024).

Informed Consent Statement: The requirement for informed consent was waived by the institutional review board of Yeungnam University Hospital owing to the retrospective nature of the study.

Data Availability Statement: The datasets generated during and/or analyzed during the current study are available from the corresponding author on reasonable request.

Conflicts of Interest: The authors declare no conflicts of interest.

Abbreviations

CNN: conventional neural network; ROI: region of interest; SMOTE: synthetic minority oversampling technique; AdamW: Adam with weight decay; ReLU: rectified linear unit; DNN: deep neural network; ROC AUC: area under the receiver operating characteristic curve.

References

1. Cavallo, F.; Mohn, A.; Chiarelli, F.; Giannini, C. Evaluation of Bone Age in Children: A Mini-Review. *Front. Pediatr.* **2021**, *9*, 580314. [CrossRef] [PubMed]
2. Jang, W.Y.; Ahn, K.S.; Oh, S.; Lee, J.E.; Choi, J.; Kang, C.H.; Kang, W.Y.; Hong, S.J.; Shim, E.; Kim, B.H.; et al. Difference between bone age at the hand and elbow at the onset of puberty. *Medicine* **2022**, *101*, e28516. [CrossRef] [PubMed]
3. Kim, J.K.; Park, D.; Chang, M.C. Assessment of Bone Age Based on Hand Radiographs Using Regression-Based Multi-Modal Deep Learning. *Life* **2024**, *14*, 774. [CrossRef] [PubMed]
4. Dimeglio, A.; Canavese, F. Progression or not progression? How to deal with adolescent idiopathic scoliosis during puberty. *J. Child. Orthop.* **2013**, *7*, 43–49. [CrossRef]
5. Hacquebord, J.H.; Leopold, S.S. In brief: The Risser classification: A classic tool for the clinician treating adolescent idiopathic scoliosis. *Clin. Orthop. Relat. Res.* **2012**, *470*, 2335–2338. [CrossRef]
6. Vira, S.; Husain, Q.; Jalai, C.; Paul, J.; Poorman, G.W.; Poorman, C.; Yoon, R.S.; Looze, C.; Lonner, B.; Passias, P.G. The Interobserver and Intraobserver Reliability of the Sanders Classification Versus the Risser Stage. *J. Pediatr. Orthop.* **2017**, *37*, e246–e249. [CrossRef] [PubMed]
7. Li, M.; Jiang, Y.; Zhang, Y.; Zhu, H. Medical image analysis using deep learning algorithms. *Front. Public Health* **2023**, *11*, 1273253. [CrossRef]
8. Thakur, G.K.; Thakur, A.; Kulkarni, S.; Khan, N.; Khan, S. Deep Learning Approaches for Medical Image Analysis and Diagnosis. *Cureus* **2024**, *16*, e59507. [CrossRef]
9. Xu, Y.; Quan, R.; Xu, W.; Huang, Y.; Chen, X.; Liu, F. Advances in Medical Image Segmentation: A Comprehensive Review of Traditional, Deep Learning and Hybrid Approaches. *Bioengineering* **2024**, *11*, 1034. [CrossRef]
10. Achararit, P.; Bongkaew, H.; Chobpenthai, T.; Nonthasaen, P. Generating accurate sex estimation from hand X-ray images using AI deep-learning techniques: A study of limited bone regions. *Leg. Med.* **2025**, *74*, 102612. [CrossRef]
11. Harris, C.E.; Liu, L.; Almeida, L.; Kassick, C.; Makrogiannis, S. Artificial intelligence in pediatric osteopenia diagnosis: Evaluating deep network classification and model interpretability using wrist X-rays. *Bone Rep.* **2025**, *25*, 101845. [CrossRef] [PubMed]
12. Oude Nijhuis, K.D.; Barvelink, B.; Prijs, J.; Zhao, Y.; Liao, Z.; Jaarsma, R.L.; FFA, I.J.; Colaris, J.W.; Doornberg, J.N.; Wijffels, M.M.E. An open source convolutional neural network to detect and localize distal radius fractures on plain radiographs. *Eur. J. Trauma Emerg. Surg. Off. Publ. Eur. Trauma Soc.* **2025**, *51*, 26. [CrossRef] [PubMed]
13. Jamaludin, A.; Kadir, T.; Zisserman, A. SpineNet: Automated classification and evidence visualization in spinal MRIs. *Med. Image Anal.* **2017**, *41*, 63–73. [CrossRef] [PubMed]
14. Liu, J.; Wang, H.; Shan, X.; Zhang, L.; Cui, S.; Shi, Z.; Liu, Y.; Zhang, Y.; Wang, L. Hybrid transformer convolutional neural network-based radiomics models for osteoporosis screening in routine CT. *BMC Med. Imaging* **2024**, *24*, 62. [CrossRef]

15. Marsilio, L.; Marzorati, D.; Rossi, M.; Moglia, A.; Mainardi, L.; Manzotti, A.; Cerveri, P. Cascade learning in multi-task encoder-decoder networks for concurrent bone segmentation and glenohumeral joint clinical assessment in shoulder CT scans. *Artif. Intell. Med.* **2025**, *165*, 103131. [CrossRef]
16. Wu, S.; Ke, Z.; Cai, L.; Wang, L.; Zhang, X.; Ke, Q.; Ye, Y. Pelvic bone tumor segmentation fusion algorithm based on fully convolutional neural network and conditional random field. *J. Bone Oncol.* **2024**, *45*, 100593. [CrossRef]
17. Han, H.; Wang, W.-Y.; Mao, B.-H. Borderline-SMOTE: A new over-sampling method in imbalanced data sets learning. In Proceedings of the International Conference on Intelligent Computing, Hefei, China, 23–26 August 2005; pp. 878–887.
18. Pedregosa, F.; Varoquaux, G.; Gramfort, A.; Michel, V.; Thirion, B.; Grisel, O.; Blondel, M.; Prettenhofer, P.; Weiss, R.; Dubourg, V.; et al. Scikit-learn: Machine learning in Python. *J. Mach. Learn. Res.* **2011**, *12*, 2825–2830.
19. Woo, S.; Debnath, S.; Hu, R.; Chen, X.; Liu, Z.; Kweon, I.S.; Xie, S. Convnext v2: Co-designing and scaling convnets with masked autoencoders. In Proceedings of the IEEE/CVF Conference on Computer Vision and Pattern Recognition, Vancouver, BC, Canada, 17–24 June 2023; pp. 16133–16142.
20. Mandrekar, J.N. Receiver operating characteristic curve in diagnostic test assessment. *J. Thorac. Oncol. Off. Publ. Int. Assoc. Study Lung Cancer* **2010**, *5*, 1315–1316. [CrossRef]
21. Takahashi, K.; Yamamoto, K.; Kuchiba, A.; Koyama, T. Confidence interval for micro-averaged F (1) and macro-averaged F (1) scores. *Appl. Intell.* **2022**, *52*, 4961–4972. [CrossRef]
22. Liu, L.; Wu, X.; Li, S.; Li, Y.; Tan, S.; Bai, Y. Solving the class imbalance problem using ensemble algorithm: Application of screening for aortic dissection. *BMC Med. Inform. Decis. Mak.* **2022**, *22*, 82. [CrossRef]
23. Ravi, V. Attention Cost-Sensitive Deep Learning-Based Approach for Skin Cancer Detection and Classification. *Cancers* **2022**, *14*, 5872. [CrossRef] [PubMed]
24. Peng, H.; Wu, C.; Xiao, Y.J.A.S. CBF-IDS: Addressing class imbalance using CNN-BiLSTM with focal loss in network intrusion detection system. *Appl. Sci.* **2023**, *13*, 11629. [CrossRef]
25. Hammond, K.E.; Dierckman, B.D.; Burnworth, L.; Meehan, P.L.; Oswald, T.S. Inter-observer and intra-observer reliability of the Risser sign in a metropolitan scoliosis screening program. *J. Pediatr. Orthop.* **2011**, *31*, e80–e84. [CrossRef] [PubMed]

bioengineering

MDPI

Article

Deep Learning in Spinal Endoscopy: U-Net Models for Neural Tissue Detection

Hyung Rae Lee [1], Wounsuk Rhee [2], Sam Yeol Chang [3], Bong-Soon Chang [3] and Hyoungmin Kim [3,*]

1 Department of Orthopedic Surgery, Korea University Anam Hospital, Seoul 02841, Republic of Korea; drhrleeos@gmail.com
2 Ministry of Health and Welfare, Government of the Republic of Korea, Sejong 30113, Republic of Korea; rhee1998@snu.ac.kr
3 Department of Orthopedic Surgery, Seoul National University College of Medicine, Seoul 03080, Republic of Korea; sam310@seoul.ac.kr (S.Y.C.); bschang@snu.ac.kr (B.-S.C.)
* Correspondence: hmkhm@snu.ac.kr

Abstract: Biportal endoscopic spine surgery (BESS) is minimally invasive and therefore benefits both surgeons and patients. However, concerning complications include dural tears and neural tissue injuries. In this study, we aimed to develop a deep learning model for neural tissue segmentation to enhance the safety and efficacy of endoscopic spinal surgery. We used frames extracted from videos of 28 endoscopic spine surgeries, comprising 2307 images for training and 635 images for validation. A U-Net-like architecture is employed for neural tissue segmentation. Quantitative assessments include the Dice-Sorensen coefficient, Jaccard index, precision, recall, average precision, and image-processing time. Our findings revealed that the best-performing model achieved a Dice-Sorensen coefficient of 0.824 and a Jaccard index of 0.701. The precision and recall values were 0.810 and 0.839, respectively, with an average precision of 0.890. The model processed images at 43 ms per frame, equating to 23.3 frames per second. Qualitative evaluations indicated the effective identification of neural tissue features. Our U-Net-based model robustly performed neural tissue segmentation, indicating its potential to support spine surgeons, especially those with less experience, and improve surgical outcomes in endoscopic procedures. Therefore, further advancements may enhance the clinical applicability of this technique.

Keywords: endoscopic spine surgery; neural tissue; image segmentation; computer vision; deep learning

1. Introduction

In spinal surgery, biportal endoscopic spine surgery (BESS) is a significant advancement over conventional open surgery owing to its advantages [1–3], which include smaller incisions, reduced muscle and bone damage, less postoperative pain, and shorter recovery times [4]. High-quality endoscopic equipment markedly enhances image clarity and provides significant assistance to surgeons during procedures. The increased magnification in modern endoscopy allows for the more detailed visualization of critical structures, further enhancing surgical precision. However, despite these advancements, complications, such as dural tears and neural tissue injuries, persist and pose significant challenges during surgery [5,6]. These complications are particularly common among younger surgeons who have not yet reached the learning curve. Among these, dural tears remain the most common and significant complication of endoscopic spinal surgery [5]. The rate of dural tears is reported to be approximately 2.7% [5]. These tears are often managed during surgery by suturing or sealing with specialized products. However, if unnoticed, patients may experience postoperative headaches, nausea, prolonged bed rest, and increased hospitalization and, in severe cases, may require revision surgery. The steep learning curve associated with these complications further limits their widespread clinical adoption, necessitating more experience and skills from surgeons.

Recently, the incorporation of artificial intelligence (AI) into healthcare has been promising, particularly in medical imaging analysis. Deep learning, a subset of AI, has demonstrated remarkable performance in clinical diagnosis and treatment owing to its self-learning capabilities and the ability to extract key features from large datasets [7–9]. Semantic segmentation, which is one of the most actively studied fields in computer vision, classifies each pixel of an image into a predefined class. Architectures such as fully convolutional networks (FCN), DeepLab, and Mask R-CNN have been developed and have shown promising results for image datasets comprising common objects [10–12]. Studies have demonstrated the effectiveness of deep learning-based segmentation in various medical imaging domains, such as retinal vessel segmentation, tumor detection [13], and instrument tip recognition in spinal surgery [14]. These studies established the foundation for our approach by illustrating the potential of U-Net and similar models for precise segmentation in challenging imaging scenarios [9,13,15].

Despite these advancements, research on the application of deep learning in spinal endoscopy remains limited. Given the critical need to minimize complications, such as dural tears and neural tissue injuries, it is necessary to develop and implement deep learning algorithms for neural tissue recognition in spinal endoscopy. In particular, U-Net and its variants have been widely adopted in biomedical imaging, particularly for small datasets [16,17]. FCN have laid the foundation for pixel-wise segmentation, whereas DeepLab and Mask R-CNN have shown robust performance in handling complex images and multi-object segmentation [15,17–19]. We chose U-Net owing to its effectiveness with small biomedical datasets and its capability to capture fine details, thereby making it suitable for neural tissue segmentation in spinal endoscopy [17,20,21].

The use of deep learning in spinal endoscopy is relatively new. Studies such as that of Cho et al. [14] focused on the automatic detection of surgical instrument tips to achieve high precision. However, challenges such as differentiating between neural tissues and surrounding structures have not been addressed. Studies on other biomedical images [16,17] have demonstrated the efficacy of U-Net architectures for segmentation, which motivated our choice of model. This study aimed to explore the feasibility of deep learning for neural tissue recognition during spinal endoscopy. By establishing a foundational understanding of how effectively deep learning can identify neural tissues, we hope to pave the way for advancements in real-time tissue recognition, ultimately enhancing the safety and efficacy of endoscopic spinal surgery.

2. Materials and Methods

2.1. Dataset

The patient cohort comprised 28 patients, including 21 with lumbar interlaminar decompressions, 5 with lumbar foraminal decompressions, and 3 with cervical foraminotomies. The procedures involved levels 1–2, with six cases involving 2-level surgeries. This dataset is diverse and encompasses a range of demographic profiles, including sex and age. Frames were extracted from each video at 10 s intervals, resulting in approximately 4000 frames. Among these, 2942 frames contained neural tissues that could be detected at the human level. Segmentation labeling was performed using LabelMe by a spinal surgeon (H.R.L., one of the authors.) with >4 years of experience in spinal endoscopic surgery. The dataset was then divided into training, validation, and test sets, with 2307 images (78%) from 22 patients (79%) and 635 images (22%) from 6 patients (21%). We performed a threefold cross-validation on the training/validation set, with each fold comprising 1538 images (52%) for training and 769 images (26%) for internal validation.

The patient demographics for each set are listed in Table 1. The training/validation and test sets did not have overlapping patients, ensuring appropriate validation and preventing the overestimation of performance measures. This study was approved by the Public Institutional Review Board (IRB) of the National Bioethics Policy Institute through the public e-IRB system. The IRB approval number and approval date for this study is "2024-1010-001" and 16 August 2024. The requirement for informed consent was waived by the IRB because of the retrospective nature of this study.

Table 1. Patient demographics for training/validation and test sets.

	Training/Validation Set	Test Set
Number of images	2307 (78%)	635 (22%)
Number of patients	22 (79%)	6 (21%)
Age (years)	65.4 ± 10.7	63.8 ± 14.1
Sex		
Male	9	3
Female	13	3

2.2. The U-Net Architecture

In this study, we trained a deep neural network resembling the U-Net architecture, which has been reported to perform well on the segmentation tasks of small image datasets [16,17]. We selected a U-Net-like architecture based on its demonstrated effectiveness in medical image segmentation, particularly with small datasets [16,17]. U-Net variants can effectively handle limited labeled data, making them suitable for application in spinal endoscopy. As shown in Figure 1, the model had an input shape of (256, 256, and 3) and an output shape of (256, 256, and 1). An input image first undergoes a down-sampling process, also known as the left branch, to extract the features. The bottommost layer or bridge of the network contains the most compressed images with the thickest layers. Subsequently, an upsampling step, or right branch, was performed to recover the original resolution and provide a set of segmentation masks. Skip connections at each level allow for the faster convergence and stability of the deep learning models.

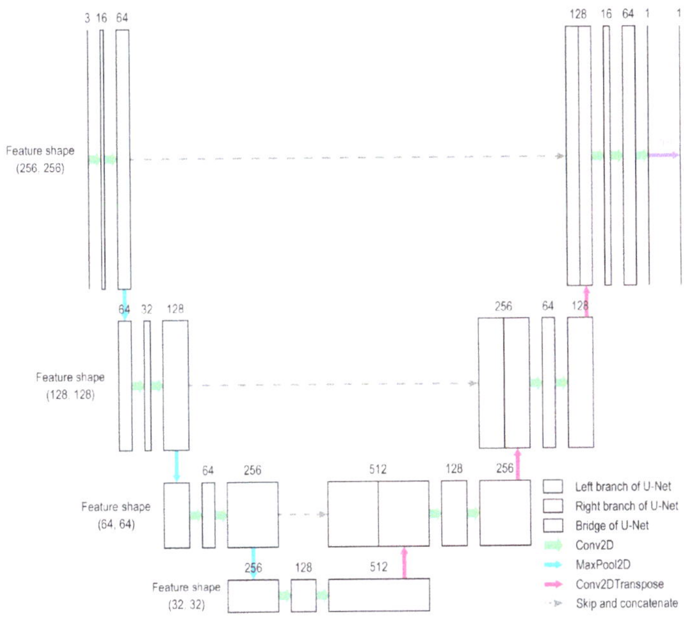

Figure 1. Architecture of the deep learning model. The model accepts an input of shape (256, 256, 3) and produces an output of shape (256, 256, 1). The number of channels is indicated above each block. This architecture is a modified version of the original U-Net, designed to reduce the number of parameters and enable faster learning.

2.3. Model Training

No preprocessing methods other than resizing or rescaling were applied. We aimed to evaluate the performance of the model under raw conditions to provide more generalized applicability across diverse clinical settings. Data augmentation, which consists of random rotation from −180 degrees to +180 degrees, random flip, and random zoom from 1.0 times to 1.2 times, was applied only during the training of each fold. No augmentation was applied during the internal validation and testing. Unlike common practice, where the training set is expanded by fivefold to tenfold, we did not expand the training set but instead applied random image transforms for each epoch, as illustrated in Figure 2, allowing the model to experience multiple random variations of the original training sample.

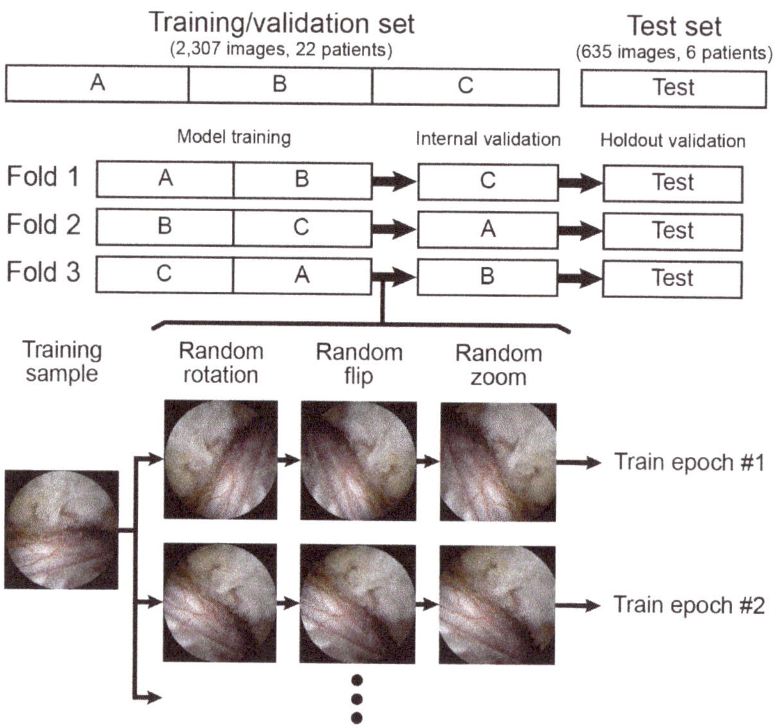

Figure 2. Threefold cross-validation and data augmentation processes with random transform are illustrated.

The convolutional layers are randomly initialized with a uniform Glorot distribution, with batch normalization applied before nonlinear activation [22,23]. The full neural network aimed to minimize dice loss, defined as Equation (1), where indices i and j refer to the indices of the rows and columns of pixels, and it was trained for a maximum of 100 epochs (the maximum number of epochs was determined empirically because most trials were terminated before completing 100 epochs owing to early stopping mechanisms) [24]. To prevent overfitting and promote adequate convergence, we incorporated early stopping and learning rate reduction mechanisms. Hyperparameter optimization was performed through a random search of 25 trials, and the search space summarized in Table 2 was determined based on initial experimentation and commonly accepted practices [25].

$$Dice\ Loss = 1 - \frac{2 \times \sum_{i,j} y_{ij}\hat{y}_{ij}}{\sum_{i,j} y_{ij} + \hat{y}_{ij}} \tag{1}$$

Table 2. The search space for a random search of hyperparameters is summarized.

Hyperparameter	Search Space
Batch size	{4, 8, 12, 16}
Initial learning rate	loguniform (0.001, 0.1)
Optimizer	{Adam, SGD}
Patience for learning rate reduction	{3, 4, 5, 6, 7}
Reducing factor for learning rate reduction	uniform (0.05, 0.15)

After training the models for each fold in the threefold cross-validation process, we generated an ensemble model that averaged the outputs of the models and measured their final performance. All training and testing were performed with TensorFlow 2.14 and Python 3.11, running on a PC with an Intel(R) Core(TM) i9-14900KF CPU, an NVIDIA RTX 4090 24GB graphics card, and 64GB of DDR5 RAM.

2.4. *Performance Assessment*

The performance of the trained model was evaluated using various methods, each of which is described in the following subsections. In this context, a true positive (TP) refers to the intersecting area of the ground truth and predicted masks, a false positive (FP) is defined as the region inside the predicted mask but outside the ground truth mask, and a false negative is the region inside the ground truth mask but outside the predicted mask. In this study, the Dice–Sorensen coefficient (DSC), Jaccard index (IoU), precision, and recall were evaluated for the test set. The image-processing time was also measured to assess the feasibility of the model for analyzing real-time video frames.

2.4.1. Dice–Sorensen Coefficient

The DSC is defined in Equation (2) and is equivalent to the F1-score of a typical two-by-two contingency table. The DSC ranged between 0 and 1, with higher values indicating better performance as the TP increased. Notably, the dice loss is a continuous analog of the negative DSC, and the Dice Loss decreases as the model performance increases.

$$DSC = \frac{2 \times TP}{2 \times TP + FP + FN} \tag{2}$$

2.4.2. Jaccard Index

The intersection over union (IoU), defined in Equation (3), is the ratio of the intersecting area of the ground truth and prediction masks to their union. Similar to the DSC, its value is always between 0 and 1, and a higher score indicates better performance.

$$IoU = \frac{TP}{TP + FP + FN} \tag{3}$$

2.4.3. Precision and Recall

Precision and recall are defined in Equations (4) and (5) and are widely adopted to measure a model's performance. Given that their values are dependent on the decision boundaries, the precision–recall curve and the area underneath were also assessed. The area under the precision–recall curve (AUPRC) is also known as average precision (AP).

$$Precision = \frac{TP}{TP + FP} \tag{4}$$

$$Recall = \frac{TP}{TP + FN} \tag{5}$$

2.4.4. Qualitative Assessment

The model performance was qualitatively assessed by exploring the prediction masks obtained from the test set images. This analysis aimed to identify the strengths and weaknesses of our model and discuss strategies for improving its performance in the future.

3. Results

3.1. Quantitative Results

Table 3 lists the sets of hyperparameters that resulted in the top-10 DSC during the holdout validation with their respective ensemble models. The model that performed the best was trained with a batch size of 12 on an Adam optimizer, with an initial learning rate of 0.00136. The learning rate was reduced by a factor of 0.079 when the loss did not decrease after 7 epochs, and the entire process was terminated when the loss did not decrease after 21 epochs. This set of hyperparameters is in line with commonly accepted practices in medical image segmentation tasks.

Table 3. Sets of hyperparameters that resulted in top-10 DSC in the holdout validation of the ensemble model are shown. Boldfaced numbers indicate the best performance among all trials.

Trial	Hyperparameters					Performance Measures (Holdout Validation)				
	Batch Size	Initial LR	Optimizer	Patience	Reduce Factor	DSC	IoU	Precision	Recall	mAP
1	12	0.00136	Adam	7	0.079	0.824	0.701	0.810	0.839	0.890
2	16	0.00868	Adam	7	0.123	0.817	0.690	0.790	0.845	0.844
3	16	0.00108	Adam	7	0.079	0.815	0.687	0.814	0.815	0.894
4	4	0.01101	SGD	7	0.107	0.814	0.687	0.786	0.845	0.864
5	12	0.00183	Adam	6	0.083	0.809	0.679	0.779	0.842	0.877
6	8	0.09321	SGD	5	0.090	0.809	0.679	0.766	0.857	0.846
7	8	0.03990	SGD	5	0.105	0.803	0.670	0.756	0.856	0.839
8	12	0.00711	Adam	6	0.149	0.798	0.664	0.759	0.842	0.820
9	12	0.01099	Adam	7	0.122	0.797	0.663	0.756	0.845	0.855
10	4	0.00103	Adam	3	0.146	0.794	0.659	0.746	0.849	0.865

Table 4 lists the performance measures evaluated from internal and holdout validation, including the performance of all three folds, as well as the ensemble model. The holdout validation performance of each fold did not significantly differ from that of internal validation, and we confirmed that the ensemble model, which is defined by averaging the outputs of models from each fold, generally outperforms each model. The ensemble model exhibited a test DSC and test IoU of 0.824 and 0.701, respectively, and a test precision and test recall of 0.810 and 0.839, respectively. Figure 3 depicts the plotting of the precision–recall curve and AUPRC of the ensemble model and models obtained from each fold.

Table 4. Internal validation and holdout validation results of the trial with the best DSC are shown. Results of models trained from each fold as well as the ensemble model are provided.

Internal Validation	DSC	IoU	Precision	Recall	AUPRC
Fold 1	0.818	0.692	0.808	0.828	0.849
Fold 2	0.815	0.688	0.821	0.809	0.868
Fold 3	0.810	0.680	0.805	0.814	0.870
Holdout validation	DSC	IoU	Precision	Recall	mAP
Fold 1	0.827	0.705	0.813	0.841	0.865
Fold 2	0.820	0.694	0.810	0.829	0.871
Fold 3	0.792	0.656	0.806	0.780	0.841
Ensemble	0.824	0.701	0.810	0.839	0.890

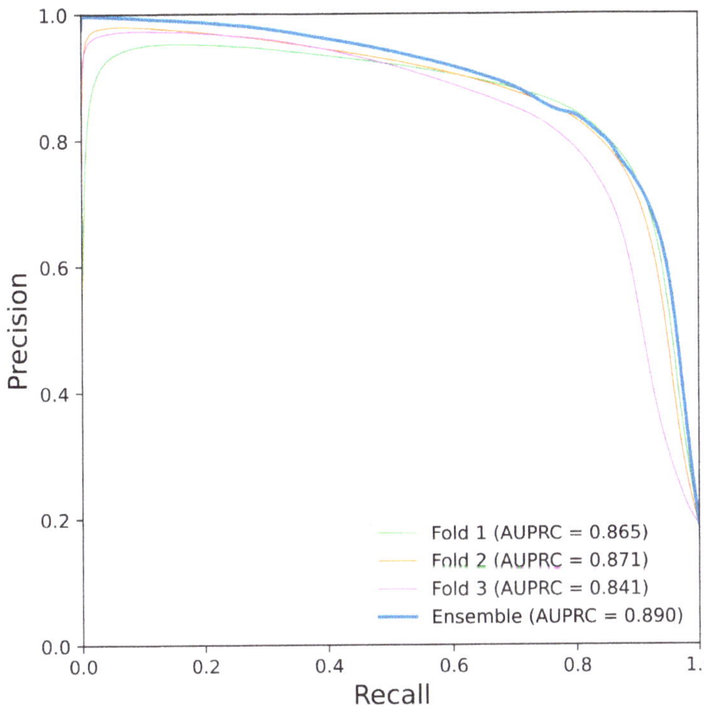

Figure 3. Precision–recall curve obtained from the best-performing trial is shown. Narrow lines indicate the performance of the models trained from each fold on the test set, and the thick line indicates that of the ensemble model.

3.2. Qualitative Results

3.2.1. Well-Performing Samples

Figure 4 shows a few well-performing test samples. In contrast to the rigid and relatively crude polygon-shaped ground truth masks generated manually using LabelMe, the prediction masks tended to be smoother and more descriptive. Moreover, Figure 4a–c show that the deep learning model effectively learned to exclude perineural fat, which often overlaps with neural tissue. Additionally, the model performed well on challenging samples, where only a small portion of the neural tissue was observed, as depicted in Figure 4d,e. Therefore, it can be concluded that the model successfully learned the distinct features of the neural tissues during spinal endoscopic surgery.

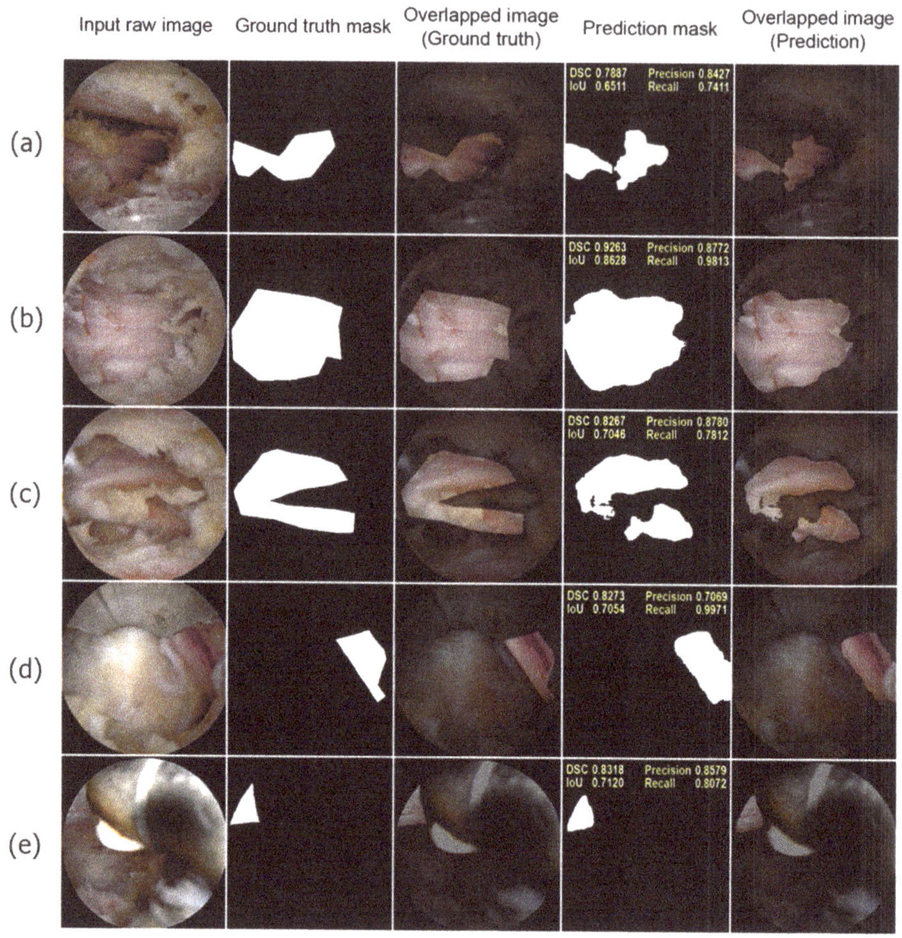

Figure 4. Well-performing test samples. For each sample, the input raw image, ground truth mask, overlapped image of the ground truth mask, prediction mask, and overlapped image of the prediction mask are shown from left to right (**a**–**c**). The deep learning model demonstrated superior accuracy and precision compared to manual annotations. The boundaries predicted by the model are significantly smoother and more precise. Notably, the model accurately identifies epidural fat tissue as non-neural tissue, a distinction that manual annotations often fail to make. This accuracy is evident in the predicted masks (**d**,**e**). Despite the neural tissue being only partially visible in the endoscopic images, the deep learning model accurately detects and represents these small segments of neural tissue. This highlights the model's impressive performance in recognizing neural tissue in challenging scenarios.

3.2.2. Poorly Performing Samples

To illustrate the limitations of the deep learning model, we present a few poorly performing samples in Figure 5. As shown in Figure 5a,b, the model mistakenly classified some parts of the surgical instruments as neural tissue. Interestingly, the FP regions often correspond to reflections of the neural tissue, suggesting that the model struggled to distinguish between the true neural tissue and its reflections, as both display similar positive features. Similar issues were observed in Figure 5c, where areas with similar morphology and texture to the neural tissue were incorrectly identified. Additionally, as shown in Figure 5d, certain surgical instruments with smooth and tubular shapes, which are typical characteristics of neural tissue, were also misidentified by the model. Furthermore, the model exhibited reduced effectiveness in scenarios with excessive bleeding, as shown in Figure 5e, which affected its overall accuracy in these exceptional cases.

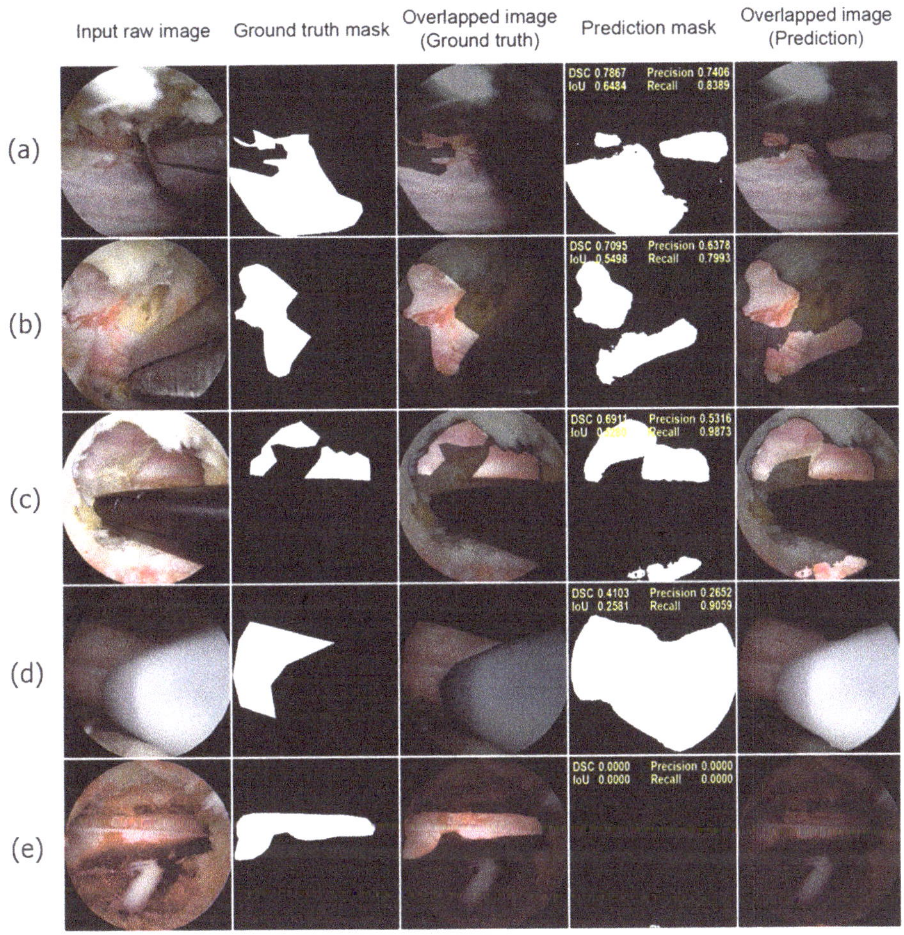

Figure 5. Poorly performing test samples. For each sample, the sequence of images is presented from left to right: the input raw image, ground truth mask, overlapped image of the ground truth mask, prediction mask, and overlapped image of the prediction mask (**a**,**b**). The model misclassified metallic surgical instruments as neural tissue owing to reflections of neural tissue on the metal surfaces (**c**). The model incorrectly identified bloody cancellous bone as neural tissue (**d**). A white instrument used for ablation was also misclassified as neural tissue (**e**). In a highly bloody surgical field, the model failed to detect neural tissue.

4. Discussion

4.1. Comparison with Related Studies

Our study highlights the potential of U-Net-based deep learning models for segmenting neural tissues in endoscopic spinal images. With a test DSC of 0.824 and IoU of 0.701, our model demonstrated competitive performance, particularly given the complexity of neural tissue recognition. In comparison to the previous study by Bu et al. [26], which employed Mask R-CNN for tissue segmentation, our U-Net-based approach achieved a higher DSC, which indicates superior neural tissue detection capabilities in endoscopic images. Despite the more challenging context of neural tissue segmentation, the higher AP in our model underscores the efficacy of our methodology. In contrast to the aforementioned study, our deep learning model identified neural tissue, which was more challenging owing to overlapping features with other tissues; therefore, we consider our results notable. Additionally, in clinical settings, accurately distinguishing neural tissue from other soft tissues, such as ligaments and fat, is crucial because they can be confused during surgery. Given the complexity of this task and the clinical necessity of accurately differentiating neural tissue from the surrounding tissues, our study is highly significant as a pilot study, highlighting the feasibility and importance of neural tissue recognition for improving surgical precision and patient outcomes.

Another study utilized Solov2 and Mask R-CNN for tissue and instrument segmentation in spinal endoscopic images, with the best mean AP of 0.735 at approximately 28 frames per second. Our model achieved a better AP with a comparable computational burden, although it may not be a fair comparison considering the differences in task objectives and image resolution. While the 23.2 frames per second achieved by our model may not be sufficient for real-time videos at 30 fps, it could be effective for videos with low sampling rates, such as 15 or 20 fps. Therefore, we conclude that the proposed model can robustly segment neural tissues in real time. Implementing such technology could greatly benefit less-experienced spinal surgeons by providing enhanced guidance during procedures, ultimately serving as an educational tool for junior surgeons.

4.2. Clinical Significance

Our qualitative analysis provides valuable insights into the ability of the model to distinguish neural tissues from other tissues, even in scenarios with limited tissue visibility. The deep learning model, trained on manually labeled ground truth masks using LabelMe, demonstrated superior accuracy by correctly excluding fat tissue, which is often mislabeled as neural tissue in manual annotations, as shown in Figure 4a–c. It also performed impressively in recognizing small segments of the neural tissue that are only partially visible in the surgical field. However, the model exhibited limitations, as shown in Figure 5a,b, where metallic surgical instruments were misclassified as neural tissue owing to the reflections of the neural tissue on the metal surfaces. This misclassification, although a shortcoming, indicates that the model has the potential to recognize complex visual patterns, including neural tissue reflections on metals, which extend beyond direct visual cues. These observations highlight the model's advanced capability in feature detection but also underscore the need for further refinement to reduce false positives associated with instrument reflections and similar tubular structures.

The high positive predictive value (PPV) demonstrates its effectiveness in accurately identifying true neural tissues, which is crucial to ensuring that neural structures are not overlooked during surgery. Our results may not be immediately acceptable for direct application in routine clinical settings. However, this study represents an early exploration of applying deep learning to neural tissue detection, a complex task with high variability in endoscopic images. Even the most skilled surgeons experience fatigue or face challenging surgical environments, which can increase the risk of errors. Our model aims to provide an additional layer of support, ultimately serving as a tool to assist surgeons in reducing preventable mistakes. With further development, including improved model performance and real-time implementation, we believe that such AI-based assistance can complement a surgeon's expertise and contribute significantly to enhancing patient safety. This high PPV is encouraged, as it reduces the risk of surgeons overlooking critical neural tissues. Therefore, despite the need for improvement in reducing false positives, as highlighted by the challenges associated with the negative predictive value (NPV), the model's current ability to reliably identify neural tissue remains clinically significant. Its existing capabilities suggest that the model is sufficiently robust to be considered for deployment in clinical settings, offering valuable support during surgical procedures.

Neural tissue recognition during surgery is particularly crucial because many surgical complications, such as dural tears or direct neural injuries, often occur when surgeons fail to detect small, partially obscured neural fibers. The ability of our model to recognize these critical but minimally visible neural structures suggests that it has substantial potential to reduce such surgical risks. Surgeons are more likely to make fewer mistakes when neural structures are fully visible and distinct from the surrounding tissues. However, errors are more common when neural structures are only slightly visible or overlap with other tissues. The success of our model in these nuanced detection tasks highlights its significance, suggesting that it can serve as a valuable tool for enhancing surgical accuracy and reducing the likelihood of complications associated with misidentification.

4.3. Limitations and Future Work

A notable limitation of our model was the low NPV, despite the high PPV. We hypothesized that this issue may be influenced by the loss function used during training. Specifically, the dice loss places a greater emphasis on TP regions and does not account for true negative (TN) areas. As a result, TN pixels may not have been adequately trained, potentially leading to a reduced NPV. Implementing binary cross-entropy loss instead of dice loss could potentially improve the NPV, although this might occur at the expense of decreased PPV. Another drawback was the relatively small dataset, which may have affected the generalizability of the model. The current focus on neural tissues limits their applicability in more complex scenarios. Enlarging the dataset by expanding the cohort is the preferred option. However, improvements can also be achieved through enhanced data preprocessing and augmentation techniques. For instance, histogram equalization methods, such as global histogram equalization and contrast-limited adaptive histogram equalization, emphasize the borders of different tissues more prominently, which can result in the improved learning of important features. Additionally, extensive augmentation techniques, such as CutMix and color jittering, may contribute to improved performance because they aid the model in learning more generalized features [24]. Diversifying label entities not only confined to neural tissue may positively affect the model's performance, because it would be able to learn complicated spatial and temporal relations among different types of objects, allowing them to "think" more like surgeons, who are also heavily dependent on anatomical clues, to distinguish between different types of tissue.

We present this study as a baseline reference and plan to extensively investigate other architectures in the future. Since the publication of U-Net, many of its variants have emerged and have produced better results in segmentation tasks [17]. Residual U-Nets manipulate skip connections within the network to enhance gradient propagation, and the utilization of recurrent convolutional blocks has been reported to improve the performance [25,27]. R2U-Net incorporates these two concepts to achieve superior results [20]. Another variant, named Attention U-Net, uses an attention mechanism to aid the neural network in learning where to "pay attention," and this method allows the model to have more explainability, which is a crucial aspect of AI, especially in the clinical setting [21].

In this study, we chose not to include preprocessing steps because our primary objective was to develop a model that could perform robustly under raw surgical conditions, thereby increasing its generalizability across diverse clinical environments. By using raw input data, we aimed to validate the model's effectiveness without relying on preprocessing, which might introduce biases or dependencies that are difficult to standardize in practice. However, in certain scenarios, preprocessing methods such as image normalization, contrast enhancement, or noise reduction could enhance the model performance, particularly for challenging or inconsistent imaging conditions. Future research could explore the addition of preprocessing techniques for specific applications where standardized imaging environments are available, and these methods could help to further improve segmentation accuracy and reduce variability.

5. Conclusions

Our study demonstrates the promising potential of U-Net-based deep learning models for neural tissue recognition in spinal endoscopy, achieving a DSC of 0.824 and a Jaccard index of 0.701. These metrics indicate competitive performance compared to similar medical image segmentation tasks. The precision and recall scores of 0.810 and 0.839, respectively, further demonstrate the robustness of our model in accurately identifying neural tissues, even in challenging surgical environments. While the results are encouraging, further research is necessary to enhance the model performance and expand its applicability to diverse tissue types. These advancements could provide significant support to spine surgeons, particularly those with less experience, and ultimately improve the surgical outcomes and patient safety during endoscopic procedures.

Author Contributions: Conceptualization, H.K.; formal analysis, H.R.L.; investigation, W.R.; writing—original draft preparation, H.R.L., W.R., S.Y.C. and H.K.; writing—review and editing, H.K., H.R.L., W.R., S.Y.C. and B.-S.C. All authors have read and agreed to the published version of the manuscript.

Funding: This research received no external funding.

Institutional Review Board Statement: This study has been approved by the Public Institutional Review Board (IRB) of the National Bioethics Policy Institute through the public e-IRB system. The IRB approval number and approval date for this study are "2024-1010-001" and 16 August 2024.

Informed Consent Statement: Informed consent was waived by the IRB due to the retrospective nature of this study.

Data Availability Statement: Data related to the findings of this study are available from the corresponding author upon reasonable request.

Acknowledgments: We thank Kuk-Jin Yoon and the graduate students of the Visual Intelligence Laboratory at the Korea Advanced Institute of Science and Technology for their efforts to review our manuscript prior to submission.

Conflicts of Interest: The authors declare no conflicts of interest.

References

1. Junjie, L.; Jiheng, Y.; Jun, L.; haixiong, L.; Haifeng, Y. Comparison of Unilateral Biportal Endoscopy Decompression and Microscopic Decompression Effectiveness in Lumbar Spinal Stenosis Treatment: A Systematic Review and Meta-analysis. *Asian Spine J.* **2023**, *17*, 418–430. [CrossRef] [PubMed]
2. Kim, J.-E.; Choi, D.-J.; Park, E.J.J.; Lee, H.-J.; Hwang, J.-H.; Kim, M.-C.; Oh, J.-S. Biportal Endoscopic Spinal Surgery for Lumbar Spinal Stenosis. *Asian Spine J.* **2019**, *13*, 334–342. [CrossRef] [PubMed]
3. Kim, S.-K.; Kang, S.-S.; Hong, Y.-H.; Park, S.-W.; Lee, S.-C. Clinical comparison of unilateral biportal endoscopic technique versus open microdiscectomy for single-level lumbar discectomy: A multicenter, retrospective analysis. *J. Orthop. Surg. Res.* **2018**, *13*, 22. [CrossRef] [PubMed]
4. Kwon, J.-W.; Moon, S.-H.; Park, S.-Y.; Park, S.-J.; Park, S.-R.; Suk, K.-S.; Kim, H.-S.; Lee, B.H. Lumbar Spinal Stenosis: Review Update 2022. *Asian Spine J.* **2022**, *16*, 789–798. [CrossRef] [PubMed]
5. Lewandrowski, K.-U.; Hellinger, S.; De Carvalho, P.S.T.; Freitas Ramos, M.R.; Soriano-SáNchez, J.-A.; Xifeng, Z.; Calderaro, A.L.; Dos Santos, T.S.; Ramírez León, J.F.; de Lima e SilvA, M.S.; et al. Dural Tears During Lumbar Spinal Endoscopy: Surgeon Skill, Training, Incidence, Risk Factors, and Management. *Int. J. Spine Surg.* **2021**, *15*, 280. [CrossRef] [PubMed]
6. Park, H.-J.; Kim, S.-K.; Lee, S.-C.; Kim, W.; Han, S.; Kang, S.-S. Dural Tears in Percutaneous Biportal Endoscopic Spine Surgery: Anatomical Location and Management. *World Neurosurg.* **2020**, *136*, e578–e585. [CrossRef] [PubMed]
7. Ryu, K.; Kitaguchi, D.; Nakajima, K.; Ishikawa, Y.; Harai, Y.; Yamada, A.; Lee, Y.; Hayashi, K.; Kosugi, N.; Hasegawa, H.; et al. Deep learning-based vessel automatic recognition for laparoscopic right hemicolectomy. *Surg. Endosc.* **2024**, *38*, 171–178. [CrossRef] [PubMed]
8. Chan, H.-P.; Samala, R.K.; Hadjiiski, L.M.; Zhou, C. Deep Learning in Medical Image Analysis. In *Deep Learning in Medical Image Analysis: Challenges and Applications*; Lee, G., Fujita, H., Eds.; Springer International Publishing: Cham, Switzerland, 2020; pp. 3–21.
9. Chen, D.; Yang, W.; Wang, L.; Tan, S.; Lin, J.; Bu, W. PCAT-UNet: UNet-like network fused convolution and transformer for retinal vessel segmentation. *PLoS ONE* **2022**, *17*, e0262689. [CrossRef] [PubMed]

10. Chen, L.C.; Papandreou, G.; Kokkinos, I.; Murphy, K.; Yuille, A.L. DeepLab: Semantic Image Segmentation with Deep Convolutional Nets, Atrous Convolution, and Fully Connected CRFs. *IEEE Trans. Pattern Anal. Mach. Intell.* **2018**, *40*, 834–848. [CrossRef] [PubMed]
11. Shelhamer, E.; Long, J.; Darrell, T. Fully Convolutional Networks for Semantic Segmentation. *IEEE Trans. Pattern Anal. Mach. Intell.* **2017**, *39*, 640–651. [CrossRef] [PubMed]
12. He, K.; Gkioxari, G.; Dollár, P.; Girshick, R. Mask R-CNN. In Proceedings of the 2017 IEEE International Conference on Computer Vision (ICCV), Venice, Italy, 22–29 October 2017; pp. 2980–2988.
13. Feng, X.; Yang, J.; Laine, A.F.; Angelini, E.D. Discriminative Localization in CNNs for Weakly-Supervised Segmentation of Pulmonary Nodules. In Proceedings of the Medical Image Computing and Computer Assisted Intervention−MICCAI 2017: 20th International Conference, Quebec City, QC, Canada, 11–13 September 2017; Volume 10435, pp. 568–576. [CrossRef]
14. Cho, S.M.; Kim, Y.G.; Jeong, J.; Kim, I.; Lee, H.J.; Kim, N. Automatic tip detection of surgical instruments in biportal endoscopic spine surgery. *Comput. Biol. Med.* **2021**, *133*, 104384. [CrossRef] [PubMed]
15. Niha, A.; Muhammad, H.; Khurram, K.; Fatima, F.; Fahad, U. An Artificial Intelligence model for implant segmentation on periapical radiographs. *J. Pak. Med. Assoc.* **2024**, *74*, S-5–S-9. [CrossRef]
16. Ronneberger, O.; Fischer, P.; Brox, T. U-Net: Convolutional Networks for Biomedical Image Segmentation. In Proceedings of the Medical Image Computing and Computer-Assisted Intervention–MICCAI 2015, Cham, Switzerland, 5–9 October 2015; pp. 234–241.
17. Siddique, N.; Paheding, S.; Elkin, C.P.; Devabhaktuni, V. U-Net and Its Variants for Medical Image Segmentation: A Review of Theory and Applications. *IEEE Access* **2021**, *9*, 82031–82057. [CrossRef]
18. He, K.; Gkioxari, G.; Dollar, P.; Girshick, R. Mask R-CNN. *IEEE Trans. Pattern Anal. Mach. Intell.* **2020**, *42*, 386–397. [CrossRef] [PubMed]
19. Kundu, S.; Karale, V.; Ghorai, G.; Sarkar, G.; Ghosh, S.; Dhara, A.K. Nested U-Net for Segmentation of Red Lesions in Retinal Fundus Images and Sub-image Classification for Removal of False Positives. *J. Digit. Imaging* **2022**, *35*, 1111–1119. [CrossRef] [PubMed]
20. Md Zahangir, A.; Chris, Y.; Mahmudul, H.; Tarek, M.T.; Vijayan, K.A. Recurrent residual U-Net for medical image segmentation. *J. Med. Imaging* **2019**, *6*, 014006. [CrossRef]
21. Oktay, O.; Schlemper, J.; Folgoc, L.L.; Lee, M.; Heinrich, M.; Misawa, K.; Mori, K.; McDonagh, S.; Hammerla, N.Y.; Kainz, B. Attention u-net: Learning where to look for the pancreas. *arXiv* **2018**, arXiv:1804.03999.
22. Xavier, G.; Yoshua, B. Understanding the difficulty of training deep feedforward neural networks. In Proceedings of the Thirteenth International Conference on Artificial Intelligence and Statistics, Sardinia, Italy, 31 March 2010; pp. 249–256.
23. Ioffe, S.; Szegedy, C. Batch normalization: Accelerating deep network training by reducing internal covariate shift. In Proceedings of the 32nd International Conference on International Conference on Machine Learning, Lille, France, 7–9 July 2015; Volume 37, pp. 448–456.
24. Yun, S.; Han, D.; Chun, S.; Oh, S.J.; Yoo, Y.; Choe, J. CutMix: Regularization Strategy to Train Strong Classifiers With Localizable Features. In Proceedings of the 2019 IEEE/CVF International Conference on Computer Vision (ICCV), Seoul, Republic of Korea, 27 October–2 November 2019; pp. 6022–6031.
25. Zhang, Z.; Liu, Q.; Wang, Y. Road Extraction by Deep Residual U-Net. *IEEE Geosci. Remote Sens. Lett.* **2018**, *15*, 749–753. [CrossRef]
26. Bu, J.; Lei, Y.; Wang, Y.; Zhao, J.; Huang, S.; Liang, J.; Wang, Z.; Xu, L.; He, B.; Dong, M.; et al. A Multi-Element Identification System Based on Deep Learning for the Visual Field of Percutaneous Endoscopic Spine Surgery. *Indian J. Orthop.* **2024**, *58*, 587–597. [CrossRef] [PubMed]
27. Wang, W.; Yu, K.; Hugonot, J.; Fua, P.; Salzmann, M. Recurrent U-Net for Resource-Constrained Segmentation. In Proceedings of the 2019 IEEE/CVF International Conference on Computer Vision (ICCV), Seoul, Republic of Korea, 27 October–2 November 2019; pp. 2142–2151.

bioengineering

MDPI

Article

Evaluation of Patients' Levels of Walking Independence Using Inertial Sensors and Neural Networks in an Acute-Care Hospital

Tatsuya Sugimoto [1,2,*], Nobuhito Taniguchi [3], Ryoto Yoshikura [3], Hiroshi Kawaguchi [3] and Shintaro Izumi [3,4]

1 Department of Rehabilitation, Japanese Red Cross Kobe Hospital, Kobe 651-0073, Japan
2 Graduate School of System Informatics, Kobe University, Kobe 657-8501, Japan
3 Graduate School of Science Technology and Innovation, Kobe University, Kobe 657-8501, Japan; shin@cs28.cs.kobe-u.ac.jp (S.I.)
4 Osaka Heat Cool Inc., Osaka 562-0035, Japan
* Correspondence: tatsuya.rgmsqz7@gmail.com

Abstract: This study aimed to evaluate walking independence in acute-care hospital patients using neural networks based on acceleration and angular velocity from two walking tests. Forty patients underwent the 10-m walk test and the Timed Up-and-Go test at normal speed, with or without a cane. Physiotherapists divided the patients into two groups: 24 patients who were monitored or independent while walking with a cane or without aids in the ward, and 16 patients who were not. To classify these groups, the Transformer model analyzes the left gait cycle data from eight inertial sensors. The accuracy using all the sensor data was 0.836. When sensor data from the right ankle, right wrist, and left wrist were excluded, the accuracy decreased the most. When analyzing the data from these three sensors alone, the accuracy was 0.795. Further reducing the number of sensors to only the right ankle and wrist resulted in an accuracy of 0.736. This study demonstrates the potential of a neural network-based analysis of inertial sensor data for clinically assessing a patient's level of walking independence.

Keywords: neural network; inertial sensor; level of walking independence; 10-m walk test; timed up-and-go test

1. Introduction

The recent global aging trend has led to an increased number of elderly patients admitted to acute-care hospitals. Consequently, many patients exhibit inherent walking impairments due to underlying illnesses and frailty [1]. Given the risk of further decline in walking function resulting from post-hospitalization treatments and prolonged bed rest, it becomes imperative to maintain or restore walking function through appropriate rehabilitation assessments and exercise therapies [2,3]. One approach to increasing ambulation practice during hospitalization involves physiotherapists allowing patients in the process of regaining ambulation to walk within the ward, either under the supervision of medical staff or independently. Thus, promoting ambulation independence at an appropriate juncture is significant for mitigating the adverse effects of rest-related disuse syndrome and facilitating early hospital discharge. However, switching to walking with a cane or without an aid can be complex for patients with advanced walking with a walker. This is because, unlike using a walker, walking with a cane or no aid increases the risk of falls owing to the reduced support surface.

The 10-m walk test (10 MWT) and Timed Up-and-Go test (TUG) are commonly used in clinical practice to assess gait function objectively. The 10 MWT involves walking 10 m in a straight line at a comfortable pace, with the time taken to calculate walking speed using a stopwatch. Previous research on community-dwelling elderly individuals has identified a 10 MWT time of 10 s or longer, corresponding to a walking speed cutoff value of 1.0 m/s or less, as a diagnostic criterion for frailty [4,5] and a predictor of long-term care needs [6].

Conversely, the TUG starts from a seated position and involves rising from the chair upon cue, walking at a comfortable or maximum speed to a designated point 3 m away, changing direction at that point, returning to the chair, and measuring the time taken to complete the task [7]. Research on community-dwelling older adults has associated a TUG cutoff value of 13.5 s or more with an increased risk of falls in daily living [8]. Therefore, shorter completion times for both tests indicated better walking and balance functions. However, it is essential to note that the hospital environment, a controlled space without steps or obstacles, may not necessarily require patients to meet these cutoff values to determine their level of walking independence. In clinical practice, physiotherapists may permit patients with slower movement speeds who do not meet the cutoff values to walk in the hospital ward after evaluating their movement techniques. Thus, the assessment of the level of walking independence considers not only movement speed but also the actual method of movement, highlighting the importance of subjective judgment by physiotherapists. However, the evaluation of the movement techniques lacks objectivity.

Various devices are available to assess movements objectively; however, inertial sensors are simple and versatile. In this approach, a small and lightweight sensor is affixed to the patient's body, and the acceleration and angular velocity are recorded during walking to evaluate movement characteristics. Numerous prior studies have utilized inertial sensors to evaluate the 10 MWT and compare healthy individuals with patients [9–11], but few studies have compared differences in physical function among patients. For instance, one study examined patients with cerebrovascular disease (CVD) within 1–6 months after illness onset [12]. In this study, patients wore inertial sensors on the head, chest, and lower back and were categorized into monitoring and independent groups based on their level of walking independence. The results indicated that patients in the monitoring group exhibited significantly lower acceleration amplitudes and symmetry in these three regions than those in the independent group. Similarly, inertial sensors have been employed in the TUG, enabling data segmentation from the lumbar and ankle regions into six sub-phases: sit-to-stand, two walking phases, two turning phases, and stand-to-sit [13]. A study comparing different fall risks in patients with CVD at least 6 months post-onset found that those requiring more than 20 s to complete the TUG exhibited significantly longer walking and turning times as well as lower angular velocities during turning [14].

Therefore, the acceleration and angular velocity data during these tests reflect the clinical fall risk and level of walking independence. Hence, inpatients with various diseases undergoing rehabilitation interventions performed the TUG at maximum speed using an inertial sensor attached to the lower back [15]. Patients were categorized into three groups based on their level of walking independence and a TUG time cutoff of 13.5 s. Results revealed that, consistent with previous findings, the monitoring and independent groups requiring more than 13.5 s demonstrated significantly longer total TUG times than those requiring less than 13.5 s. However, differences in walking time and angular velocity during turning were only observed between the monitoring group and the independent group, which required less than 13.5 s, with no significant differences observed between the latter and the independent group, which required more than 13.5 s. This suggests that, even among patients with slower movement speeds, distinctions based on their level of walking independence were discernible.

In recent years, acceleration and angular velocity data analysis using machine learning, especially neural networks (NN), have been increasingly used for further data analysis. This approach allows for a more comprehensive and detailed evaluation of gait function, including the interrelationships among different measurement items. In a previous study involving healthy subjects, smartwatches with built-in inertial sensors were worn on the left and right wrists [16]. The participants were instructed to perform a 15-m walk at normal speed with and without visual field restrictions. The classification accuracies of these conditions were compared using four methods: random forest (RF), support vector machine (SVM), convolutional neural network (CNN), and recurrent neural network (RNN). The results indicated that the CNN and RNN models outperformed traditional machine learning methods. Another study investigated the use of NN to predict differences in fall risk among community-dwelling elderly individuals aged 65 years or older [17]. The participants performed the TUG with inertial sensors attached to their necks and feet. The data were analyzed using SVMs and CNN, with the CNN model showing higher sensitivity, particularly when analyzing the angular velocity of the neck. Similarly, in another study, a 55-year-old community resident performed the TUG with an inertial sensor attached to the waist [18]. The fall risk level classification accuracy was compared among machine learning methods such as RF, SVM, and CNN. The CNN model exhibited the highest accuracy.

These findings suggest that NN-based analysis can be applied to classify walking independence among hospitalized patients, as the acceleration and angular velocity during walking tasks vary depending on the patient's physical function and fall risk. However, no such studies have been conducted to date. Therefore, this study aimed to develop an NN model to evaluate the level of walking independence of patients admitted to an acute-care hospital based on acceleration and angular velocity data collected during the 10 MWT and TUG. The anticipated outcome was that the model's accuracy would be comparable to that of judgments made by physiotherapists.

2. Materials and Methods

2.1. Patients

A total of 40 patients (mean age 78.2 years, range 52–94 years) were enrolled in this study, comprising 19 men and 21 women. These patients were admitted to the acute-care hospital for emergency or surgical purposes related to medical and surgical conditions and subsequently received rehabilitation intervention. The inclusion criteria were as follows: (1) patients who were independently ambulating with a cane or unaided before admission; (2) patients who were capable of ambulating with a walker, at least independently, at the time of measurement; and (3) patients who had initiated practicing walking with a cane or no aid within one week. The exclusion criteria included evident cognitive decline, comorbidities, or medical history that would impede gait practice or measurement.

Patients were classified into two groups: the "Walking Acquired" (WA group) comprised those who ambulated with a cane or unaided within the ward, with or without monitoring, while the "Not Acquired" (NA group) included patients who still required a walker for ambulation.

2.2. Measurement Procedure

Before testing, using Velcro bands, eight inertial sensors (Xsens DOT, Xsens) equipped with built-in triaxial acceleration and angular velocity sensors were attached to the patient's body. The sensors were affixed to the chest over the sternum lower back at the level of the third lumbar vertebra, above the right and left wrists, midfront of the right and left thighs, and above the right and left ankles. These sensors had a measurement range of 16 G for acceleration and 2000 °/s for angular velocity, with a sampling frequency of 120 Hz. Six acceleration and angular velocity signals were continuously recorded for each sensor during both 10 MWT and TUG. The signals include three acceleration axes: anterior-posterior acceleration (X-axis), mediolateral acceleration (Y-axis), and vertical acceleration (Z-axis), and three angular velocity axes: roll, which is the rotation around the X-axis; pitch, which is the rotation around the Y-axis; and yaw, which is the rotation around the Z-axis. The sensors were connected to a tablet device (iPad Mini, Apple) via Bluetooth and operated using a dedicated application.

After explaining the method of each test to the subjects, we commenced the 10 MWT. A straight line of 16 m, including acceleration and deceleration paths of 3 m each, was used, and the time required to cover the central 10 m was measured using a stopwatch. Subsequently, the TUG was performed. The TUG used a chair with a seat height of 43 cm and one cone. Using a stopwatch, we measured the time required to stand up from the chair, walk 3 m, turn at the cone, return, and sit down again. Figure 1 shows an actual TUG measurement scene with an attached inertial sensor. Both tests were conducted twice at normal speed, and the patients were instructed to walk with or without a cane. The decision regarding the mode of walking was made in consultation with the physiotherapists in charge and the patients themselves. Other physical functions assessed included grip strength and the Frailty Screening Index (FSI) [19]. Patients were also asked about any falls they may have experienced in the past year.

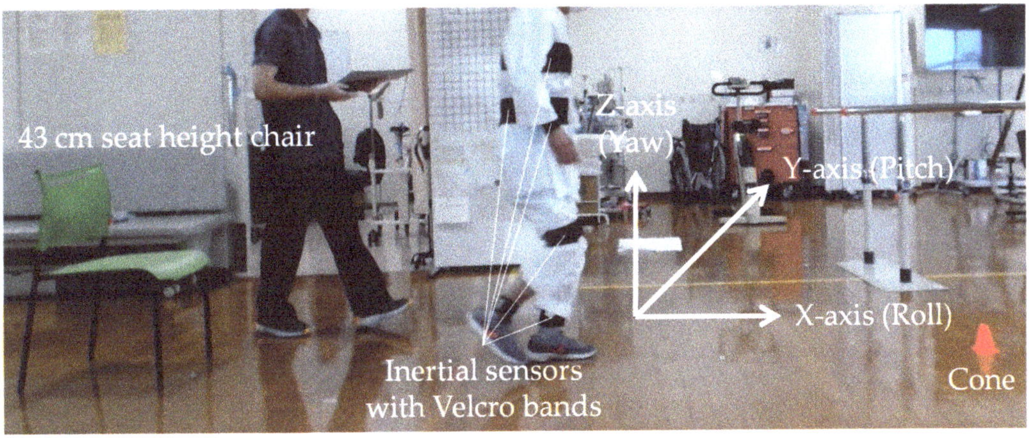

Figure 1. Sensor attachment sites and TUG measurement scene.

2.3. Signal Processing

After the measurement, the data from each sensor were transferred to a laptop using dedicated software to synchronize the data between the sensors. The 10 MWT data from both trials were analyzed, excluding the first and last steps and including data from the acceleration and deceleration paths. The TUG followed the method of a previous study [13], with the sub-phases of sit-to-stand and stand-to-sit, as well as the start and end points of the two turning phases, identified. Specifically, the sit-to-stand and stand-to-sit phases were identified by the maximum and minimum values of the pitch angle of the lumbar angular velocity, respectively (see the pitch angle in the lower part of Figure 2). Additionally, the two turning phases were identified as the maximum absolute value of the yaw angle, followed by locating the range before or after this value and below a threshold value of 0.1 (see the yaw angle in the lower part of Figure 2). The first walking phase was defined as the period from the end of the sit-to-stand phase to the start of the first turn. The second walking phase was defined as the period from the end of the first turn to the start of the second turn. In this study, only these walking phases were used in both tests to analyze the data while walking in conjunction with the 10 MWT.

Pre-processing for use with the NN input data was performed as follows: First, the acceleration data were high-pass filtered at 1 Hz to exclude the effects of gravitational acceleration. Next, to use the data for each gait cycle, the combined accelerations of the right and left ankles, as shown in Equation (1), were calculated, respectively. These calculations were then differentiated from one sample neighbor, and the periodic peak value was defined as the initial contact (IC) for each cycle (Figure 3). For example, if the right gait cycle is 4 steps in the first walking phase of the TUG and three steps in the second phase, seven data sets for the right gait cycle were obtained. This study used left gait cycle data in the analysis because more left gait cycle datasets were obtained than right.

$$Combined\ Acceleration = \sqrt{Acceleration^2_{X-axis} + Acceleration^2_{Y-axis} + Acceleration^2_{Z-axis}} \quad (1)$$

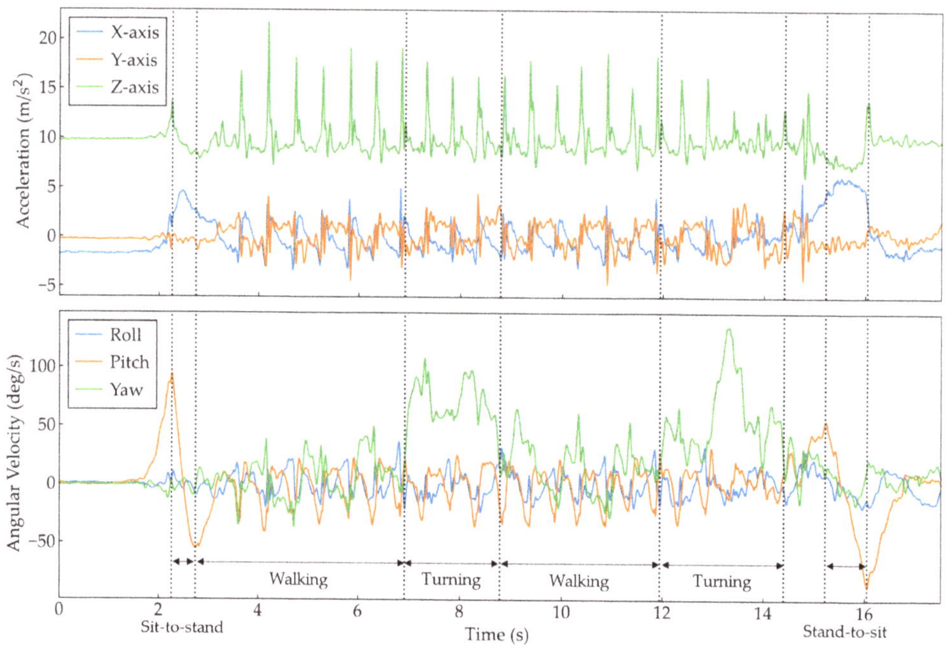

Figure 2. Example of acceleration and angular velocity of the lumbar during TUG.

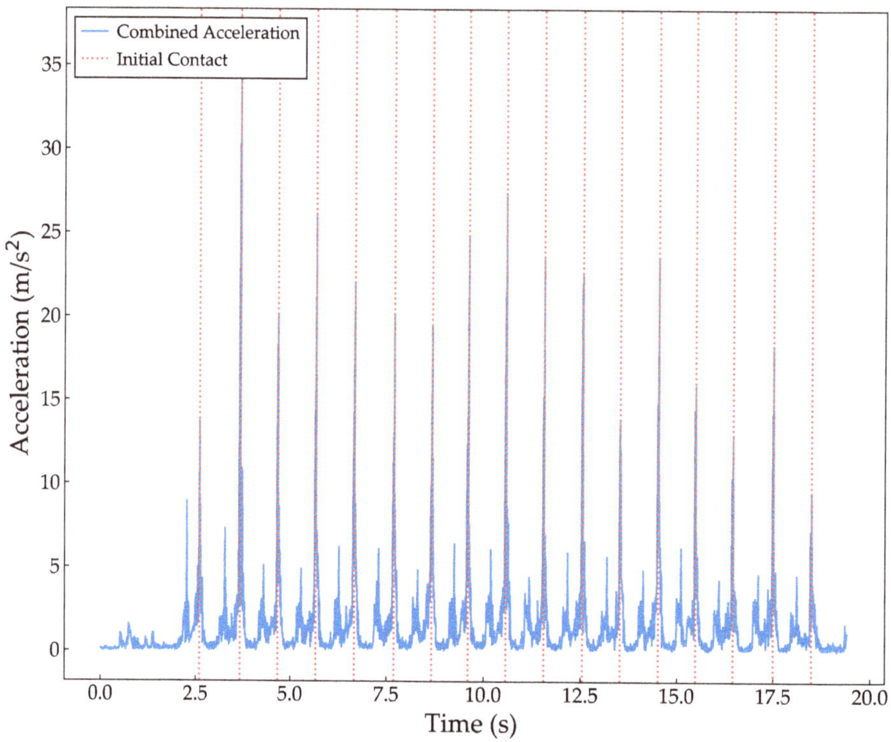

Figure 3. Example of identifying ICs from the combined acceleration of the ankle during 10 MWT.

Furthermore, as a method of normalization, the acceleration and angular velocity were set to a range of 0 to 1 so that the baseline of each dataset was 0.5, as they varied in both the positive and negative directions. Specifically, for each of the three axes of acceleration and angular velocity for each subject, the value of each sensor was divided by the maximum absolute value of all sensor values, then by 2, and a 0.5 was added. Depending on whether the maximum value used for the division is positive or negative, the normalized data will satisfy either a minimum value of zero or a maximum value of one for any sensor in any gait cycle within a trial. Finally, to align the lengths of all data sets, a 0.5 was added to the end of the data set shorter than 276, the longest walking cycle (Figure 4). All the data processing steps were performed using Python and its libraries.

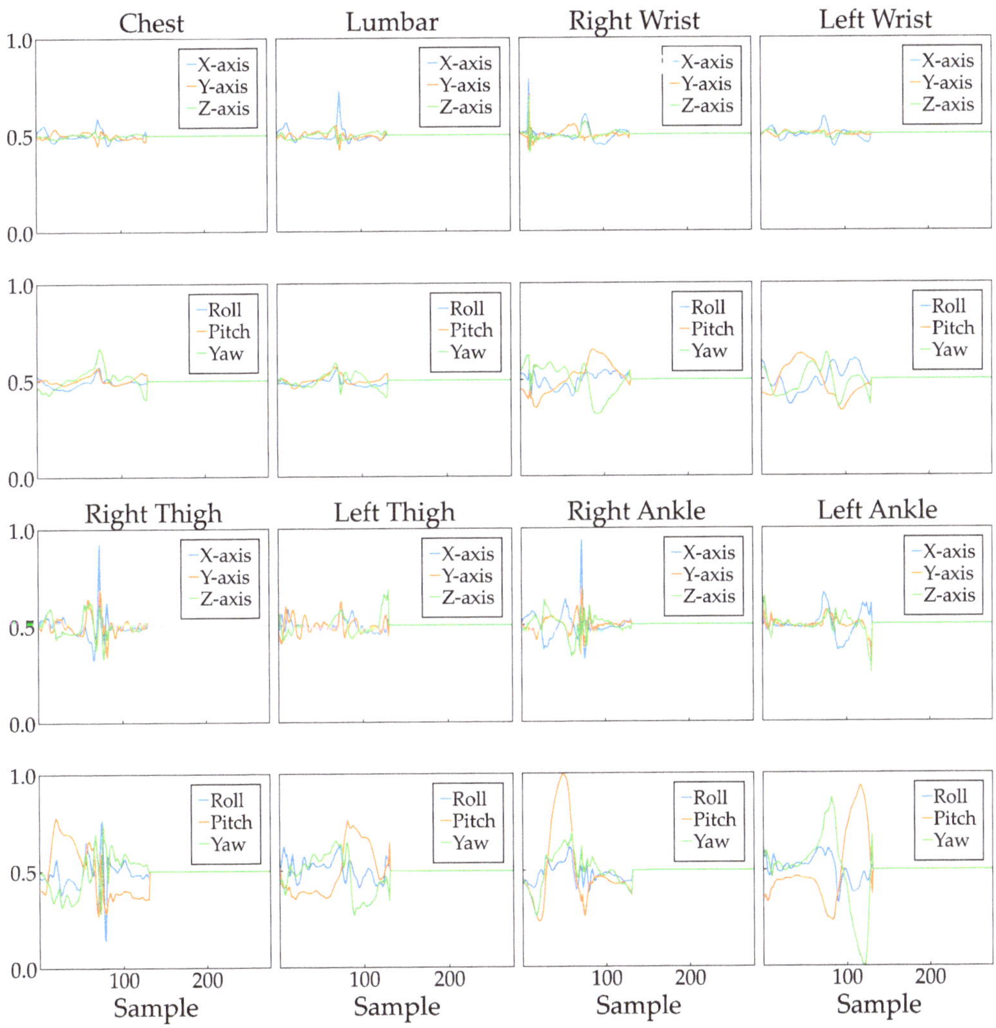

Figure 4. Example of normalized data for all 48 channels in one left gait cycle.

2.4. Neural Network

Transformer was implemented using PyTorch version 2.0.0, a Python library. The Transformer is a machine-learning model [20] known for its strong performance in natural language processing and image recognition tasks. It is built around an attention mechanism (attention) that selectively highlights important feature information by computing the association between each input element and the other elements. This enabled the model to effectively capture long-distance dependencies and flexibly learn feature combinations at different locations. The architecture of the Transformer model used in this study included an input layer, Input Embedding, Positional Encoding, Transformer Block, Fully Connected (FC) layer, Softmax Function, and an output layer. The Transformer Block comprises a multihead attention module, feed-forward module, Layer Normalization, and residual connection, which were repeated five times in this study for deeper learning. The program defined a class using nn.Module and nn.TransformerEncoder, which incorporated the embedding layer, Positional Encoding layer, Transformer's encoder layer, and FC layer. The structure of the Transformer network is illustrated in Figure 5, and the specifics of the parameters for each network layer are listed in Table 1. The input and output sizes from the input data to the Transformer Block in Table 1 represent the batch size, data length, and number of channels, respectively. Details regarding the batch size and number of channels are described below.

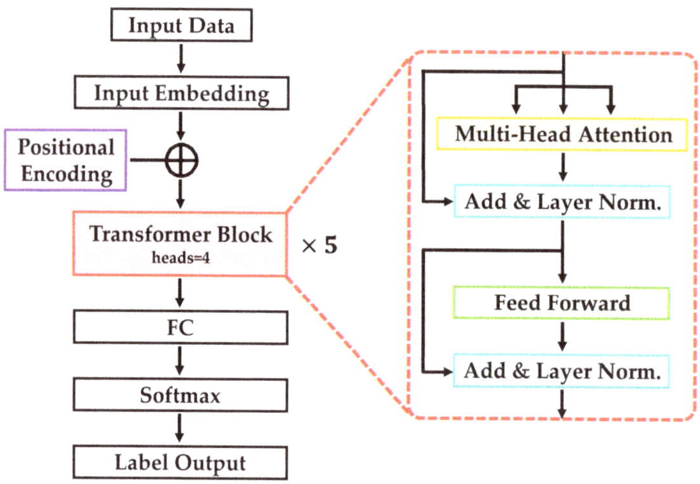

Figure 5. Transformer network architecture diagram.

Table 1. Detailed parameters for each network layer.

Layer	Input	Output
Input Embedding	(64, 276, 48)	(64, 276, 48)
Positional Encoding	(64, 276, 48)	(64, 276, 48)
Transformer Block	(64, 276, 48)	(64, 276, 48)
FC	(64, 13248)	(64, 2)

To augment the total input data, this study included the original dataset and four additional datasets, each with random noise ranging from −0.1 to 0.1 added to every value. This approach resulted in a five-fold increase in data points compared with the original dataset. The data ratio between the two groups was balanced in the training and test datasets, with a test data ratio of 0.1. The training process utilized 130 epochs, a batch size of 64, and a learning rate of 1×10^{-5}. The final accuracies of the training and test datasets were recorded. For evaluation, the leave-one-out-of-one cross-validation (LOOCV) method was employed, wherein each subject was iteratively excluded from the training, and the resulting model was used to predict the omitted subject. This process yielded 40 models, corresponding to the number of subjects in the dataset. A confusion matrix was generated for each inference according to Table 2, and the accuracy, sensitivity, and specificity, as expressed in Equations (2)–(4), were calculated. In the present study, the NA group was defined as positive.

$$Accuracy = \frac{TP + TN}{TP + TN + FP + FN} \tag{2}$$

$$Sensitivity = \frac{TP}{TP + FN} \tag{3}$$

$$Specificity = \frac{TN}{TN + FP} \tag{4}$$

Table 2. Confusion matrix.

True Label	Predicted Label	
	Positive (NA Group)	Negative (WA Group)
Positive (NA group)	True Positive (TP)	False Negative (FN)
Negative (WA group)	False Positive (FP)	True Negative (TN)

The input data consisted of 48 channels comprising six axes of acceleration and angular rate meters for each of the eight sensors per subject. To propose a more straightforward method for clinical applications, this study assessed the model's performance with a reduced number of sensors. Specifically, the average accuracy of LOOCV was evaluated by excluding one sensor at a time. When excluded, five sensors were identified as important sites based on a significant decline in accuracy. Subsequently, two to five sensors were used for validation. All excluded sensor data were replaced with a value of 0.5 to maintain consistency.

2.5. Statistical Analysis

Statistical methods were used to compare basic information between the groups. The chi-square or Fisher's exact test was used to compare categorical variables such as sex ratio, outcome (discharge or transfer), and history of falls in the past year. For other items, an unpaired *t*-test or Mann-Whitney U-test was used after checking each data point's normal distribution and homogeneity of variance for group comparison. Statistical analyses were performed using a two-tailed test with Modified R Commander version 4.2.2 [21]. The level of statistical significance was set at a p value < 0.05. Descriptive statistics (means and standard deviations) were used to summarize the results.

3. Results

All trials were completed without adverse events in 26 and 14 patients in the WA and NA groups, respectively. The patient characteristics for each group are shown in Table 3. The diseases included spinal compression fractures, postoperative femoral neck fractures, postoperative knee or hip osteoarthritis (OA), postoperative lumbar spinal canal stenosis (LCS), CVD, and other medical conditions. The WA group was significantly younger than the NA group, had a significantly higher proportion of patients discharged home as the outcome destination, and the 10 MWT and TUG times were significantly shorter. The walking speeds calculated from the 10 MWT times of the WA and NA groups averaged 0.85 m/s and 0.61 m/s, respectively. There were no differences in the number of days from admission to measurement or the length of hospital stay between the groups.

Table 3. Basic information for each group (M: male, F: female). Data are shown as the mean (standard deviation) except where noted. *p* values less than 0.05 are highlighted in bold.

	WA Group (n = 26)	NA Group (n = 14)	p Values
Age (years)	76.4 (10.3)	81.6 (3.8)	**0.029**
Gender	14 M, 12 F	5 M, 9 F	0.270
Height (cm)	158.1 (10.0)	156.5 (11.7)	0.671
Weight (kg)	56.5 (13.5)	58.4 (13.7)	0.672
Measurement since admission (days)	16.8 (8.5)	19.8 (7.1)	0.254
Total length of stay (days)	23.2 (8.1)	29.1 (10.2)	0.072
Discharge and transfer	22, 4	1, 13	**<0.001**
Diseases:			
Postoperative LCS	6	2	
Postoperative femoral neck fracture	2	6	
Postoperative knee or hip OA	5	1	
CVD	1	3	
Others	12	2	
10MWT time (s)	12.4 (2.8)	18.1 (6.4)	**0.006**
TUG time (s)	14.7 (2.9)	21.2 (6.6)	**0.003**
Grip strength (kg)	22.4 (8.8)	19.2 (10.4)	0.339
FSI (from 0 to 5)	1.5 (1.2)	2.1 (1.3)	0.148
Faller, %	5, 19.2	7, 50.0	0.071

Because two patients had missing TUG measurement data, we analyzed 40 patients for the 10 MWT and 38 patients for the TUG. The total number of gait cycles analyzed was 1684, with 981 in the WA and 703 in the NA groups. The dataset size was increased fivefold at each training iteration, resulting in approximately 8000 datasets. When trained with all eight sensors, the accuracy, sensitivity, and specificity were 0.836, 0.876, and 0.780, respectively. The confusion matrix and inference results for each subject are shown in Figure 6. Most subjects had an accuracy of 0.5 or better, but subjects 18 in the WA group and 1 and 3 in the NA group did not improve with further changes in the hyperparameters during learning. Next, we checked accuracy by excluding one sensor at a time to identify the critical sensor attachment sites for learning and inference. The results show that the accuracy decreased significantly for the right ankle (0.709), left wrist (0.730), right wrist (0.735), right thigh (0.801), and chest (0.812), as shown in Figure 7. Training with these five sensors yielded a slightly lower accuracy of 0.830, whereas the specificity improved to 0.821 compared to all eight sensors (Figure 8). Using three sensors (right ankle, left wrist, and right wrist) resulted in an accuracy of 0.795, which was lower than that achieved using five sensors (Figure 9). Finally, when comparing the accuracies of the two sensor combinations (right ankle/left wrist and right ankle/right wrist), the latter was superior, with an accuracy of 0.736 (Figure 10). The four LOOCV performance metrics are listed in Table 4.

Table 4. LOOCV performance metrics for each input data.

Input Data	Accuracy	Sensitivity	Specificity
All 8 sensors	0.836	0.876	0.780
5 sensors (right ankle, left wrist, right wrist, right thigh, and chest)	0.830	0.837	0.821
3 sensors (right ankle, left wrist, and right wrist)	0.795	0.784	0.809
2 sensors (right ankle and right wrist)	0.736	0.728	0.748

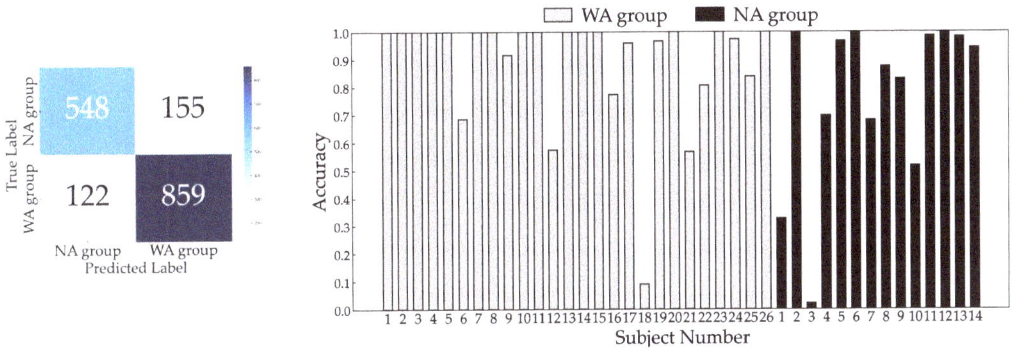

(a) (b)

Figure 6. Confusion matrix (**a**) and individual inference results (**b**) of LOOCV using all sensors.

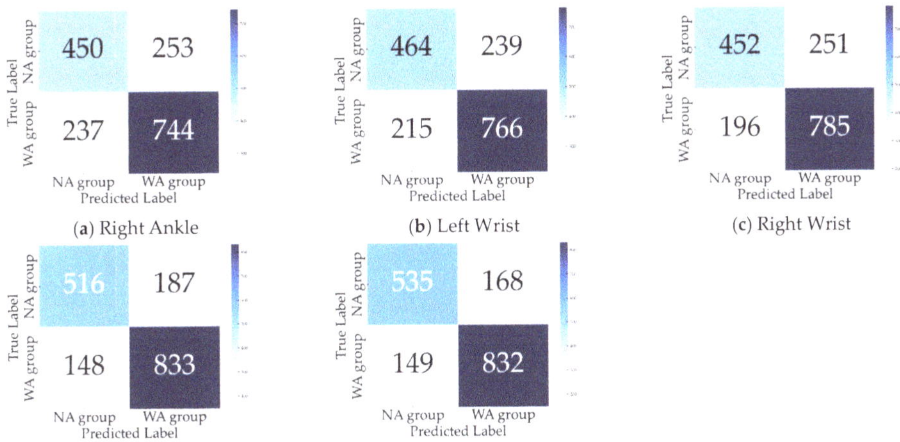

(**a**) Right Ankle (**b**) Left Wrist (**c**) Right Wrist

(**d**) Right Thigh (**e**) Chest

Figure 7. Confusion matrix by excluding (**a**) right ankle, (**b**) left wrist, (**c**) right wrist, (**d**) right thigh, and (**e**) chest.

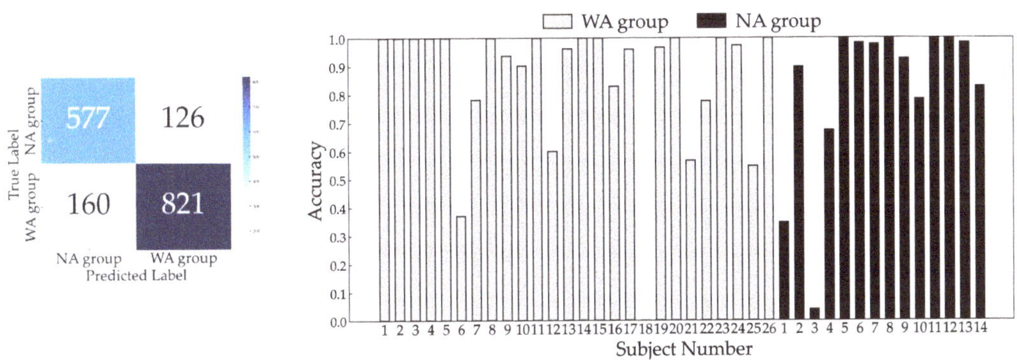

(a) (b)

Figure 8. Confusion matrix (**a**) and individual inference results (**b**) of LOOCV using five sensors: right ankle, left wrist, right wrist, right thigh, and chest.

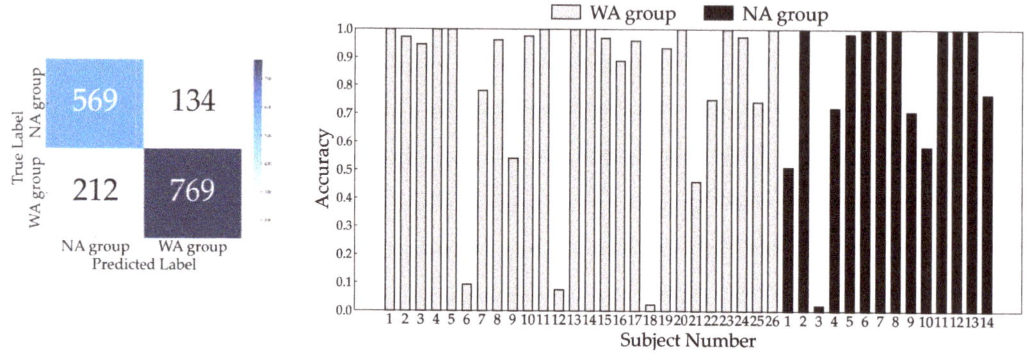

(a) (b)

Figure 9. Confusion matrix (**a**) and individual inference results (**b**) of LOOCV using three sensors: right ankle, left wrist, and right wrist.

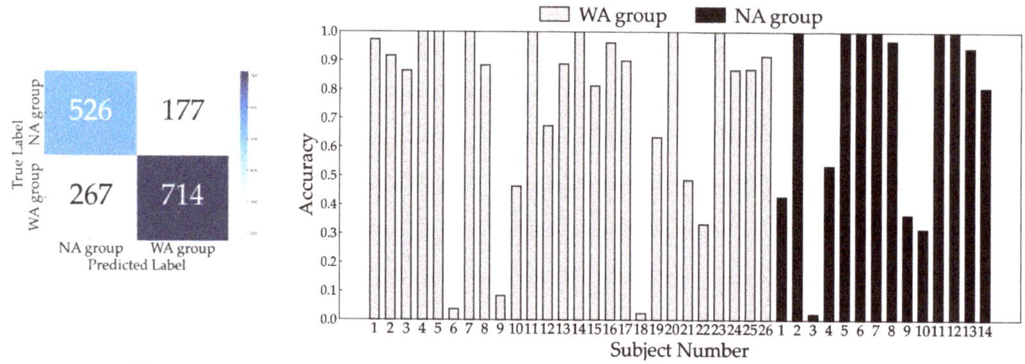

(a) (b)

Figure 10. Confusion matrix (**a**) and individual inference results (**b**) of LOOCV using two sensors: right ankle and right wrist.

4. Discussion

In this study, 40 patients admitted to an acute-care hospital in the early stages of gait practice after beginning cane or unassisted walking were fitted with eight inertial sensors to perform the 10 MWT and TUG. Acceleration and angular velocity while walking were measured to evaluate the patient's level of walking independence using Transformer. The results showed that the accuracy was 0.836 using all sensors, although this was not as good as the evaluation by the physiotherapists. Even when the number of sensor sites was reduced to three and two, the accuracies remained at 0.795 and 0.736, respectively.

In a previous study analyzing inertial sensor data using an NN, 101 community-dwelling elderly people with an average age of approximately 75 years were assessed by clinicians for fall risk, achieving an accuracy of 0.865 based on the angular velocity of the neck during the TUG using a CNN [17]. Additionally, in predicting the occurrence of falls in 73 nursing home residents with an average age of approximately 83 years, a CNN achieved an accuracy of 0.750 using the acceleration and angular velocity of the lower back during a 6-min walk test [22]. Despite the small sample size of the present study (40 patients) and the comparable mean age, the achieved accuracy was similar to that of these studies. On the other hand, the physiotherapists' assessment of the patient's level of walking independence was based on an overall assessment of the time required for the two walking tasks and the actual method of movement. Nevertheless, there were significant group differences in age and time required for the 10 MWT and TUG. This reflects the physical functional decline due to aging and suggests that minimal walking speed may also be important for the possibility of independence.

Additional analyses were conducted for three subjects, 18 in the WA group and one and three in the NA group, who exhibited poor accuracy even with all sensors. Specifically, the first half of the walking phase of these three subjects (corresponding to the first half of the total number of steps of the 10 MWT and the first walking phase of the TUG) and data from all other subjects were used for training. In contrast, the second half of the walking phase of these three subjects (representing the second half of the total number of steps of the 10 MWT and the second walking phase of the TUG) was used to assess accuracy. Although the data extraction points differed, both training and inference involved information from the same subjects. Consequently, the accuracy of the number 18 in the WA group and number 1 in the NA group notably improved, whereas the accuracy of the number 3 in the NA group remained largely unchanged. This suggests that the poor accuracy of the two subjects may be due to the limited sample size. Conversely, it is possible that the motor skills of subject #3 in the NA group were sufficiently high to enable him to practice walking in the ward; however, this capability may not have been recognized. This oversight could be partly attributed to the limited time for physiotherapists to conduct repeated assessments. This study relied on data collected within the first week of walking practice, reflecting the participants' level of walking independence at that specific time.

When the accuracy of LOOCV was examined by excluding one sensor at a time, a significant decrease in accuracy was observed, particularly when the sensors attached to the right foot, left hand, and right hand were excluded. This decrease can be attributed to the crucial role of the right lower limb in the left gait cycle. Specifically, in the left gait cycle, the right lower limb underwent an initial swing phase, followed by the IC and stance phases [23]. The range of motion was greater during the swing phase than during the stance phase because of the forward swing of the limb. The IC phase also involved the lower leg muscles, which supported the floor reaction force [23]. Hence, it is plausible that the acceleration and angular velocity of the contralateral lower limb, encompassing these phases and the transitional phase with a significant range of motion and floor reaction force, are pivotal in determining the level of walking independence. In contrast, the transition of the left lower limb from the stance to the swing phase appeared less critical. This finding is consistent with the fact that instability during gait tends to occur at the IC or shortly after that in clinical situations. Although the ankle is a common site analyzed in previous studies [10,11,15,17], including its relationship with the gait cycle is a novel finding.

Similar to the results for the ankle sensors, the accuracy decreased when sensors attached to the left and right wrists were excluded; however, this could be attributed to the fact that the wrists are also endpoints with a considerable range of motion. The arms swing during walking, as calculated from the inertial sensor data attached to the wrists, decreases with slower walking speed [24] and aging [25]. Additionally, individuals with a history of falls may not increase their arm swing in response to increased walking speed [26]. Therefore, wrist data can reflect a person's gait function. However, most previous studies that analyzed the inertial sensor data using NN in elderly individuals and patients focused on sensors attached to the waist or feet. To our knowledge, only one study validated wrist sensor data conducted on healthy young adults [19]. This study achieved a classification accuracy of 0.889 for the two visibility conditions, although no sensors were worn at other locations. Therefore, the results of our study suggest that wrist acceleration and angular velocity may be essential factors in determining a patient's level of walking independence.

In contrast, data from the lower back, which has been a focal point in prior studies [18,22], exhibited less significance in determining the level of gait independence in this study than data from the wrist and ankle. This discrepancy can be attributed to the normalization method employed in this study. Specifically, the maximum value among all eight normalization sensors consistently originated from the wrist or ankle across all subjects. Consequently, relatively minor acceleration and angular velocity fluctuations were observed in the chest and lower back, as illustrated in Figure 4. This normalization method was selected based on the premise that the interplay between acceleration and angular velocity across different anatomical sites plays a crucial role in determining walking independence. Therefore, modifying the normalization method, such as by adopting regional normalization, may yield diverse outcomes in future investigations.

The limitations of this study include an insufficient sample size and the fact that only walking cycles were used. Concerning the former, further validation with a larger sample size is needed before the results of this study can be generalized. In particular, the latter excluded the sit-to-stand, two-turn, and stand-to-sit sub-phases, which could have provided more critical information. However, focusing on the walking cycle allowed us to consider which body parts were crucial for the classification and why. As in previous studies, future analyses based solely on TUG data should encompass all phases.

5. Conclusions

Through the utilization of eight inertial sensors on hospitalized patients and the analysis of data from the 10 MWT and TUG walking phases with Transformer, one of the NN, we achieved notable accuracy in determining the patient's level of walking independence, with an accuracy of 0.836. This accuracy closely approximated the evaluation accuracy achieved by physiotherapists. Furthermore, the accuracy was maintained at 0.795, even when the number of sensors was limited to three, positioned at both wrists and right ankle. This approach is valuable for mitigating the patient burden during measurements.

Based on the results of this study, this analysis method can support physiotherapists in clinical settings. Specifically, the inference results of the model can supplement the assessment findings of physiotherapists who struggle with deciding whether to allow patients to practice walking in the ward. Additionally, it can be beneficial when a different or less experienced physiotherapist than the one in charge evaluates a patient's walking.

Author Contributions: Conceptualization, T.S., H.K. and S.I.; methodology, T.S., N.T., R.Y. and S.I.; software, T.S., N.T., R.Y. and S.I.; validation, T.S.; formal analysis, T.S.; investigation, T.S.; writing—original draft preparation, T.S.; writing—review and editing, T.S. and S.I.; visualization, T.S.; supervision, H.K. and S.I.; project administration, T.S. and S.I.; funding acquisition, S.I. All authors have read and agreed to the published version of the manuscript.

Funding: This study was partially funded by the Japan Science and Technology Agency (grant number: JPMJPF2115, awarded to S. I.).

Institutional Review Board Statement: This study was conducted in accordance with the Declaration of Helsinki and approved by the Medical Ethics Committee of the Japanese Red Cross Kobe Hospital (registry number: 300).

Informed Consent Statement: Informed consent was obtained from all participants involved in the study.

Data Availability Statement: The datasets presented in this article are not readily available because they are part of an ongoing study. Requests to access the datasets were directed to the first authors' e-mail addresses.

Conflicts of Interest: Author Shintaro Izumi was employed by the company Osaka Heat Cool Inc. The remaining authors declare that the research was conducted in the absence of any commercial or financial relationships that could be construed as a potential conflict of interest.

References

1. Basile, G.; Catalano, A.; Mandraffino, G.; Maltese, G.; Alibrandi, A.; Ciancio, G.; Brischetto, D.; Morabito, N.; Lasco, A.; Cesari, M. Frailty Modifications and Prognostic Impact in Older Patients Admitted in Acute Care. *Aging Clin. Exp. Res.* **2019**, *31*, 151–155. [CrossRef] [PubMed]
2. Martínez-Velilla, N.; Casas-Herrero, A.; Zambom-Ferraresi, F.; Sáez de Asteasu, M.L.; Lucia, A.; Galbete, A.; García-Baztán, A.; Alonso-Renedo, J.; González-Glaría, B.; Gonzalo-Lázaro, M.; et al. Effect of Exercise Intervention on Functional Decline in Very Elderly Patients during Acute Hospitalization: A Randomized Clinical Trial. *JAMA Intern. Med.* **2019**, *179*, 28–36. [CrossRef]

3. Sáez de Asteasu, M.L.; Martínez-Velilla, N.; Zambom-Ferraresi, F.; Casas-Herrero, Á.; Lucía, A.; Galbete, A.; Izquierdo, M. Physical Exercise Improves Function in Acutely Hospitalized Older Patients: Secondary Analysis of a Randomized Clinical Trial. *J. Am. Med. Dir. Assoc.* **2019**, *20*, 866–873. [CrossRef]
4. Satake, S.; Arai, H. The Revised Japanese Version of the Cardiovascular Health Study Criteria (revised J-CHS Criteria). *Geriatr. Gerontol. Int.* **2020**, *20*, 992–993. [CrossRef] [PubMed]
5. Tsutsumimoto, K.; Doi, T.; Makizako, H.; Hotta, R.; Nakakubo, S.; Makino, K.; Suzuki, T.; Shimada, H. Association of Social Frailty with Both Cognitive and Physical Deficits Among Older People. *J. Am. Med. Dir. Assoc.* **2017**, *18*, 603–607. [CrossRef]
6. Shimada, H.; Suzuki, T.; Suzukawa, M.; Makizako, H.; Doi, T.; Yoshida, D.; Tsutsumimoto, K.; Anan, Y.; Uemura, K.; Ito, T.; et al. Performance-Based Assessments and Demand for Personal Care in Older Japanese People: A Cross-Sectional Study. *BMJ Open* **2013**, *3*, e002424. [CrossRef] [PubMed]
7. Podsiadlo, D.; Richardson, S. The Timed "Up & Go": A Test of Basic Functional Mobility for Frail Elderly Persons. *J. Am. Geriatr. Soc.* **1991**, *39*, 142–148.
8. Shumway-Cook, A.; Brauer, S.; Woollacott, M. Predicting the Probability for Falls in Community-Dwelling Older Adults Using the Timed Up & Go Test. *Phys. Ther.* **2000**, *80*, 896–903. [PubMed]
9. Garcia, F.D.V.; da Cunha, M.J.; Schuch, C.P.; Schifino, G.P.; Balbinot, G.; Pagnussat, A.S. Movement Smoothness in Chronic Post-Stroke Individuals Walking in an Outdoor Environment-A Cross-Sectional Study Using IMU Sensors. *PLoS ONE* **2021**, *16*, e0250100. [CrossRef]
10. Voisard, C.; de l'Escalopier, N.; Vienne-Jumeau, A.; Moreau, A.; Quijoux, F.; Bompaire, F.; Sallansonnet, M.; Brechemier, M.-L.; Taifas, I.; Tafani, C.; et al. Innovative Multidimensional Gait Evaluation Using IMU in Multiple Sclerosis: Introducing the Semiogram. *Front. Neurol.* **2023**, *14*, 1237162. [CrossRef]
11. Madsalae, T.; Thongprong, T.; Chaikeeree, N.; Boonsinsukh, R. Changes in Gait Performances during Walking with Head Movements in Older Adults with Chronic Neck Pain. *Front. Med.* **2024**, *11*, 1324375. [CrossRef] [PubMed]
12. Bergamini, E.; Iosa, M.; Belluscio, V.; Morone, G.; Tramontano, M.; Vannozzi, G. Multi-Sensor Assessment of Dynamic Balance during Gait in Patients with Subacute Stroke. *J. Biomech.* **2017**, *61*, 208–215. [CrossRef] [PubMed]
13. Weiss, A.; Mirelman, A.; Buchman, A.S.; Bennett, D.A.; Hausdorff, J.M. Using a Body-Fixed Sensor to Identify Subclinical Gait Difficulties in Older Adults with IADL Disability: Maximizing the Output of the Timed up and Go. *PLoS ONE* **2013**, *8*, e68885. [CrossRef] [PubMed]
14. Spina, S.; Facciorusso, S.; D'Ascanio, M.C.; Morone, G.; Baricich, A.; Fiore, P.; Santamato, A. Sensor Based Assessment of Turning during Instrumented Timed up and Go Test for Quantifying Mobility in Chronic Stroke Patients. *Eur. J. Phys. Rehabil. Med.* **2023**, *59*, 6–13. [CrossRef] [PubMed]
15. Sugimoto, T.; Yoshikura, R.; Kawaguchi, H.; Izumi, S. Quantitative Evaluation Method of Timed up and Go Test for Hospitalized Patients Using Inertial Sensors. In Proceedings of the 2023 IEEE 19th International Conference on Body Sensor Networks (BSN), Boston, MA, USA, 9–11 October 2023; IEEE: Piscataway, NJ, USA, 2023; pp. 1–4.
16. Kiprijanovska, I.; Gjoreski, H.; Gams, M. Detection of Gait Abnormalities for Fall Risk Assessment Using Wrist-Worn Inertial Sensors and Deep Learning. *Sensors* **2020**, *20*, 5373. [CrossRef] [PubMed]
17. Roshdibenam, V.; Jogerst, G.J.; Butler, N.R.; Baek, S. Machine Learning Prediction of Fall Risk in Older Adults Using Timed up and Go Test Kinematics. *Sensors* **2021**, *21*, 3481. [CrossRef] [PubMed]
18. Pedrero-Sánchez, J.-F.; De-Rosario-Martínez, H.; Medina-Ripoll, E.; Garrido-Jaén, D.; Serra-Añó, P.; Mollà Casanova, S.; López-Pascual, J. The Reliability and Accuracy of a Fall Risk Assessment Procedure Using Mobile Smartphone Sensors Compared with a Physiological Profile Assessment. *Sensors* **2023**, *23*, 6567. [CrossRef] [PubMed]
19. Yamada, M.; Arai, H. Predictive Value of Frailty Scores for Healthy Life Expectancy in Community-Dwelling Older Japanese Adults. *J. Am. Med. Dir. Assoc.* **2015**, *16*, 1002.e7–1002.e11. [CrossRef] [PubMed]
20. Vaswani, A.; Shazeer, N.; Parmar, N.; Uszkoreit, J.; Jones, L.; Gomez, A.N.; Kaiser, Ł.U.; Polosukhin, I. Attention Is All You Need. In *Proceedings of the Advances in Neural Information Processing Systems*; Guyon, I., Luxburg, U.V., Bengio, S., Wallach, H., Fergus, R., Vishwanathan, S., Garnett, R., Eds.; Curran Associates, Inc.: Red Hook, NY, USA, 2017; Volume 30.
21. Modified R Commander. Available online: https://personal.hs.hirosaki-u.ac.jp/pteiki/research/stat/R/ (accessed on 27 May 2023).
22. Buisseret, F.; Catinus, L.; Grenard, R.; Jojczyk, L.; Fievez, D.; Barvaux, V.; Dierick, F. Timed up and Go and Six-Minute Walking Tests with Wearable Inertial Sensor: One Step Further for the Prediction of the Risk of Fall in Elderly Nursing Home People. *Sensors* **2020**, *20*, 3207. [CrossRef]
23. Perry, J.; Judith, B. *Gait Analysis: Normal and Pathological Function*, 2nd ed.; Slack Inc.: Thorofare, NJ, USA, 2010; pp. 3–47.
24. Warmerdam, E.; Romijnders, R.; Welzel, J.; Hansen, C.; Schmidt, G.; Maetzler, W. Quantification of Arm Swing during Walking in Healthy Adults and Parkinson's Disease Patients: Wearable Sensor-Based Algorithm Development and Validation. *Sensors* **2020**, *20*, 5963. [CrossRef]

25. Fang, X.; Jiang, Z. Three-Dimensional Thoracic and Pelvic Kinematics and Arm Swing Maximum Velocity in Older Adults Using Inertial Sensor System. *PeerJ* **2020**, *8*, e9329. [CrossRef] [PubMed]
26. Shishov, N.; Gimmon, Y.; Rashed, H.; Kurz, I.; Riemer, R.; Shapiro, A.; Debi, R.; Melzer, I. Old Adult Fallers Display Reduced Flexibility of Arm and Trunk Movements When Challenged with Different Walking Speeds. *Gait Posture* **2017**, *52*, 280–286. [CrossRef] [PubMed]

bioengineering

MDPI

Article

Deep Learning Method for Precise Landmark Identification and Structural Assessment of Whole-Spine Radiographs

Sung Hyun Noh [1,2,*,†], Gaeun Lee [3,†], Hyun-Jin Bae [3], Ju Yeon Han [1], Su Jeong Son [1], Deok Kim [1], Jeong Yeon Park [1], Seung Kyeong Choi [1], Pyung Goo Cho [1], Sang Hyun Kim [1], Woon Tak Yuh [4], Su Hun Lee [5], Bumsoo Park [6], Kwang-Ryeol Kim [7], Kyoung-Tae Kim [8] and Yoon Ha [9]

1 Department of Neurosurgery, Ajou University College of Medicine, Suwon 16499, Republic of Korea
2 Department of Neurosurgery, Yonsei University College of Medicine, Seoul 03722, Republic of Korea
3 Promedius Inc., Seoul 05609, Republic of Korea
4 Department of Neurosurgery, Hallym University Dongtan Sacred Heart Hospital, Hwaseong-si 18450, Republic of Korea
5 Department of Neurosurgery, Pusan National University Yangsan Hospital, Busan 50612, Republic of Korea
6 Department of Neurosurgery, Bon Hospital, Daejeon 34188, Republic of Korea
7 Department of Neurosurgery, Daegu Catholic University College of Medicine, Daegu 42400, Republic of Korea
8 Department. of Neurosurgery, School of Medicine, Kyungpook National University, Kyungpook National University Hospital, Daegu 41944, Republic of Korea
9 Department of Neurosurgery, Spine and Spinal Cord Institute, Severance Hospital, Yonsei University College of Medicine, Seoul 03722, Republic of Korea
* Correspondence: juwuman12@gmail.com; Tel.: +82-31-219-5230; Fax: +82-31-219-5232
† These authors contributed equally to this work.

Abstract: This study measured parameters automatically by marking the point for measuring each parameter on whole-spine radiographs. Between January 2020 and December 2021, 1017 sequential lateral whole-spine radiographs were retrospectively obtained. Of these, 819 and 198 were used for training and testing the performance of the landmark detection model, respectively. To objectively evaluate the program's performance, 690 whole-spine radiographs from four other institutions were used for external validation. The combined dataset comprised radiographs from 857 female and 850 male patients (average age 42.2 ± 27.3 years; range 20–85 years). The landmark localizer showed the highest accuracy in identifying cervical landmarks (median error 1.5–2.4 mm), followed by lumbosacral landmarks (median error 2.1–3.0 mm). However, thoracic landmarks displayed larger localization errors (median 2.4–4.3 mm), indicating slightly reduced precision compared with the cervical and lumbosacral regions. The agreement between the deep learning model and two experts was good to excellent, with intraclass correlation coefficient values >0.88. The deep learning model also performed well on the external validation set. There were no statistical differences between datasets in all parameters, suggesting that the performance of the artificial intelligence model created was excellent. The proposed automatic alignment analysis system identified anatomical landmarks and positions of the spine with high precision and generated various radiograph imaging parameters that had a good correlation with manual measurements.

Keywords: artificial intelligence; deep learning; radiography; spine

1. Introduction

Recently, there has been a remarkable surge in the availability of biomedical data, presenting challenges and opportunities for healthcare research. This wealth of data includes extensive collections of medical images, such as computed tomography (CT) scans, magnetic resonance imaging (MRI), and radiographs, which play a crucial role in various medical tasks, such as pathology detection and classification, as well as pinpointing vital anatomical landmarks. Spine imaging, in particular, holds significant clinical importance as it enables the precise characterization of spinal alignment through angles, distances, and shapes, proving invaluable for tasks such as surgical planning and monitoring of deformity progression [1]. Traditionally, these parameters are measured either manually using tools such as rulers and protractors on physical images or with specialized software for digital images [2]. However, this approach is prone to inaccuracies and inconsistencies due to variations in measurements by different observers.

To address these challenges, there has been a growing emphasis on developing computer-aided diagnosis systems over the past few years. These systems aim to reduce errors and enhance the efficiency of image analysis; however, they often require manual input [3]. The advent of fully automated software tools promises to eliminate these shortcomings and revolutionize both medical research and clinical practice. Recent advancements in deep learning (DL) technologies, coupled with the high computational capabilities of graphics processing units (GPUs), have made it feasible to develop tools capable of autonomously measuring spinal parameters [4,5]. These technological advances not only streamline the analysis process but also enhance its accuracy, paving the way for more precise and reliable medical diagnostics and treatments.

In medical imaging, the integration of artificial intelligence, particularly DL, has significantly increased in recent times, often surpassing the expertise of human observers in terms of performance. One notable advancement was the development of an automatic tool for identifying vertebrae in CT scans [6]. This tool accurately pinpointed vertebral centroids but fell short of providing practical clinical applications. In a study by Jacobsen et al., DL was employed for the automatic segmentation of cervical vertebrae [7]. However, their methodology exhibited non-negligible errors in locating the vertebral corners, and the focus was limited to the cervical area with a relatively small dataset, hindering its practicality in routine clinical environments.

To address the limitations of these studies, we aimed to develop an artificial intelligence model to accurately identify points from which to perform key measurements on whole-spine radiographs. This study aimed to measure each parameter automatically by accurately marking the point for measuring each parameter on whole-spine radiographs.

2. Materials

2.1. Dataset

Between January 2020 and December 2021, a comprehensive collection of 1017 sequential lateral whole-spine radiographs was retrospectively gathered. In adherence to the guidelines of our hospital's institutional review board (IRB no. 2023218), a waiver for informed consent was granted for this study. A leading radiologist meticulously reviewed the entire set of images and excluded several categories: (1) insufficient length, failing to capture either the C2 dens or both femoral heads; (2) anatomical variances, such as spinal columns with less or more than the standard 25 vertebrae; and (3) compromise by suboptimal contrast, hindering clear identification of pelvic structures.

Of the 1017 radiographs, data from 819 and 198 were used for training and testing the performance of the landmark detection model, respectively. To objectively evaluate the performance of the program, 690 whole-spine radiographs from four other institutions were used for external validation. The annotated landmarks contained 26 points, as shown in Table 1 and Figure 1. The demographic profile for these 1707 annotated images revealed a mean patient age of 42.2 $\pm$ 27.3 years (age range: 20–85 years) at the time of the radiographic examinations.

Table 1. Names and descriptions of landmarks annotated on whole-spine lateral X-ray.

Name	Description
FH_1	Center of the Femur head
FH_2	Center of the Femur head
S_1	Anterior point of the upper endplate of the sacrum

Table 1. *Cont.*

Name	Description
S_2	Posterior point of the upper endplate of the sacrum
L1_1	Anterior point of the upper endplate of the L1 vertebra
L1_2	Posterior point of the upper endplate of the L1 vertebra
L4_1	Anterior point of the upper endplate of the L4 vertebra
L4_2	Posterior point of the upper endplate of the L4 vertebra
T4_1	Anterior point of the upper endplate of the T4 vertebra
T4_2	Posterior point of the upper endplate of the T4 vertebra
T12_1	Anterior point of the lower endplate of the T12 vertebra
T12_2	Posterior point of the lower endplate of the T12 vertebra
T1	Center of the T1 vertebral body
Forehead	Forehead
FM_1	Anterior point of the foramen magnum
FM_2	Posterior point of the foramen magnum
ODT	Odontoid
Jaw	Jaw
C2_1	Anterior point of the lower endplate of the C2 vertebra
C2_2	Posterior point of the lower endplate of the C2 vertebra
C7	Center of the C7 vertebral body
C7_1	Anterior point of the lower endplate of the C7 vertebra
C7_2	Posterior point of the lower endplate of the C7 vertebra
C7_3	Posterior point of the upper endplate of the C7 vertebra
T1_1	Anterior point of the upper endplate of the T1 vertebra
T1_2	Posterior point of the upper endplate of the T1 vertebra

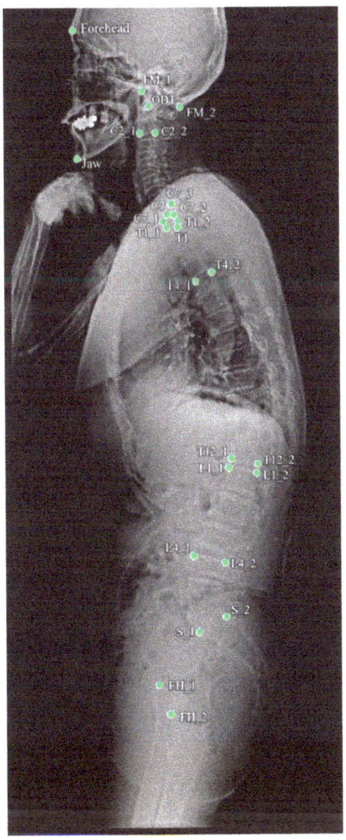

Figure 1. Landmarks annotated on a whole-spine lateral radiograph.

2.2. Learning of Heatmap-Based Landmark Detection

The model for detecting landmarks used U-Net [8], and learning was conducted based on a heatmap. The heatmap-based method indirectly learns coordinates through heatmaps instead of directly learning them. This method is widely used in landmark detection for pose estimation [9] or face landmark detection [10]. Heatmap-based learning is slower than the direct prediction of coordinates, but it is less sensitive to slight differences that may occur owing to human annotations because it accepts the surroundings of coordinates more generously. The proposed heatmap-based landmark detection model used a Gaussian heatmap generated around landmark coordinates as the ground truth (Figure 2), and the dice coefficient loss ($\mathcal{L}_{dice}$) and weighted L1 loss ($\mathcal{L}_{wl}$) were used as the loss functions [11].

$$\mathcal{L} = \alpha\mathcal{L}_{dice} + \beta\mathcal{L}_{wl} \tag{1}$$

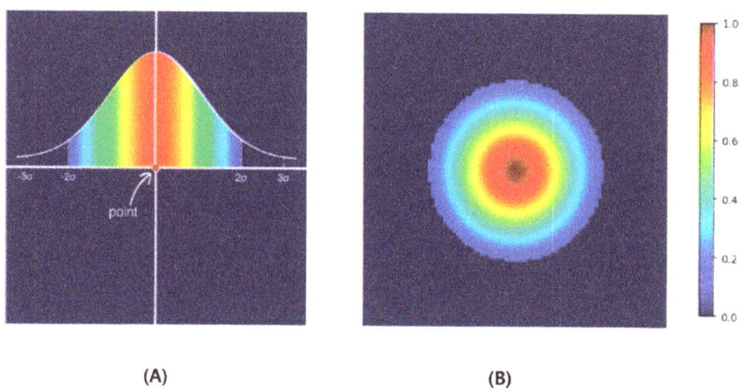

Figure 2. As an example, if the point located in the center of 100 × 100 as in (**A**) is expanded to Gaussian values and normalized to values 0 to 1, a heatmap like (**B**) is created. In this example, σ was set to 10, thresholded in the ±2σ range, and visualized with a jet colormap.

L1 loss, which is the absolute difference between the ground truth and the prediction, leads to a predicted heatmap ($\hat{Y}$) similar to the ground truth (Y). However, compared with the overall image size, a single point is very small. Therefore, we categorized the area of the point as the foreground and the area outside the point as the background. Subsequently, we applied the weighted L1 loss by assigning weights that were inversely proportional to each foreground and background area. The background (bg) and foreground (fg) were determined based on 2σ of the simulated Gaussian.

$$\begin{gathered} fg(x) = \begin{cases} 0, & x \le 2\sigma \\ 1, & x > 2\sigma \end{cases} \\ bg(x) = \begin{cases} 1, & x \le 2\sigma \\ 0, & x > 2\sigma \end{cases} \\ \mathcal{L}_{wl} = \sum\left(W * \left|Y - \hat{Y}\right|\right) \\ W = fg(Y)/\sum(fg(Y)) + bg(Y)/\sum(bg(Y)) \end{gathered} \tag{2}$$

Dice loss was added to bring the predicted heat map closer to the ground-truth Gaussian-distributed heat map. This loss is inversely related to the dice similarity coefficient (DSC), which measures the similarity between two samples.

$$\begin{gathered} y = fg(Y) * Y \\ \hat{y} = fg(\hat{Y}) * \hat{Y} \\ \mathcal{L}_{dice} = 1 - DSC(y, \hat{y}) \end{gathered} \tag{3}$$

DSC has a value between 0 and 1. The higher the similarity, the closer it is to 1, and the lower the similarity, the closer it is to 0. DSC calculates only the foreground area of each sample, and in this case, the foreground is an area divided by 2σ as a boundary, similar to weighted L1 loss.

$$DSC(y, \hat{y}) = \frac{\sum[(y+\hat{y}) * (y * \hat{y} > 0)]}{\sum y + \sum \hat{y}} \tag{4}$$

Finally, the landmark coordinate outputs from the model were the center points of the maximum values from the predicted heatmap.

2.3. Workflow of the Landmark Detection in Whole-Spine Lateral Radiographs

The landmark detection model in whole-spine lateral radiographs was divided into two steps: detection of the upper cervical area above T1 and the lower thoracic–femur area (Figure 3). This aimed to achieve precise detection of densely clustered landmarks in the cervical area, which have a higher density than the resolution of the entire image. The detection of the cervical area was further divided into two steps. First, the cervical region of interest (ROI) within a whole-spine radiograph was identified. The cervical ROI range was specified with a margin of 30% of the horizontal margin in a tightly bound box from 13 landmarks above T1 detected on the whole-spine radiograph. In the second step, detection was performed at a higher resolution in the cervical ROI. Finally, the predicted landmarks of the whole-spine radiograph were derived by combining the prediction points of the detection model in the thoracic–femur area and the detection model in the cervical ROI.

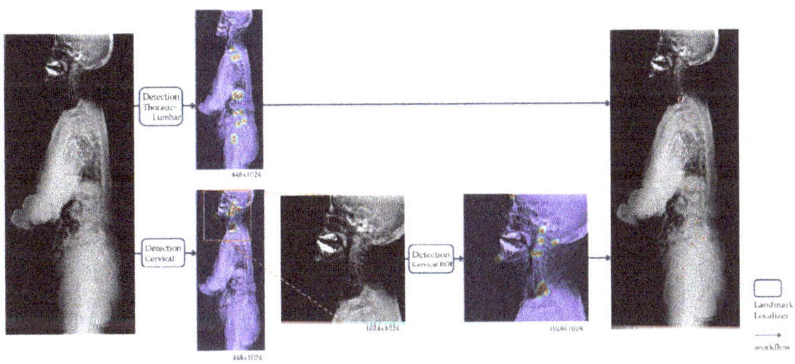

Figure 3. Operational flow of the landmark detection model in whole-spine lateral radiographs. For automatic landmark detection in a single radiograph, the thoracic–lumbar and cervical spine are localized separately. The outputs of landmark localizers for each image input are all heatmaps, and the final output of the model is the coordinates (orange points) restored to match the original image resolution derived from the heatmaps.

2.4. Training Details

The input image size was set to 448 × 1024, whereas the cervical ROI training model used a 1024 × 1024 resolution image as the input. All the inputs were resized while maintaining the aspect ratio (height/width), and pixel values were rescaled by referring to the windowing information in the whole spine radiograph DICOM header, after which contrast limited adaptive histogram equalization (CLAHE) was applied. All inputs were resized by maintaining the aspect ratio and then rescaled and inputted after applying CLAHE. Augmentation during training was shift (±10%), zoom (±10%), and rotation (±10°). The sigma (σ) for heatmap generation was set to 10 and 15 for the whole-spine lateral radiograph and cervical ROI, respectively. Dice loss could be applied after a certain amount of training, so the α in the loss function started from 0 and increased by 0.002 per epoch, while β was set as $1-\alpha$. All models were trained in an Ubuntu 22.04.4 LTS, Intel® Core™ i9-9900X CPU @ 3.50GHz x4ea, a single GPU environment [Quadro RTX 8000

(48 GB)], and the TensorFlow 2.11 version was used as a framework. Of the 819 training sets, 794 were used to update the model's weights, and 25 were used as validation sets during training. After running 300 epochs with a batch size of 10, the weight at the epoch with the lowest average validation loss in the cumulative 10 epochs was selected as the final weight of the detection model. Figure 4 shows the loss and accuracy graph monitored for each 100 steps during the learning process.

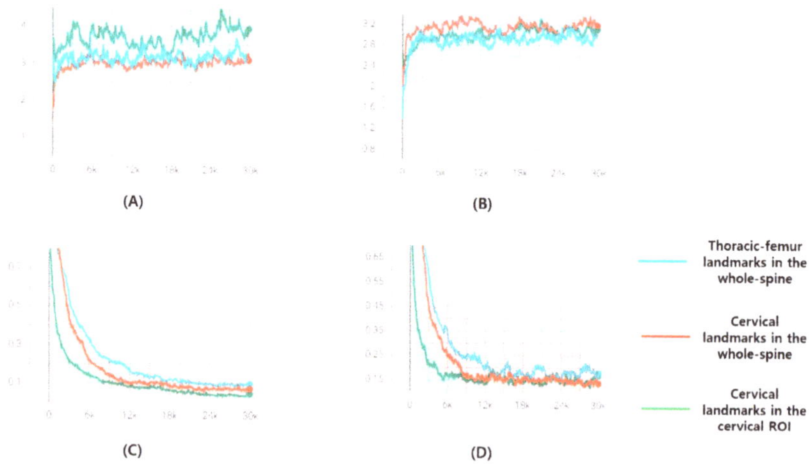

Figure 4. These are loss and accuracy curve graphs for 300 epochs of the training set and validation set: (**A**) Accuracy curve graphs of training set; (**B**) accuracy curve graphs of validation set; (**C**) loss curve graphs of training set; (**D**) loss curve graphs of validation set. The *x*-axis represents steps and is plotted at every 100 steps. Blue is the curve of the model that finds thoracic–femur landmarks in the whole spine, orange is the curve of the model that finds cervical landmarks in the whole spine, and green is the curve of the model that finds cervical landmarks in the cervical ROI.

2.5. Measurement of Spinal Parameters

Fifteen spinal parameters were measured from the landmarks detected in whole-spine lateral radiographs using the landmark detection model. The names and measurement methods for these parameters are listed in Table 2.

Table 2. Names and measurement methods of spinal parameters measured from landmarks detected in whole-spine lateral X-ray.

	Name	Measurement
PI	Pelvic Incidence	The angle between the line connecting the center of femur heads and the center of the sacrum's upper endplate, and the perpendicular line of the sacrum's upper endplate.
PT	Pelvic Tilt	The angle between the line connecting the center of the femur heads and the center of the sacrum's upper endplate, and the vertical.
SS	Sacral Slope	The angle between the sacrum's upper endplate and the horizontal.
LL	Lumbar Lordosis	The angle between the upper endplate of L1 and the endplate of the sacrum.
L4S1	L4S1 Lordosis	The angle between the upper endplate of L4 and the endplate of the sacrum.
TK	Thoracic Kyphosis	The angle between the upper endplate of T4 and the lower endplate of T12.
TPA	T1pelvic Angle	The angle between the line connecting the center of the T1 vertebral body and the center of the femur heads, and the line connecting the center of the femur heads and the center of the sacrum's upper endplate.
CBVA	Chin-Brow Vertical Angle	The angle between the line connecting the forehead and chin, and the vertical.
C2C7	C2C7 Angle (Cervical Lordosis Angle)	The angle between the lower endplate of C2 and the lower endplate of C7.

Table 2. *Cont.*

	Name	Measurement
TS	T1 Slope	The angle between the upper endplate of T1 and the horizontal.
TS-CL	T1 Slope—Cervical Lordosis	T1 slope minus cervical lordosis.
ODHA	Odontoid hip axis angle	The angle between the line connecting the odontoid to the center of femur heads, and the vertical.
PI-LL	Pelvic Incidence—Lumbar Lordosis	Pelvic Incidence minus Lumbar Lordosis
SSA	Spino-Sacral Angle	The angle between the line connecting the center of the C7 body and the center of the sacrum's upper endplate, and sacrum's upper endplate.
SVA	Sagittal Vertical Axis	Distance between the vertical line at the center of the C7 body and a posterior point of the sacrum's upper endplate.

2.6. Statistical Analysis

The landmark localization errors were used to evaluate the performance of the trained landmark localizer. Interrater reliability was used to determine the level of agreement among the following three raters:

Rater 1 (R1): Senior neurosurgeon

Rater 2 (R2): Junior neurosurgeon

Proposed DL model (landmark localizer and numerical algorithm)

In this study, Pearson correlation coefficients were employed to assess the relationships between the predicted radiographic parameters using a DL model and the actual ground truth values. To determine the numerical discrepancies between the model predictions and ground truth, Wilcoxon signed-rank tests were utilized, with a p-value threshold of <0.05 indicating statistical significance. Furthermore, the intraclass correlation coefficient (ICC) was used to measure the interobserver reliability of three human evaluators (junior resident, spine fellow, and senior surgeon), the DL model, and ground truth. This analysis was based on a dataset of 198 images specifically chosen for interobserver reliability evaluation. The reliability was categorized into four levels based on the ICC value: excellent (0.9–1.0), high (0.7–0.9), moderate (0.5–0.7), and low (0.25–0.5). All statistical analyses and procedures in this research were performed using SPSS version 25.0 (SPSS Inc, Chicago, IL, USA)

3. Results

3.1. Dataset Demographic

The dataset comprised radiographs from 857 female and 850 male patients, with an average age of 42.2 ± 27.3 (range: 20–85) years. In this dataset, spinal implants were present in 170 images (approximately 10%), with the range of instrumentation extending from C4 to the ilium, averaging 8.2 ± 3.0 levels per image.

3.2. Performance of the Landmark Localizer

The landmark localizer showed the highest accuracy in identifying cervical landmarks, with a median error of 1.5–2.4 mm. This was followed by the lumbosacral landmarks, which exhibited a median error of 2.1–3.0 mm. In contrast, the thoracic landmarks displayed larger localization errors, with median values of 2.4–4.3 mm, indicating slightly reduced precision compared with the cervical and lumbosacral regions. Figure 5 shows a visualization of localized landmarks in the test set.

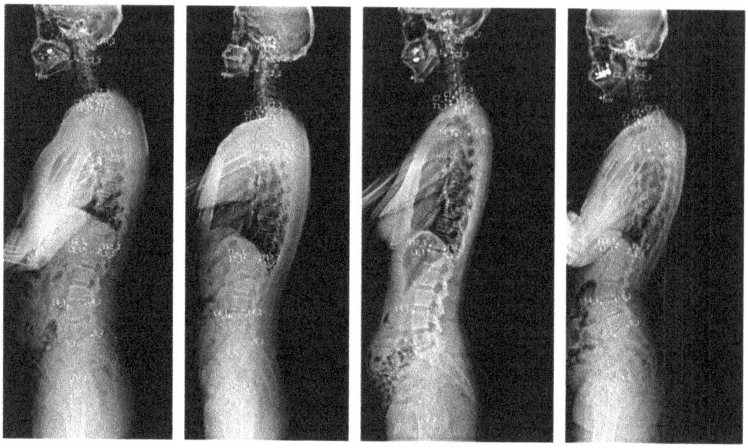

Figure 5. Examples of landmarks automatically localized in the test set.

3.3. Inter-Rater Reliability between the Two Human Experts and Developed Deep Learning Model

Table 3 shows the inter-rater reliability of the spinal curvature characteristics between the two human experts and the developed DL model. The consistency in measurements between the senior and junior neurosurgeons was outstanding across all spinal curvature characteristics, with all ICCs exceeding 0.9, indicating excellent agreement. When compared with the evaluations made by human experts, the proposed DL model showed slightly lower reliability in accurately predicting the cervicothoracic junction point and the degree of thoracic kyphosis. However, its performance in determining the thoracolumbar junction, cervical and lumbar points, and lumbar lordosis was comparable with that of human experts. Overall, the agreement between the DL model and the two experts ranged from good to excellent, with ICC values exceeding 0.88.

Table 3. Inter-rater reliability between the two human experts and developed deep learning model.

Parameters	R1 versus R2	DL versus R1	DL versus R2
PI (°)	0.978	0.891	0.889
PT (°)	0.981	0.923	0.915
SS (°)	0.962	0.905	0.897
LL (°)	0.957	0.921	0.915
L4S1 (°)	0.961	0.901	0.894
TK (°)	0.979	0.945	0.931
TPA (°)	0.945	0.894	0.884
CBVA (°)	0.951	0.907	0.901
C2C7 (°)	0.947	0.887	0.881
TS (°)	0.923	0.915	0.909
TS-CL (°)	0.914	0.909	0.897
ODHA (°)	0.928	0.903	0.891
PI-LL (°)	0.927	0.896	0.884
SSA (°)	0.944	0.945	0.925
SVA (mm)	0.957	0.912	0.902

PI, pelvic incidence; PT, pelvic tilt; SS, sacral slope; LL, lumbar lordosis; L4S1, L4S1 lordosis; TK, thoracic kyphosis; TPA, T1 pelvic angle; CBVA, chin-brow vertical angle; C2C7, C2C7 angle; TS, T1 slope; TS-CL, T1 slope—cervical lordosis; ODHA, odontoid hip axis angle; PI-LL, pelvic incidence—lumbar lordosis; SSA, spino-sacral angle; SVA, sagittal vertical axis.

3.4. Performance Evaluation of the Spinal Parameters of the Deep Learning Model

The performance of the DL model in estimating spinopelvic parameters was rigorously evaluated using a test dataset comprising 198 spinal radiographic images. The results, outlined in Table 4, show mean errors for these parameters, considering the non-normal distribution of error values. The mean errors were accompanied by the standard deviation.

Table 4. Performance evaluation of the spinal parameters of the deep learning model.

Parameters	Ground Truth	Parameter Error	Correlation Analysis		Wilcoxon Signed-Rank Test
			R	*p* Value	*p* Value
PI (°)	53.8 ± 18.8°	2.6 ± 3.1°	0.982	<0.001 *	0.497
PT (°)	14.8 ± 11.3°	1.8 ± 2.2°	0.917		0.512
SS (°)	39.4 ± 7.9°	2.2 ± 3.4°	0.912		0.459
LL (°)	41.2 ± 17.3°	5.7 ± 3.5°	0.991		0.279
L4S1 (°)	30.7 ± 11.6°	4.5 ± 2.8°	0.857		0.247
TK (°)	27.2 ± 11.2°	5.5 ± 4.5°	0.812		0.078
TPA (°)	24.9 ± 23.2°	1.8 ± 1.1°	0.792		0.758
CBVA (°)	1.8 ± 5.2°	0.7 ± 0.6°	0.984		0.678
C2C7 (°)	13.6 ± 9.7°	5.5 ± 6.5°	0.845		0.598
TS (°)	22.8 ± 10.2°	5.7 ± 6.2°	0.784		0.084
TS-CL (°)	9.8 ± 2.4°	4.1 ± 5.9°	0.809		0.097
ODHA (°)	4.3 ± 5.4°	0.2 ± 0.2°	0.978		0.594
PI-LL (°)	12.1 ± 7.5°	3.0 ± 4.5°	0.962		0.596
SSA (°)	120.1 ± 12.4°	3.3 ± 2.5°	0.927		0.492
SVA (mm)	22.1 ± 19.2 mm	3.0 ± 2.9 mm	0.986		0.745

PI, pelvic incidence; PT, pelvic tilt; SS, sacral slope; LL, lumbar lordosis; L4S1, L4S1 lordosis; TK, thoracic kyphosis; TPA, T1 pelvic angle; CBVA, chin-brow vertical angle; C2C7, C2C7 angle; TS, T1 slope; TS-CL, T1 slope—cervical lordosis; ODHA, odontoid hip axis angle; PI-LL, pelvic incidence—lumbar lordosis; SSA, spino-sacral angle; SVA, sagittal vertical axis; * p value < 0.05.

All predicted radiographic parameters demonstrated significant correlations with the ground truth values, with p-values less than 0.001. For core spinopelvic parameters, the mean error varied from 0.16° for odontoid hip axis angle (ODHA) to 5.69° for lumbar lordosis. Notably, no significant differences were found between the model predictions and ground truth values, as evidenced by all p-values > 0.05 in the Wilcoxon signed-rank tests. The predicted Chin-Brow Vertical Angle (CBVA) and pelvic incidence (PI) were particularly well correlated with the ground truth, exhibiting Pearson correlation coefficients (R) > 0.9. When examining regional spinal parameters, performance varied across anatomical regions. In the cervicothoracic region, the mean errors spanned from 0.66° for cervical CBVA to 5.66° for T1 slope (TS). In the thoracic region, the mean errors for thoracic kyphosis were 5.53°. For the lumbosacral parameters, the mean errors were 1.87° for pelvic tilt (PT) and 5.69° for the lumbar lordosis angle.

3.5. Predicted Spinal Parameters of the External Validation Dataset

A comparative analysis was performed with four external validation datasets (Table 5). There were no statistical differences between datasets in all parameters, suggesting that the performance of the artificial intelligence model created was excellent.

Table 5. Predicted spinal parameters of the external validation dataset.

Parameters	Ground Truth	Parameter Error	External-Validation Dataset 1 Error	External-Validation Dataset 2 Error	External-Validation Dataset 3 Error	External-Validation Dataset 4 Error	*p*-Value
PI (°)	53.8 ± 18.8°	2.7 ± 3.1°	3.3 ± 2.1°	2.2 ± 3.9°	4.2 ± 2.4°	3.6 ± 2.1°	0.479
PT (°)	14.8 ± 11.3°	1.9 ± 2.2°	2.7 ± 2.0°	2.2 ± 2.7°	2.5 ± 1.2°	2.3 ± 1.3°	0.545
SS (°)	39.4 ± 7.9°	2.2 ± 3.4°	2.3 ± 3.3°	3.6 ± 2.2°	3.8 ± 2.4°	3.6 ± 3.0°	0.471
LL (°)	41.2 ± 17.3°	5.7 ± 3.5°	5.1 ± 3.0°	6.2 ± 4.4°	5.6 ± 3.6°	4.2 ± 3.3°	0.784
L4S1 (°)	30.7 ± 11.6°	4.5 ± 2.8°	5.2 ± 2.5°	4.2 ± 2.6°	4.4 ± 3.1°	5.0 ± 2.4°	0.612
TK (°)	27.2 ± 11.2°	5.5 ± 4.5°	5.9 ± 4.4°	5.9 ± 5.2°	4.2 ± 3.8°	5.0 ± 4.4°	0.274

Table 5. *Cont.*

Parameters	Ground Truth	Parameter Error	External-Validation Dataset 1 Error	External-Validation Dataset 2 Error	External-Validation Dataset 3 Error	External-Validation Dataset 4 Error	*p*-Value
TPA (°)	24.9 ± 23.2°	1.8 ± 1.1°	1.4 ± 1.8°	1.9 ± 1.7°	1.9 ± 1.9°	1.5 ± 1.1°	0.798
CBVA (°)	1.8 ± 5.2°	0.7 ± 0.6°	0.6 ± 0.4°	0.4 ± 0.2°	0.8 ± 1.4°	0.8 ± 1.0°	0.571
C2C7 (°)	13.6 ± 9.7°	5.5 ± 6.5°	4.6 ± 4.4°	5.4 ± 5.2°	4.8 ± 5.4°	5.8 ± 4.0°	0.435
TS (°)	22.8 ± 10.2°	5.7 ± 6.2°	4.4 ± 4.4°	5.1 ± 6.1°	5.7 ± 4.6°	5.4 ± 6.4°	0.645
TS-CL (°)	9.8 ± 2.4°	4.1 ± 5.9°	4.5 ± 6.3°	4.1 ± 5.3°	3.9 ± 4.4°	3.7 ± 4.8°	0.421
ODHA (°)	4.3 ± 5.4°	0.2 ± 0.2°	0.1 ± 0.4°	0.1 ± 0.2°	0.1 ± 0.3°	0.3 ± 0.9°	0.764
PI-LL (°)	12.1 ± 7.5°	3.0 ± 4.5°	3.1 ± 4.9°	2.0 ± 2.7°	2.4 ± 4.8°	2.1 ± 3.2°	0.841
SSA (°)	120.1 ± 12.4°	3.3 ± 2.5°	3.2 ± 2.6°	4.0 ± 2.48°	3.1 ± 2.4°	3.9 ± 2.5°	0.623
SVA (mm)	22.1 ± 19.2 mm	3.0 ± 2.9 mm	2.0 ± 2.5 mm	2.9 ± 2.5 mm	2.7 ± 1.1 mm	2.9 ± 1.5 mm	0.812

PI, pelvic incidence; PT, pelvic tilt; SS, sacral slope; LL, lumbar lordosis; L4S1, L4S1 lordosis; TK, thoracic kyphosis; TPA, T1 pelvic angle; CBVA, chin-brow vertical angle; C2C7, C2C7 angle; TS, T1 slope; TS-CL, T1 slope—cervical lordosis; ODHA, odontoid hip axis angle; PI-LL, pelvic incidence—lumbar lordosis; SSA, spino-sacral angle; SVA, sagittal vertical axis.

4. Discussion

Adult spinal deformity (ASD) affects a significant proportion of the elderly population, with 32–68% of individuals over 65 experiencing this condition [12–14]. The causes of ASD are diverse, including conditions such as de novo scoliosis, progressive adolescent idiopathic scoliosis, degenerative hyperkyphosis, and iatrogenic flat back deformity [15]. A comprehensive radiographic assessment of the entire spine, including the hip joints, is crucial for evaluating sagittal balance in ASD. Various studies have established the relationship between key spinopelvic parameters and health-related quality of life outcomes, as well as the success of ASD corrective surgeries [16]. These parameters, both regional and global, are vital for disease classification and preoperative planning, offering insights into the overall sagittal balance by considering factors such as cervical hyperlordosis, thoracic hypokyphosis, and pelvic retroversion, independent of postural changes and body size differences [17]. However, manually measuring these parameters can be time-consuming and subject to interobserver variability. Our study introduced a DL model that shows performance comparable to that of human observers in accurately measuring 15 critical sagittal spinal parameters across various spinal conditions.

Numerous studies have applied DL techniques to analyze plain radiographs of the lateral spine automatically. For instance, in a study conducted by Weng et al. [18], a DL model based on an advanced ResUNet architecture was developed for the automatic measurement of the sagittal vertical axis (SVA), demonstrating exceptional reliability compared with human expert assessments. The scope of automatic measurements in whole-spine lateral radiographs has been broadened to include various spinopelvic parameters, such as pelvic incidence, sacral slope, and PT. These measurements have shown not only acceptable error margins but also robust correlations with ground truth values [19]. Further, a study by Yeh et al. [20] reported that the automatic predictions of spinopelvic parameters utilizing a sophisticated two-stage DL model were on par with the reliability of human experts, even in cases involving complex spinal disorders. This underscores the increasing efficacy and reliability of DL applications in spinal radiographic analyses. Galbusera et al. attempted to calculate the spine angles automatically using standardized biplanar images from the EOS system [19]. Despite standardization, this approach also demonstrated the potential for improvement in angle calculation. Other initiatives have focused on 3D spinal reconstruction using both automatic and semiautomatic models. One such study applied a statistical model and a convolutional neural network to reconstruct the shape of the spine precisely, assessing the model accuracy through the Euclidean distance between predictions and actual measurements. Manual intervention was required before the relevant parameters could be calculated.

A key benefit of DL in medical imaging is its ability to provide rapid, objective, and consistent interpretations. Despite advancements in Picture Archiving and Communication Systems (PACS) and specialized commercial software, such as Surgimap (Nemaris, MA, USA), manual identification of points still requires significant professional input and considerable time. While a few studies have reported automatic curvature feature analyses in various spinal imaging modalities [21], these have not been widespread. A notable advancement in this area is the use of annotated vertebral centers for spline-based curve angle measurements. As demonstrated in a recent study [22], this approach yields higher intrarater and interrater reliability than traditional manual Cobb angle measurements, especially in anteroposterior spinal radiographs. However, it is important to note that much of this research has predominantly concentrated on analyzing the frontal plane curvature, with less emphasis on the sagittal plane, highlighting a potential area for development in spinal imaging analysis.

Weng et al. created an artificial intelligence model that analyzed the curvature of the entire spine by detecting the inflection points and apices [23]. Point detection in spinal sagittal curvatures has been the subject of extensive research in both healthy and pathological contexts [24]. Biomechanically, inflection points signify transitional areas between different sagittal curves, while apices influence the distribution of lumbar lordosis [25]. Therefore, achieving accurate relocation of the inflection points and apices and restoring the ideal sagittal profile are critical for spinal surgical procedures. However, because it does not find points to accurately measure parameters, it has the limitation of estimating parameters using a virtual curvature line through inflection points and apices. In this study, we increased the efficiency of angle measurements by directly detecting the points required for angle measurement using artificial intelligence. Although our DL model significantly reduces manual labeling efforts, incorporating a human review process into real clinical settings is advisable.

This study had some limitations. First, although radiological examinations from a multicenter study were used for external validation, the overall dataset size was small. Second, images with atypical vertebral counts were excluded, implying that the model may not accurately predict cases with anomalies such as lumbosacral transitional vertebrae. Third, the predictions were based solely on lateral radiographs, whereas a biplanar EOS system with 3D reconstruction might offer more comprehensive assessments of spinal deformities. Fourth, the performance of the DL model may vary across different spinal conditions as radiographs include a wide range of spinal issues. Despite these limitations, our DL model demonstrated the ability to interpret sagittal spinal curves automatically and consistently.

5. Conclusions

The landmark localizer showed the highest accuracy in identifying cervical landmarks, with a median error of 1.5–2.4 mm. External validation was performed using data from four other institutions and good results were obtained. The proposed automatic alignment analysis system identified the positions of the anatomical landmarks of the spine with high precision and generated various radiograph imaging parameters that had a good correlation with manual measurements.

Author Contributions: Conceptualization, S.H.N.; methodology, S.H.N.; software, S.H.N., G.L. and H.-J.B.; validation, S.H.N., P.G.C., S.H.K., W.T.Y., S.H.L., B.P., K.-R.K., K.-T.K. and Y.H.; formal analysis, S.H.N., G.L. and H.-J.B.; investigation, S.H.N.; resources, S.H.N.; data curation, J.Y.H., S.J.S., D.K., J.Y.P. and S.K.C.; writing—original draft preparation, S.H.N. and G.L.; writing—review and editing, S.H.N. and G.L.; visualization, S.H.N. and G.L.; supervision, S.H.N., P.G.C., S.H.K., W.T.Y., S.H.L., B.P., K.-R.K., K.-T.K. and Y.H.; project administration, S.H.N. All authors have read and agreed to the published version of the manuscript.

Funding: This research received no external funding.

Institutional Review Board Statement: Not applicable.

Informed Consent Statement: Not applicable.

Data Availability Statement: Data are contained within the article.

Conflicts of Interest: Gaeun Lee and Hyun-Jin Bae were employed by the company Promedius Inc. The remaining authors declare that the research was conducted in the absence of any commercial or financial relationships that could be construed as a potential conflict of interest.

References

1. Le Huec, J.C.; Charosky, S.; Barrey, C.; Rigal, J.; Aunoble, S. Sagittal imbalance cascade for simple degenerative spine and consequences: Algorithm of decision for appropriate treatment. *Eur. Spine J.* **2011**, *20* (Suppl. S5), 699–703. [CrossRef] [PubMed]
2. Carman, D.L.; Browne, R.H.; Birch, J.G. Measurement of scoliosis and kyphosis radiographs. Intraobserver and interobserver variation. *J. Bone Jt. Surg. Am.* **1990**, *72*, 328–333. [CrossRef]
3. Summers, R.M. Deep learning and computer-aided diagnosis for medical image processing: A personal perspective. In *Deep Learning and Convolutional Neural Networks for Medical Image Computing*; Lu, L., Zheng, Y., Carneiro, G., Yang, L., Eds.; Springer International Publishing AG: Cham, Switzerland, 2017; pp. 3–10. [CrossRef]
4. Sun, H.; Zhen, X.; Bailey, C.; Rasoulinejad, P.; Yin, Y.; Li, S. *Direct Estimation of Spinal Cobb Angles by Structured Multi-Output Regression*; Springer International Publishing: Cham, Switzerland, 2017; pp. 529–540. [CrossRef]
5. Wu, H.; Bailey, C.; Rasoulinejad, P.; Li, S. Automated comprehensive adolescent idiopathic scoliosis assessment using MVC-Net. *Med. Image Anal.* **2018**, *48*, 1–11. [CrossRef] [PubMed]
6. Levine, M.; De Silva, T.; Ketcha, M.D.; Vijayan, R.; Doerr, S.; Uneri, A.; Vedula, S.; Theodore, N.; Siewerdsen, J.H. Automatic vertebrae localization in spine CT: A deep-learning approach for image guidance and surgical data science. In Proceedings of the SPIE 10951, Medical Imaging 2019: Image-Guided Procedures, Robotic Interventions, and Modeling, 109510S (8 March 2019), San Diego, CA, USA, 17–19 February 2019. [CrossRef]
7. Jakobsen, I.M.G.; Plocharski, M. Automatic detection of cervical vertebral landmarks for fluoroscopic joint motion analysis. In *Image Analysis. SCIA 2019. Lecture Notes in Computer Science*; Felsberg, M., Forssén, P.E., Sintorn, I.M., Unger, J., Eds.; Springer: Cham, Switzerland, 2019; Volume 11482, pp. 209–220. [CrossRef]
8. Isensee, F.; Petersen, J.; Klein, A.; Zimmerer, D.; Jaeger, P.F.; Kohl, S.; Wasserthal, J.; Koehler, G.; Norajitra, T.; Wirkert, S.; et al. Abstract: nnU-Net: Self-adapting framework for U-Net-based medical image segmentation. In *Bildverarbeitung für die Medizin*; Springer Fachmedien Wiesbaden: Wiesbaden, Germany, 2019; Volume 22. [CrossRef]
9. Alejandro, N.; Yang, K.; Deng, J. Stacked hourglass networks for human pose estimation. In Proceedings of the Computer Vision–ECCV 2016: 14th European Conference, Amsterdam, The Netherlands, 11–14 October 2016; Proceedings Part VIII 14. Springer International Publishing: Cham, Switzerland, 2016.
10. Kumar, H.; Marks, T.K.; Mou, W.; Wang, Y.; Jones, M.; Cherian, A.; Koike-Akino, T.; Liu, X.; Feng, C. Luvli face alignment: Estimating landmarks' location, uncertainty, and visibility likelihood. In Proceedings of the IEEE/CVF Conference on Computer Vision and Pattern Recognition, Seattle, WA, USA, 13–19 June 2020.
11. Zhang, Z.; Chai, K.; Yu, H.; Majaj, R.; Walsh, F.; Wang, E.; Mahbub, U.; Siegelmann, H.; Kim, D.; Rahman, T. Neuromorphic high-frequency 3D dancing pose estimation in dynamic environment. *Neurocomputing* **2023**, *547*, 126388. [CrossRef]
12. Kebaish, K.M.; Neubauer, P.R.; Voros, G.D.; Khoshnevisan, M.A.; Skolasky, R.L. Scoliosis in adults aged forty years and older: Prevalence and relationship to age, race, and gender. *Spine* **2011**, *36*, 731–736. [CrossRef] [PubMed]
13. Noh, S.H.; Lee, H.S.; Park, G.E.; Ha, Y.; Park, J.Y.; Kuh, S.U.; Chin, D.K.; Kim, K.S.; Cho, Y.E.; Kim, S.H.; et al. Predicting mechanical complications after adult spinal deformity operation using a machine learning based on modified global alignment and proportion scoring with body mass index and bone mineral density. *Neurospine* **2023**, *20*, 265–274. [CrossRef] [PubMed]
14. Noh, S.H.; Ha, Y.; Park, J.Y.; Kuh, S.U.; Chin, D.K.; Kim, K.S.; Cho, Y.E.; Lee, H.S.; Kim, K.H. Modified global alignment and proportion scoring with body mass index and bone mineral density analysis in global alignment and proportion score of each 3 categories for predicting mechanical complications after adult spinal deformity surgery. *Neurospine* **2021**, *18*, 484–491. [CrossRef] [PubMed]
15. Diebo, B.G.; Shah, N.V.; Boachie-Adjei, O.; Zhu, F.; Rothenfluh, D.A.; Paulino, C.B.; Schwab, F.J.; Lafage, V. Adult spinal deformity. *Lancet* **2019**, *394*, 160–172. [CrossRef] [PubMed]
16. Le Huec, J.C.; Thompson, W.; Mohsinaly, Y.; Barrey, C.; Faundez, A. Sagittal balance of the spine. *Eur. Spine J.* **2019**, *28*, 1889–1905. [CrossRef] [PubMed]
17. Barrey, C.; Jund, J.; Noseda, O.; Roussouly, P. Sagittal balance of the pelvis-spine complex and lumbar degenerative diseases. A comparative study about 85 cases. *Eur. Spine J.* **2007**, *16*, 1459–1467. [CrossRef] [PubMed]
18. Weng, C.H.; Wang, C.L.; Huang, Y.J.; Yeh, Y.C.; Fu, C.J.; Yeh, C.Y.; Tsai, T.T. Artificial intelligence for automatic measurement of sagittal vertical axis using ResUNet framework. *J. Clin. Med.* **2019**, *8*, 1826. [CrossRef] [PubMed]
19. Galbusera, F.; Niemeyer, F.; Wilke, H.J.; Bassani, T.; Casaroli, G.; Anania, C.; Costa, F.; Brayda-Bruno, M.; Sconfienza, L.M. Fully automated radiological analysis of spinal disorders and deformities: A deep learning approach. *Eur. Spine J.* **2019**, *28*, 951–960. [CrossRef] [PubMed]
20. Yeh, Y.C.; Weng, C.H.; Huang, Y.J.; Fu, C.J.; Tsai, T.T.; Yeh, C.Y. Deep learning approach for automatic landmark detection and alignment analysis in whole-spine lateral radiographs. *Sci. Rep.* **2021**, *11*, 7618. [CrossRef] [PubMed]

21. Zhou, G.; Jiang, W.; Lai, K.; Zheng, Y. Automatic measurement of spine curvature on 3-D ultrasound volume projection image with phase features. *IEEE Trans. Med Imaging* **2017**, *36*, 1250–1262. [CrossRef]
22. Bernstein, P.; Metzler, J.; Weinzierl, M.; Seifert, C.; Kisel, W.; Wacker, M. Radiographic scoliosis angle estimation: Spline-based measurement reveals superior reliability compared to traditional COBB method. *Eur. Spine J.* **2021**, *30*, 676–685. [CrossRef] [PubMed]
23. Weng, C.H.; Huang, Y.J.; Fu, C.J.; Yeh, Y.C.; Yeh, C.Y.; Tsai, T.T. Automatic recognition of whole-spine sagittal alignment and curvature analysis through a deep learning technique. *Eur. Spine J.* **2022**, *31*, 2092–2103. [CrossRef] [PubMed]
24. Roussouly, P.; Gollogly, S.; Berthonnaud, E.; Dimnet, J. Classification of the normal variation in the sagittal alignment of the human lumbar spine and pelvis in the standing position. *Spine* **2005**, *30*, 346–353. [CrossRef] [PubMed]
25. Pan, C.; Wang, G.; Sun, J.; Lv, G. Correlations between the inflection point and spinal sagittal alignment in asymptomatic adults. *Eur. Spine J.* **2020**, *29*, 2272–2280. [CrossRef] [PubMed]

bioengineering

MDPI

Article

Automatic Osteoporosis Screening System Using Radiomics and Deep Learning from Low-Dose Chest CT Images

Xiaoyu Tong †, Shigeng Wang †, Jingyi Zhang, Yong Fan, Yijun Liu and Wei Wei *

Department of Radiology, First Affiliated Hospital of Dalian Medical University, Dalian 116014, China; wangshigeng9855@163.com (S.W.); fyfan_yong@163.com (Y.F.)
* Correspondence: weiweidy1988@163.com; Tel.: +86-180-9887-6987
† These authors contributed equally to this work.

Abstract: Objective: Develop two fully automatic osteoporosis screening systems using deep learning (DL) and radiomics (Rad) techniques based on low-dose chest CT (LDCT) images and evaluate their diagnostic effectiveness. Methods: In total, 434 patients who underwent LDCT and bone mineral density (BMD) examination were retrospectively enrolled and divided into the development set (n = 333) and temporal validation set (n = 101). An automatic thoracic vertebra cancellous bone (TVCB) segmentation model was developed. The Dice similarity coefficient (DSC) was used to evaluate the segmentation performance. Furthermore, the three-class Rad and DL models were developed to distinguish osteoporosis, osteopenia, and normal bone mass. The diagnostic performance of these models was evaluated using the receiver operating characteristic (ROC) curve and decision curve analysis (DCA). Results: The automatic segmentation model achieved excellent segmentation performance, with a mean DSC of 0.96 ± 0.02 in the temporal validation set. The Rad model was used to identify osteoporosis, osteopenia, and normal BMD in the temporal validation set, with respective area under the receiver operating characteristic curve (AUC) values of 0.943, 0.801, and 0.932. The DL model achieved higher AUC values of 0.983, 0.906, and 0.969 for the same categories in the same validation set. The Delong test affirmed that both models performed similarly in BMD assessment. However, the accuracy of the DL model is 81.2%, which is better than the 73.3% accuracy of the Rad model in the temporal validation set. Additionally, DCA indicated that the DL model provided a greater net benefit compared to the Rad model across the majority of the reasonable threshold probabilities Conclusions: The automated segmentation framework we developed can accurately segment cancellous bone on low-dose chest CT images. These predictive models, which are based on deep learning and radiomics, provided comparable diagnostic performance in automatic BMD assessment. Nevertheless, it is important to highlight that the DL model demonstrates higher accuracy and precision than the Rad model.

Keywords: bone mineral density; osteoporosis; deep learning; tomography; X-ray computed; radiomics

1. Introduction

Osteoporosis, a commonly occurring musculoskeletal disease, is characterized by a decrease in bone mineral density (BMD) and damage to the microstructure of bone tissue, leading to heightened bone fragility and an increased risk of fractures [1]. Often termed a "silent disease", osteoporosis typically exhibits no discernible signs or symptoms until fractures manifest [2]. Notably, osteoporosis-related fractures are the primary cause of morbidity and mortality in the elderly. It is estimated that globally, approximately 9 million new cases of osteoporosis-related fractures occur annually, leading to a substantial burden on public health systems [3,4]. Given these circumstances, it is imperative to prioritize early warning and screening for osteoporosis.

Radiomics (Rad), a quantitative technique that utilizes high-throughput radiomics features, has provided substantial evidence in assessing diseases. Specifically, it has been shown that radiomics can effectively extract BMD information from thoracic vertebrae within chest CT images, enabling the provision of quantitative heterogeneity measures [5]. This approach holds promise for opportunistic and preventive osteoporosis screening, as it eliminates the need for additional costs and radiation exposure. In addition, there is growing concern regarding the radiation risks associated with CT scans, given the increasing utilization of CT imaging and the public's heightened awareness of radiation protection [6,7]. Low-dose chest CT (LDCT), particularly with a tube voltage of 80 kVp, has been widely applied in clinical practice for lung cancer screening among the high-risk population, as well as routine physical examination [8,9]. However, it is worth noting that modifying the tube voltage setting can potentially impact the stability of the radiomics model [10–12]. To the best of our knowledge, the Rad model of BMD assessment based on 80 kVp images has not been well established.

Recently, the field of artificial intelligence has witnessed a surge of interest in deep learning (DL) techniques. DL utilizes deep convolutional neural networks (CNN) to automatically extract high-dimensional features from CT images, enabling end-to-end learning without requiring manual feature extraction [13,14]. DL has exhibited remarkable performance in image analysis and has proven advantages in differentiating between benign and malignant vertebral compression fractures [15]. Although both Rad and DL methods have demonstrated promising diagnostic capabilities in relevant aspects, there exists a dearth of studies comparing their performance in BMD assessment based on chest LDCT images, especially 80 kVp CT images. Can the novel deep learning network surpass traditional radiomics models in accurately diagnosing bone density?

It is worth noting that both Rad and DL methods require manual delineation of the region of interest, which can be a burdensome workload for radiologists and may introduce observer variability that can impact image analysis. Fortunately, advancements in deep learning architectures have enabled the development of automatic segmentation models that can mitigate these challenges and provide satisfactory segmentation results [16,17]. Therefore, this study had dual objectives. Firstly, we endeavored to train an automatic segmentation model using VB-Net architecture specifically for thoracic vertebra cancellous bone (TVCB). Secondly, we aimed to develop and compare the diagnostic performance of two predictive models—a deep learning-based model (DL model) and a radiomics-based model (Rad model)—for BMD assessment based on low-dose chest CT images acquired at 80 kVp. We hypothesize that the novel DL model may outperform traditional Rad models in accurately assessing bone mineral density.

2. Materials and Methods

This retrospective study received approval from the Ethics Committee, which also waived the requirement for informed patient consent (IRB No. PJ-KS-KY-2023-276).

2.1. Study Population

A total of 687 patients who underwent chest LDCT scans and BMD examination were retrospectively retrieved from the picture archiving and communication system from May 2021 to April 2023. Patients with the following conditions were excluded: (1) the time interval between LDCT and BMD was more than one month (n = 138); (2) the scanning range failed to cover the required thoracic vertebra (n = 9); (3) a history of surgery and metal implants in the lower thoracic vertebrae (n = 36); (4) bone metastasis of malignant tumors (n = 38); (5) abnormal vertebral morphology in the lower thoracic vertebrae, such as compression fracture, severe degenerative changes or deformities (n = 29); and (6) recent use of drugs affecting bone metabolism (n = 3). Eventually, 434 patients were enrolled and divided into a development set (n = 333, examined between May 2021 and June 2022) and a temporal validation set (n = 101, examined between July 2022 and April 2023) according to the examination time. This development set was utilized for training automatic segmentation models as well as BMD assessment models. During the training of the BMD assessment models (Rad and DL model), the development set was randomly partitioned into two subsets for BMD assessment models training and internal evaluation, with 80% allocated for the internal training set and the remaining 20% for the testing set. The temporal validation set was used to evaluate the performance of all models. A detailed enrollment flowchart is shown in Figure 1, and the overall workflow of this study is illustrated in Figure 2. The automatic segmentation framework construction, Rad model, and DL model were developed and validated on the uAI Research Portal V1.1 (United Imaging Intelligence, Co., Ltd. (Shanghai, China)). The design of uAI Research Portal architecture takes a modular and layered approach [18]: (1) The lower level is composed of hardware drivers, such as graphics processing unit (GPU) accelerated using NVIDIA CUDA, and cloud servers, such as Amazon web services (AWS); (2) At the middle level, there is an application programming interface (API), primarily Python and C++, contributing a range of algorithms (e.g., segmentation, classification); (3) the higher level presents build blocks to the end users for domain-specific analysis.

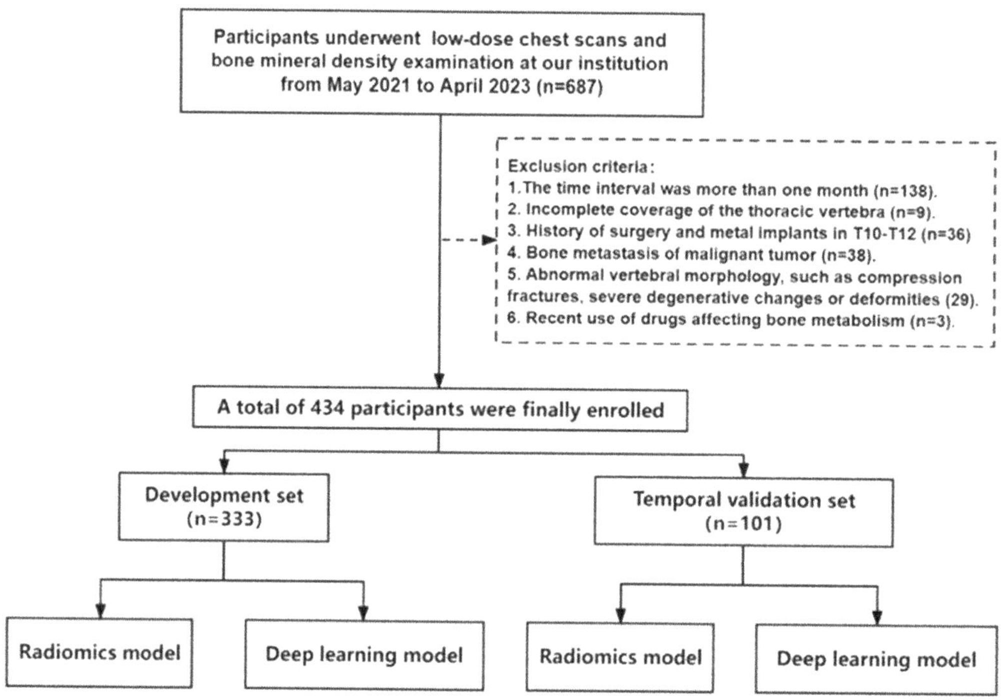

Figure 1. A detailed flowchart of patient enrollment.

2.2. Image Acquisition and BMD Assessment

All CT images were acquired on a 256-row CT scanner (Revolution CT, GE HealthCare, Milwaukee, WI, USA). The chest LDCT scans were acquired using a low tube voltage of 80 kV, smart mA (noise index: 10, 50–400 mA), rotation speed of 0.5 s/rot, detector width of 80 mm, pitch of 0.992, and scanning slice thickness and slice interval of 5 mm. The scan coverage started from the lung apexes to 2 cm below the diaphragm. All images were reconstructed using the standard kernel, adaptive statistical iterative reconstruction-Veo (ASIR-V) at 40% strength, and reconstruction thickness and interval of 1.25 mm.

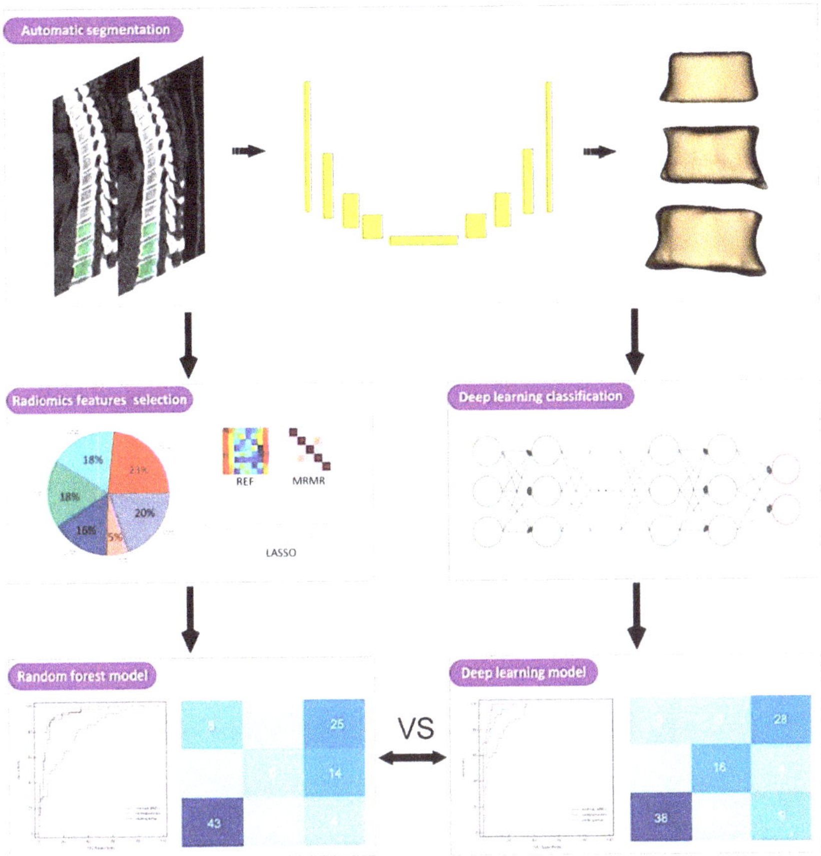

Figure 2. The overall flowchart of this study. The construction of the radiomics model utilizes a random forest classifier, while the deep learning model adopts the Res-Net architecture. REF, Recursive Feature Elimination; MRMR, Minimum Redundancy Maximum Relevance; LASSO, the Least Absolute Shrinkage and Selection Operator.

BMD examinations were performed using a standardized protocol following the manufacturer's guidelines for the quantitative computed tomography (QCT) workstation. The details of the QCT scanning protocol can be found in Supplementary S1. Patient abdominal data were transferred to a QCT Pro workstation (version 6.1, Mindways Software, Inc. (Austin, TX, USA)), and BMD measurements were taken at two consecutive vertebral bodies (L1 and L2). Compared to conventional methods, QCT measures volumetric BMD, reflecting BMD in different regions (trabecular and cortical) of the skeleton. This gives QCT an advantage in assessing osteoporosis severity, guiding treatment strategies, and monitoring treatment efficacy. According to clinical guidelines for BMD assessment [19], osteoporosis was defined as a BMD below 80 mg/cm^3, osteopenia as a BMD between 80 and 120 mg/cm^3, and normal status as a BMD above 120 mg/cm^3. For this study, the diagnostic performance was analyzed through the construction of receiver operating characteristic (ROC) curves, employing QCT data as the diagnostic standard. The ROC curve assesses a classification or diagnostic model's performance by plotting the true positive (sensitivity) and false positive rate (1-specificity) against various thresholds [20]. This provides an overview of the model's performance in predicting bone status.

2.3. TVCB Auto-Segmentation Framework and VOI Delineation

Budoff et al. suggested that the cancellous bone of the lower thoracic vertebrae (TVCB), specifically T10–12, closely correlates with lumbar vertebrae in providing information about bone mineral density (BMD), making it a viable target for BMD assessment [21]. Therefore, the volume of interest (VOI) of TVCB was manually delineated on the axial images and carefully avoided vertebral venous plexuses and cortical bone. The boundary was placed along the inner edge of the vertebral cortex. In addition, 100 patients were randomly selected to assess the interobserver repeatability in the manual segmentation, and VOI was independently delineated on CT images by two readers (W. Wei and Y. Liu, with 5 and 12 years of experience in musculoskeletal radiology, respectively). The Dice similarity coefficient (DSC) was employed to assess the consistency of inter-observer segmentation. If a satisfactory agreement was achieved, the junior radiologist would complete the remaining cases under the supervision of the senior radiologist.

For the auto-segmentation framework, we trained a cascade model with two VB-Nets based on the coarse-to-fine principle, including a coarse-scale segmentation network for rapidly locating the target area and a fine-scale segmentation network for precisely delineating target and optimization. The detailed architecture of the VB-Net is shown in Supplementary Figure S1. In pre-processing, it was normalized by subtracting the window level (WL: 100) and dividing by the window width (WW: 300). For training the coarse-scale segmentation network, global sampling was used. The images were resampled to $3 \times 3 \times 3$ mm using B-Spline interpolation. In the fine-scale segmentation network, images were resampled to crop high-resolution local images with a resampling voxel size of $1 \times 1 \times 1$ mm, and mask sampling was used. The learning rate was 1×10^{-4}, the batch size was 8, the number of epochs was set to 1001, and the optimizer was Adam. We used the focal loss function to monitor the convergence of the training model and optimize the network. The detailed settings of the coarse-scale segmentation network are given in Supplementary S2. DSC and volume difference (VD) were used to evaluate the segmentation performance of the model. The DSC coefficient is a measure of similarity between the segmentation results and the reference criteria. Its calculation method is based on the overlapping area between the segmentation result and the reference standard. The VD was defined as the absolute value of the manually segmented volume minus the automatically segmented volume.

2.4. Radiomics Model Construction

After establishing the auto-segmentation model, the model was used for automatic cancellous bone segmentation in the development and temporal validation sets.

2.4.1. Radiomics Features Extraction

All images were normalized using Z-score and resampled, the voxel spacing to $1 \times 1 \times 1$ mm using B-Spline interpolation, and the image gray level was discretized with 25 binwidth. Z-score normalization is a widely utilized technique for standardizing data to make it comparable across different features. This is accomplished by subtracting the mean from each data point and dividing it by the standard deviation of the feature's data within the given sample. A total of 90 features in six categories were extracted from the original images, including first-order features and texture features. Details of the extracted radiomics features are provided in Supplementary Table S1.

2.4.2. Features Selection and Model Construction

The development set was randomly divided into the internal training and testing sets at a ratio of 8:2. The Z-score normalization was conducted to pre-process the features and ensure the comparability between the data before the feature selection and Rad model construction. A step-wise feature selection strategy was used to determine the optimal features (Supplementary S3).

Finally, random forest was performed to establish a three-classification model to distinguish osteoporosis, osteopenia, and normal BMD. Random forest is a widely used ensemble technique in radiomics classification tasks. It is based on a collection of decision trees, forming a "forest", and incorporates random feature selection and bootstrap sampling during training and prediction. The ROC curve was conducted to evaluate the efficacy of the Rad model in diagnosing osteoporosis, osteopenia, and normal BMD. The area under the receiver operating characteristic curve (AUC), sensitivity, specificity, precision, and accuracy were calculated to evaluate the performance of training, internal test, and temporal validation set.

2.5. Deep Learning Network Construction

The DL model was trained using the residual network (Res-Net), which integrates residual learning to prevent gradient dispersion and precision loss in deep networks, achieving enhanced accuracy as the network depth increases [22]. The Res-Net is composed of four simple residual blocks, which enable the network to learn more efficiently and effectively; each residual block consists of two convolutional layers followed by a skip connection, which can effectively learn both low-level and high-level features simultaneously. During the training process, all images were resampled with voxel spacing of $1 \times 1 \times 1$ mm and normalized by min-max normalization. Figure 3 shows the detailed architecture of the Res-Net. The batch size was set to 8, and the IO threads were set to 4. The focal loss function and Adam optimizer were used to monitor the convergence of the model with an initial learning rate of 1×10^{-4}, and the "step" learning rate strategy was applied to accelerate convergence. The diagnostic performance of the deep learning classification model was evaluated on the internal test and temporal validation sets using ROC analysis.

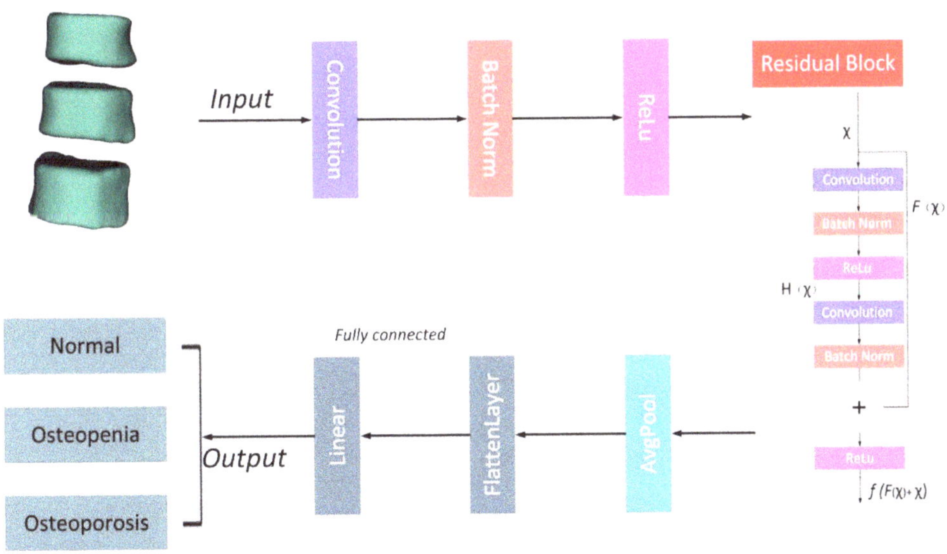

Figure 3. The Residual Network Structure.

2.6. Statistical Analysis

SPSS version 24.0 (IBM Corp., Armonk, NY, USA) and MedCalc version 20.022 (MedCalc Ltd., Ostend, Belgium) were used for statistical analysis. The data were tested for normality using the Kolmogorov–Smirnov test, and continuous variables were expressed as mean ± standard deviation or medians (25–75th percentile). The chi-square test was used for gender and bone status distribution in development and temporal validation sets.

An independent sample *t*-test was used to test the age difference between the development and the temporal validation sets. The DeLong test was used to assess the difference in diagnostic performance between the Rad model and the DL model. The clinical application value of the Rad model and the DL model was evaluated in the temporal validation set by constructing decision curve analysis (DCA).

3. Results

3.1. Participant Demographics

A total of 434 patients were enrolled in the study, including 333 patients in the development set (mean age: 62.89 ± 11.55 years) and 101 patients in the temporal validation set (mean age: 60.76 ± 10.41 years). In both sets, there were no significant differences in the distributions of age, gender, and BMD distribution. The detailed demographic characteristics are shown in Table 1.

Table 1. Participant demographics.

Characteristic	Development Set	Temporal Validation Set	*p*-Value
All (*n*)	333	101	
Male (*n*)	170	57	
Female (*n*)	163	44	0.404
All (years)	62.89 ± 11.55	60.76 ± 10.41	0.098
Male (years)	65.37 ± 10.37	62.60 ± 9.14	0.073
Female (years)	60.30 ± 12.17	58.39 ± 11.54	0.350
Osteoporosis (*n*)	84	20	
Osteopenia (*n*)	134	34	
Normal BMD (*n*)	115	47	0.094

Data are presented as the number of patients except for mean ± standard deviation for age.

3.2. Automatic Segmentation Model

The cancellous bone segmentation was in good agreement between the two observers, with a mean DSC of 0.96 ± 0.02. The automatic segmentation model demonstrated excellent performance with a mean DSC of 0.96 ± 0.02 in the temporal validation set. The detailed distribution of DSC is shown in Figure 4. The VD did not exceed 1 cm^3 with a mean of 0.50 (0.17, 0.69). The segmentation performance of TVCB for different BMD populations is illustrated in Table 2.

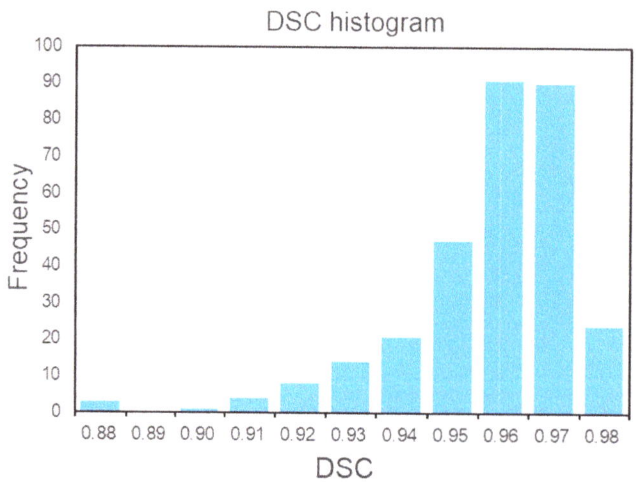

Figure 4. Histogram of the DSC. DSC, Dice similarity coefficient.

Table 2. The Dice similarity coefficient and volume difference of manual and automatic segmentation.

Category	DSC	VD (cm^3)
All	0.96 ± 0.02	0.50 (0.17, 0.69)
Osteoporosis	0.97 ± 0.01	0.44 (0.09, 0.68)
Osteopenia	0.96 ± 0.02	0.53 (0.19, 0.63)
Normal BMD	0.96 ± 0.02	0.50 (0.18, 0.80)

DSC, Dice similarity coefficient; VD, volume difference; BMD, bone mineral density.

3.3. The Comparison of the Rad Model and DL Model

In the Rad model, 6 radiomics features were selected, including 1 first-order feature and 5 texture features (Supplementary Table S2). The AUCs in predicting osteoporosis, osteopenia, and normal BMD were 0.919, 0.873, and 0.976, respectively, in the internal test set. In the temporal validation set, the AUCs were 0.943, 0.801, and 0.932, respectively.

As for the DL model, the AUCs in predicting osteoporosis, osteopenia, and normal BMD were 0.942, 0.866, and 0.972, respectively, in the internal test set. In the temporal validation set, the AUCs were 0.983, 0.906, and 0.969, respectively.

The two models achieved similar performance in distinguishing osteoporosis, osteopenia, and normal BMD for the temporal validation set, with no significant difference demonstrated by the DeLong test. The results of more detailed metrics are summarized in Table 3, and the ROC curves are shown in Figures 5 and 6. DCA showed that the DL model had a higher net benefit than the Rad model across the majority of the range of reasonable threshold probabilities in the temporal validation set, indicating that the DL model has good clinical utility (Figure 7).

Table 3. Overall performance of BMD assessment for the Rad model and DL model.

Model	Set	Category	AUC	95%CI	Sensitivity (%)	Specificity (%)	Precision (%)	Accuracy (%)
Rad Model	Internal training set	Osteoporosis	0.959	0.927–0.979	88.1	92.0	88.9	
		Osteopenia	0.881	0.835–0.917	90.7	75.5	67.3	
		Normal BMD	0.977	0.95–0.991	84.8	98.9	96.3	
		Overall						79.0
	Internal test set	Osteoporosis	0.919	0.826–0.971	88.2	86.0	71.4	
		Osteopenia	0.873	0.769–0.942	81.5	85.0	60.0	
		Normal BMD	0.976	0.906–0.998	100.0	93.2	90.0	
		Overall						70.2
	Temporal validation set	Osteoporosis	0.943	0.878–0.979	90.0	90.1	85.7	
		Osteopenia	0.801	0.709–0.874	82.4	67.2	58.1	
		Normal BMD	0.932	0.864–0.972	93.6	85.2	84.3	
		Overall						73.3
DL Model	Internal training set	Osteoporosis	0.975	0.948–0.990	95.5	96.5	87.7	
		Osteopenia	0.936	0.900–0.962	89.7	95.6	93.2	
		Normal BMD	0.972	0.944–0.988	96.7	94.8	95.6	
		Overall						92.5
	Internal test set	Osteoporosis	0.942	0.857–0.985	100.0	76.0	75.0	
		Osteopenia	0.866	0.760–0.937	74.1	85.0	71.4	
		Normal BMD	0.972	0.900–0.997	100.0	90.9	87.0	
		Overall						77.6
	Temporal validation set	Osteoporosis	0.983	0.935–0.998	100.0	92.6	84.2	
		Osteopenia	0.906	0.831–0.955	85.3	80.6	68.3	
		Normal BMD	0.969	0.914–0.993	95.7	85.2	92.7	
		Overall						81.2

DL, deep learning; Rad, radiomics; AUC, area under the receiver operating characteristic curve; CI, confidence interval; BMD, bone mineral density.

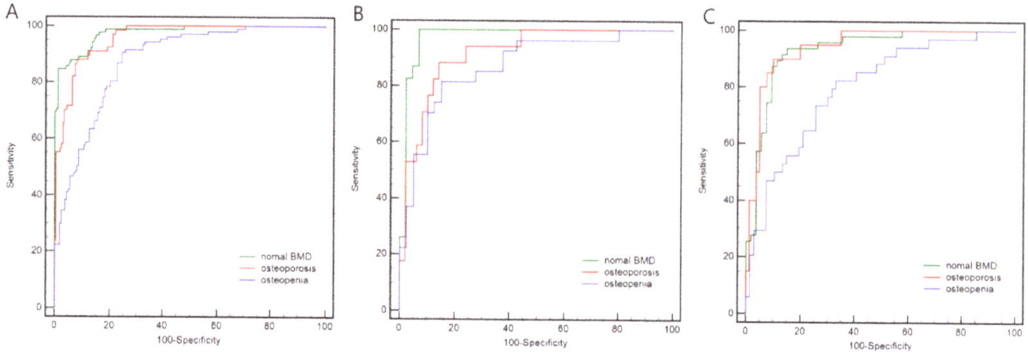

Figure 5. The receiver operating characteristic curves of the radiomics model on the internal training (**A**), the internal testing set (**B**), and the temporal validation set (**C**). The AUC values of the radiomics model on the internal training set for osteoporosis, osteopenia, and normal BMD were 0.959, 0.881, and 0.977, respectively. As for the internal testing set, these values were 0.919, 0.873, and 0.976, respectively. As for the temporal validation set, these values were 0.943, 0.801, and 0.932, respectively. The red, blue, and green lines represent predicted osteoporosis, osteopenia, and normal BMD, respectively. AUC, area under the receiver operating characteristic curve; BMD, bone mineral density.

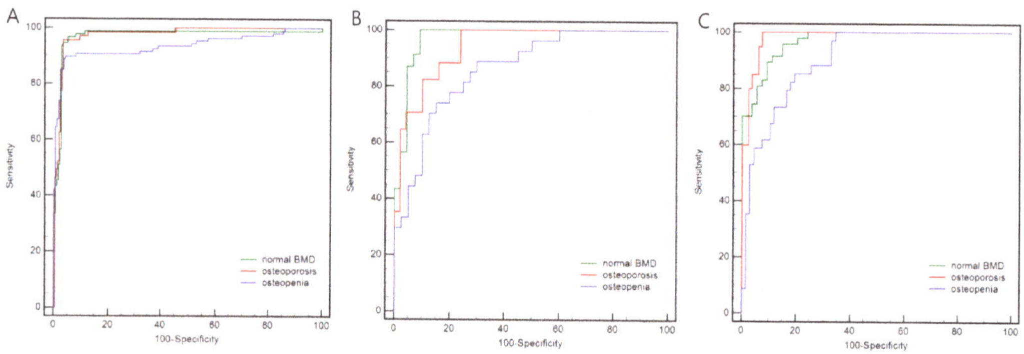

Figure 6. The receiver operating characteristic curves of the deep learning model on the internal training (**A**), the internal testing set (**B**), and the temporal validation set (**C**). The AUC values of the radiomics model on the internal training set for osteoporosis, osteopenia, and normal BMD were 0.975, 0.936, and 0.972, respectively. As for the internal testing set, these values were 0.942, 0.866, and 0.972, respectively. As for the temporal validation set, these values were 0.983, 0.906, and 0.969, respectively. The red, blue, and green lines represent predicted osteoporosis, osteopenia, and normal BMD, respectively. AUC, area under the receiver operating characteristic curve; BMD, bone mineral density.

Furthermore, we compared the performance of the proposed method with several benchmark methods. The comparison reveals that our DL model demonstrates superior performance in detecting osteoporosis, osteopenia, and normal BMD (Table 4).

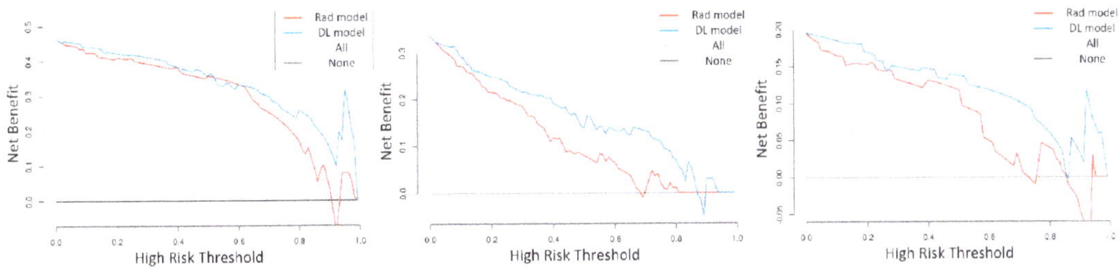

(A) (B) (C)

Figure 7. DCAs of the Rad model and DL model in the temporal validation set. (**A**) DCA of the Rad model and DL model in predicting abnormal BMD. (**B**) DCA of the Rad model and DL model in predicting osteopenia. (**C**) DCA of the Rad model and DL model in predicting osteoporosis. Rad model, radiomics model; DL model, deep learning model; DCA, decision curve analysis; BMD, bone mineral density.

Table 4. The performance of our proposed method is compared with several benchmark methods.

Authors(methods)	Key Findings	AUC	Sensitivity (%)	Specificity (%)	Accuracy (%)
Xue et al. (Radiomics) [23]	Detecting abnormal BMD	0.944	95.8	-	-
	Detecting osteoporosis	0.866	83.3	-	-
Chen et al. (Radiomics) [24]	Detecting abnormal BMD	0.960	93.0	89.0	91.0
	Detecting osteoporosis	0.980	95.0	93.0	94.0
Wang et al. (Radiomics) [25]	Detecting osteoporosis	0.914	90.7	75.0	89.8
Ours (Radiomics)	Detecting abnormal BMD	0.932	93.6	85.2	
	Detecting osteopenia	0.801	82.4	67.5	73.3
	Detecting osteoporosis	0.943	90.0	90.1	
Yang et al. (Deep learning) [5]	Detecting osteopenia	0.831	73.6	80.5	-
	Detecting osteoporosis	0.972	95.6	88.0	
Ours (Deep learning)	Detecting abnormal BMD	0.969	95.7	85.2	
	Detecting Osteopenia	0.906	85.3	80.6	81.2
	Detecting osteoporosis	0.983	100	92.6	

BMD, bone mineral density.

4. Discussion

In this study, we developed an automatic TVCB segmentation model using the VB-Net network architecture and a coarse-to-fine cascade training strategy based on 80 kVp chest LDCT images. The model achieved segmentation accuracy comparable to that of manual depiction, with mean DSC surpassing 0.90. In addition, we compared the classification performance between the Rad and DL models for BMD assessment. The AUCs of the Rad and DL models were 0.943 and 0.983 for predicting osteoporosis, 0.801 and 0.906 for predicting osteopenia, and 0.932 and 0.969 for predicting normal BMD in the validation set, respectively. The Delong test showed that for diagnostic performance, there was no statistically significant difference between the Rad and DL models. However, the DL model demonstrated superior sensitivity, specificity, precision, and overall accuracy in evaluating various performance metrics compared to the traditional Rad model. In addition, the end-to-end learning strategy employed in the DL model eliminated intermediate steps such as Rad model data pre-processing, feature extraction, and classifier selection, which reduces human intervention and improves the efficiency of model construction and the objectivity of the results.

LDCT is primarily accomplished by reducing the tube current or tube voltage. As the radiation dose is directly proportional to the square of the tube voltage, reducing the tube voltage can effectively decrease the radiation dose [26]. This is particularly advantageous for the Asian population, which typically has smaller body sizes. Lower tube voltage scans do not significantly compromise diagnostic confidence but provide more cost-effective and radiation-dose-efficient imaging for patients [27].

To the best of our knowledge, no attempt has been made to establish automatic segmentation of TVCB on LDCT using 80 kVp. Previous segmentation models have been constructed using 120 kVp images in a complex or error-prone manner. Chen et al. initially used CNN networks to identify the entire thoracic vertebrae and subsequently applied an erosion algorithm to remove the bone cortex [24]. However, the working process of this method to obtain TVCB was complex. Wang et al. used a fixed-size cylindrical shape to identify TVCB, leading to incomplete segmentation in cancellous bone and introducing bias in the BMD assessment [28]. In our study, we employed the VB-Net to construct an automatic segmentation model for TVCB. The VB-Net is a modified version of CNN that incorporates a bottleneck structure in place of convolutional, normalization, and activation layers. This modification not only reduces the number of model parameters but also improves inference efficiency and robustness [28]. The VB-Net has been demonstrated to produce satisfactory segmentation results, with established applications in cervical and lung cancer segmentation [29,30]. Additionally, the uneven distribution of BMD in the thoracic vertebrae can reduce the sensitivity of osteoporosis assessment if the entire vertebrae are segmented. However, some researchers found that utilizing the lower thoracic vertebrae (T10–12) for BMD assessment yields high levels of accuracy and repeatability [21]. Therefore, we used a cascade approach utilizing VB-Net in this work. The 10-12th vertebrae were initially identified at a "coarse" resolution to achieve accurate spatial localization, followed by the detailed delineation of bony cortex and cancellous bone at a "fine" resolution. It is worthwhile to emphasize the advantages of our method, as it efficiently and accurately identifies the TVCB in chest LDCT images. Our method achieved DSC results exceeding 0.90 in the temporal validation set.

Radiomics encompasses the extraction of high-dimensional tissue data from medical images, which can be further integrated with machine learning techniques to establish radiomics signatures. The radiomics features extracted from TVCB can reflect the transformation of bone microstructure and accurately assess BMD [31]. Notably, Chen et al. pointed out that the performance of radiomics in assessing BMD significantly decreased in the external validation set, with a 20% lower accuracy compared to the internal validation set [24]. This phenomenon occurs because the stability of radiomics features depends on image acquisition parameters. Altering factors such as tube voltage or slice thickness can indeed impact the effectiveness of existing radiomics models [32]. Therefore, we deem it imperative to establish a novel Rad model in 80 kVp chest CT images for BMD assessment. To ensure the stability of the feature selection process and the generalization ability of the Rad model, we employed a step-wise feature selection strategy to select 6 highly effective features. Encouragingly, these 6 features have been closely related to bone quantity, microstructure, and loss in relevant studies [23,25]. Our Rad model could provide valuable information in BMD assessment and demonstrate comparable or superior performance compared to recent research results.

Deep learning has emerged as a highly promising approach for achieving accurate diagnostic outcomes in medical imaging. Recent advancements in artificial intelligence have been crucial in driving this progression. Mehdi et al. developed a DL model that was capable of distinguishing tumor invasiveness, achieving accuracy comparable to pathology results [33]. Li et al. developed a DL model based on CT images using Res-Net, achieving faster convergence and high accuracy in diagnosing vertebral fractures [34]. Kitamura et al. [35] discovered that Res-Net convolutional neural networks demonstrated strong performance in ankle fracture detection with small sample sizes. Therefore, we selected Res-Net to build a three-classification BMD assessment model. The core concept of Res-Net is to learn residuals, which involves the network learning the difference between inputs and outputs. To tackle the challenges of vanishing and exploding gradients in training deep neural networks, Res-Net introduces "residual blocks" [34]. These blocks enable the network to efficiently capture the disparity between input and output through shortcut connections, resulting in faster convergence and improved accuracy [36]. With this innovative network architecture, Res-Net empowers models to train deeper neural networks, effectively addressing complex visual tasks like image classification, object detection, and semantic segmentation.

In our study, the DL model utilized automatic segmentation of TVCB as an input, eliminating the need for time-consuming, manually segmented regions of interest. Furthermore, the DL model enabled the extraction and analysis of high-level semantic features in an end-to-end manner, facilitating the automatic learning of pertinent and robust features without human intervention. Consequently, the overall approach mitigated human bias arising from artificial features. Our DL model yielded satisfactory outcomes in BMD assessment.

Previous studies have compared the performance of Rad and DL models across various tasks. Mehdi et al. [33] discovered that the Rad model outperformed the DL model in predicting malignancy of pulmonary nodules from chest LDCT images. Li et al. [37] observed that their DL model outperformed the Rad model in classifying molecular subtypes of diffuse gliomas. In our study, we developed Rad and DL models based on relatively large samples. To the best of our knowledge, this is the first study to investigate and compare the performance of DL networks against traditional Rad models in assessing BMD. The main findings of our study demonstrate that the novel DL model outperformed the traditional Rad model in the precise assessment of BMD. The DL model exhibited enhanced sensitivity, specificity, precision, and overall accuracy across various performance metrics relative to the traditional Rad model. Zhou et al. [37] obtained similar results when distinguishing between benign and malignant breast lesions using Rad and DL models. In the Rad model, it is necessary to determine the most suitable features for the BMD assessment task in advance. In contrast, the DL model does not require predefined features and can automatically determine the nuanced features of the target task with almost no human intervention, ensuring objectivity and efficient classification performance. Consequently, our results indicate that deep learning has the potential to serve as a diagnostic tool for BMD assessment in clinical practice. The improved performance of the DL model can provide enhanced diagnostic accuracy, thus leading to better clinical decision-making and improving patient outcomes. By accurately predicting BMD status, clinicians can identify individuals at high risk of fractures and tailor intervention strategies accordingly. This approach can lead to early interventions that prevent or mitigate the progression of bone diseases, ultimately improving patient outcomes and reducing healthcare costs. Furthermore, the successful application of DL networks in assessing BMD highlights the potential for similar approaches in other medical domains.

This study has some limitations. Firstly, our proposed Rad and DL models were developed using chest LDCT images acquired from a single center, which may restrict their applicability of the models to the LDCT in other institutions. Additionally, while residual networks have shown significant success in enhancing performance, the architecture can also suffer from black-box effects stemming from the complexity caused by convolutional layers and non-linear activation functions. Finally, the selection of the random forest classifier, although informed by a comprehensive literature review, was not accompanied by comparative analysis against other potential classifiers in our study, which leaves room for exploration regarding optimal classification strategies.

5. Conclusions

In conclusion, we developed and evaluated a model for automatic TVCB segmentation using 80 kVp chest LDCT images, which laid the foundation for future fully automated BMD assessment programs. In addition, we developed deep learning-based and radiomics-based predictive models, which provided similar excellent diagnostic performance in BMD assessment. Nevertheless, it is important to highlight that the deep learning model demonstrates higher accuracy and precision compared to the radiomics model. Future research should investigate whether variations in CT scan parameters would affect the performance of DL models in assessing bone mineral density.

Supplementary Materials: The following supporting information can be downloaded at: https://www.mdpi.com/article/10.3390/bioengineering11010050/s1, Supplementary S1: The BMD scanning protocol and measurement; Supplementary S2: The detailed settings of the coarse-scale segmentation network; Supplementary S3: Radiomic features extraction methods; Figure S1: VB-Net architecture. VB-Net is a variant segmentation network structure of V-Net that utilizes a bottleneck structure (B stands for bottleneck) instead of the convolution, normalization, and activation layers within the Down Block and Up block. A bottleneck structure in a neural network has fewer neurons than its adjacent layers, which helps compress feature representations to fit in the available vector space. The bottleneck structure consists of three convolutional layers. The first and third convolutional layers use the unit convolution kernel and match the dimensions of the preceding and succeeding layers, respectively. The second convolution layer performs spatial convolution on the feature image that has been reduced in dimension by the first convolution layer. This reduction in dimensionality helps reduce the number of model parameters, leading to increased efficiency; Table S1: Radiomics features extracted from original images; Table S2: Selected features for constructing radiomics model.

Author Contributions: Conceptualization, X.T., S.W. and W.W.; methodology, X.T. and S.W.; software, S.W. and J.Z.; validation, X.T. and Y.F.; investigation, X.T. and S.W.; resources, W.W. and Y.L.; data curation, Y.L.; writing—original draft preparation, X.T. and S.W.; writing—review and editing, J.Z.; visualization, Y.F.; supervision, W.W.; project administration, Y.L. All authors have read and agreed to the published version of the manuscript.

Funding: This research received no external funding.

Institutional Review Board Statement: The study was conducted in accordance with the Declaration of Helsinki and approved by the Institutional Review Board (or Ethics Committee) of First Affiliated Hospital of Dalian Medical University (protocol code PJ-KS-KY-2023-276. Approval date 12 June 2023).

Informed Consent Statement: Patient consent was waived due to the retrospective nature of the study.

Data Availability Statement: The raw data supporting the conclusions of this article will be made available by the authors without undue reservation.

Acknowledgments: We express our sincere appreciation to Jingjing Cui and Jianying Li for their invaluable contributions in proofreading the manuscript and offering insightful suggestions.

Conflicts of Interest: The authors declare no conflicts of interest.

References

1. Gruenewald, L.D.; Koch, V.; Martin, S.S.; Yel, I.; Eichler, K.; Gruber-Rouh, T.; Lenga, L.; Wichmann, J.L.; Alizadeh, L.S.; Albrecht, M.H.; et al. Diagnostic accuracy of quantitative dual-energy CT-based volumetric bone mineral density assessment for the prediction of osteoporosis-associated fractures. *Eur. Radiol.* **2022**, *32*, 3076–3084. [CrossRef]
2. Chang, Q.; Huang, J.; He, L.; Xi, F. Simple immunosensor for ultrasensitive electrochemical determination of biomarker of the bone metabolism in human serum. *Front. Chem.* **2022**, *10*, 940795. [CrossRef] [PubMed]
3. Del Real, Á.; Valero, C.; Olmos, J.M.; Hernández, J.L.; Riancho, J.A. Pharmacogenetics of Osteoporosis: A Pathway Analysis of the Genetic Influence on the Effects of Antiresorptive Drugs. *Pharmaceutics* **2022**, *14*, 776. [CrossRef] [PubMed]
4. Si, L.; Winzenberg, T.M.; Jiang, Q.; Chen, M.; Palmer, A.J. Projection of osteoporosis-related fractures and costs in China: 2010–2050. *Osteoporos. Int.* **2015**, *26*, 1929–1937. [CrossRef] [PubMed]
5. Yang, J.; Liao, M.; Wang, Y.; Chen, L.; He, L.; Ji, Y.; Xiao, Y.; Lu, Y.; Fan, W.; Nie, Z.; et al. Opportunistic osteoporosis screening using chest CT with artificial intelligence. *Osteoporos. Int.* **2022**, *33*, 2547–2561. [CrossRef]
6. Yoon, H.J.; Chung, M.J.; Hwang, H.S.; Moon, J.W.; Lee, K.S. Adaptive Statistical Iterative Reconstruction-Applied Ultra-Low-Dose CT with Radiography-Comparable Radiation Dose: Usefulness for Lung Nodule Detection. *Korean J. Radiol.* **2015**, *16*, 1132–1141. [CrossRef]
7. Xiao, M.; Zhang, M.; Lei, M.; Lin, F.; Chen, Y.; Chen, J.; Liu, J.; Ye, J. Diagnostic accuracy of ultra-low-dose CT compared to standard-dose CT for identification of non-displaced fractures of the shoulder, knee, ankle, and wrist. *Insights Into Imaging* **2023**, *14*, 40. [CrossRef]
8. Wood, D.E.; Kazerooni, E.A.; Baum, S.L.; Eapen, G.A.; Ettinger, D.S.; Hou, L.; Jackman, D.M.; Klippenstein, D.; Kumar, R.; Lackner, R.P.; et al. Lung Cancer Screening, Version 3.2018, NCCN Clinical Practice Guidelines in Oncology. *J. Natl. Compr. Cancer Netw. JNCCN* **2018**, *16*, 412–441. [CrossRef]

9. Aberle, D.R.; Adams, A.M.; Berg, C.D.; Black, W.C.; Clapp, J.D.; Fagerstrom, R.M.; Gareen, I.F.; Gatsonis, C.; Marcus, P.M.; Sicks, J.D. Reduced lung-cancer mortality with low-dose computed tomographic screening. *N. Engl. J. Med.* **2011**, *365*, 395–409. [CrossRef]
10. Jin, S.; Zhang, B.; Zhang, L.; Li, S.; Li, S.; Li, P. Lung nodules assessment in ultra-low-dose CT with iterative reconstruction compared to conventional dose CT. *Quant. Imaging Med. Surg.* **2018**, *8*, 480–490. [CrossRef]
11. Sun, J.; Zhang, Q.; Hu, D.; Shen, Y.; Yang, H.; Chen, C.; Zhou, Z.; Peng, Y. Feasibility study of using one-tenth mSv radiation dose in young children chest CT with 80 kVp and model-based iterative reconstruction. *Sci. Rep.* **2019**, *9*, 12481. [CrossRef] [PubMed]
12. Reiazi, R.; Abbas, E.; Famiyeh, P.; Rezaie, A.; Kwan, J.Y.Y.; Patel, T.; Bratman, S.V.; Tadic, T.; Liu, F.F.; Haibe-Kains, B. The impact of the variation of imaging parameters on the robustness of Computed Tomography radiomic features: A review. *Comput. Biol. Med.* **2021**, *133*, 104400. [CrossRef] [PubMed]
13. Gu, B.; Meng, M.; Bi, L.; Kim, J.; Feng, D.D.; Song, S. Prediction of 5-year progression-free survival in advanced nasopharyngeal carcinoma with pretreatment PET/CT using multi-modality deep learning-based radiomics. *Front. Oncol.* **2022**, *12*, 899351. [CrossRef] [PubMed]
14. Guo, Y.; Gao, Y.; Shen, D. Deformable MR Prostate Segmentation via Deep Feature Learning and Sparse Patch Matching. *IEEE Trans. Med. Imaging* **2016**, *35*, 1077–1089. [CrossRef] [PubMed]
15. Duan, S.; Hua, Y.; Cao, G.; Hu, J.; Cui, W.; Zhang, D.; Xu, S.; Rong, T.; Liu, B. Differential diagnosis of benign and malignant vertebral compression fractures: Comparison and correlation of radiomics and deep learning frameworks based on spinal CT and clinical characteristics. *Eur. J. Radiol.* **2023**, *165*, 110899. [CrossRef] [PubMed]
16. Wu, K.; Gu, D.; Qi, P.; Cao, X.; Wu, D.; Chen, L.; Qu, G.; Wang, J.; Pan, X.; Wang, X.; et al. Evaluation of an automated intracranial aneurysm detection and rupture analysis approach using cascade detection and classification networks. *Comput. Med. Imaging Graph.* **2022**, *102*, 102126. [CrossRef]
17. Lin, M.; Lin, N.; Yu, S.; Sha, Y.; Zeng, Y.; Liu, A.; Niu, Y. Automated Prediction of Early Recurrence in Advanced Sinonasal Squamous Cell Carcinoma With Deep Learning and Multi-parametric MRI-based Radiomics Nomogram. *Acad. Radiol.* **2023**, *30*, 2201–2211. [CrossRef]
18. Wu, J.; Xia, Y.; Wang, X.; Wei, Y.; Liu, A.; Innanje, A.; Zheng, M.; Chen, L.; Shi, J.; Wang, L.; et al. uRP: An integrated research platform for one-stop analysis of medical images. *Front. Radiol.* **2023**, *3*, 1153784. [CrossRef]
19. Engelke, K.; Lang, T.; Khosla, S.; Qin, L.; Zysset, P.; Leslie, W.D.; Shepherd, J.A.; Shousboe, J.T. Clinical Use of Quantitative Computed Tomography-Based Advanced Techniques in the Management of Osteoporosis in Adults: The 2015 ISCD Official Positions-Part III. *J. Clin. Densitom.* **2015**, *18*, 393–407. [CrossRef]
20. Quaia, E.; Grisi, G.; Baratella, E.; Cuttin, R.; Poillucci, G.; Kus, S.; Cova, M.A. Diagnostic imaging costs before and after digital tomosynthesis implementation in patient management after detection of suspected thoracic lesions on chest radiography. *Insights Into Imaging* **2014**, *5*, 147–155. [CrossRef]
21. Budoff, M.J.; Malpeso, J.M.; Zeb, I.; Gao, Y.L.; Li, D.; Choi, T.Y.; Dailing, C.A.; Mao, S.S. Measurement of phantomless thoracic bone mineral density on coronary artery calcium CT scans acquired with various CT scanner models. *Radiology* **2013**, *267*, 830–836. [CrossRef] [PubMed]
22. Ardakani, A.A.; Kanafi, A.R.; Acharya, U.R.; Khadem, N.; Mohammadi, A. Application of deep learning technique to manage COVID-19 in routine clinical practice using CT images: Results of 10 convolutional neural networks. *Comput. Biol. Med.* **2020**, *121*, 103795. [CrossRef] [PubMed]
23. Xue, Z.; Huo, J.; Sun, X.; Sun, X.; Ai, S.T.; Zhang, L.; Liu, C. Using radiomic features of lumbar spine CT images to differentiate osteoporosis from normal bone density. *BMC Musculoskelet. Disord.* **2022**, *23*, 336. [CrossRef] [PubMed]
24. Chen, Y.C.; Li, Y.T.; Kuo, P.C.; Cheng, S.J.; Chung, Y.H.; Kuo, D.P.; Chen, C.Y. Automatic segmentation and radiomic texture analysis for osteoporosis screening using chest low-dose computed tomography. *Eur. Radiol.* **2023**, *33*, 5097–5106. [CrossRef]
25. Wang, J.; Zhou, S.; Chen, S.; He, Y.; Gao, H.; Yan, L.; Hu, X.; Li, P.; Shen, H.; Luo, M.; et al. Prediction of osteoporosis using radiomics analysis derived from single source dual energy CT. *BMC Musculoskelet. Disord.* **2023**, *24*, 100. [CrossRef]
26. Kim, S.Y.; Cho, J.Y.; Lee, J.; Hwang, S.I.; Moon, M.H.; Lee, E.J.; Hong, S.S.; Kim, C.K.; Kim, K.A.; Park, S.B.; et al. Low-Tube-Voltage CT Urography Using Low-Concentration-Iodine Contrast Media and Iterative Reconstruction: A Multi-Institutional Randomized Controlled Trial for Comparison with Conventional CT Urography. *Korean J. Radiol.* **2018**, *19*, 1119–1129. [CrossRef]
27. Takafuji, M.; Kitagawa, K.; Ishida, M.; Goto, Y.; Nakamura, S.; Nagasawa, N.; Sakuma, H. Myocardial Coverage and Radiation Dose in Dynamic Myocardial Perfusion Imaging Using Third-Generation Dual-Source CT. *Korean J. Radiol.* **2020**, *21*, 58–67. [CrossRef]
28. Beckmann, N.M. The Rising Utilization of Opportunistic CT Screening and Machine Learning in Bone Mineral Density. *Can. Assoc. Radiol. J.* **2023**, *74*, 616–617. [CrossRef]
29. Ma, C.Y.; Zhou, J.Y.; Xu, X.T.; Guo, J.; Han, M.F.; Gao, Y.Z.; Du, H.; Stahl, J.N.; Maltz, J.S. Deep learning-based auto-segmentation of clinical target volumes for radiotherapy treatment of cervical cancer. *J. Appl. Clin. Med. Phys.* **2022**, *23*, e13470. [CrossRef]
30. Dong, H.; Yin, L.; Chen, L.; Wang, Q.; Pan, X.; Li, Y.; Ye, X.; Zeng, M. Establishment and validation of a radiological-radiomics model for predicting high-grade patterns of lung adenocarcinoma less than or equal to 3 cm. *Front. Oncol.* **2022**, *12*, 964322. [CrossRef]
31. Pan, Y.; Shi, D.; Wang, H.; Chen, T.; Cui, D.; Cheng, X.; Lu, Y. Automatic opportunistic osteoporosis screening using low-dose chest computed tomography scans obtained for lung cancer screening. *Eur. Radiol.* **2020**, *30*, 4107–4116. [CrossRef] [PubMed]

32. Berenguer, R.; Pastor-Juan, M.D.R.; Canales-Vázquez, J.; Castro-García, M.; Villas, M.V.; Mansilla Legorburo, F.; Sabater, S. Radiomics of CT Features May Be Nonreproducible and Redundant: Influence of CT Acquisition Parameters. *Radiology* **2018**, *288*, 407–415. [CrossRef] [PubMed]
33. Astaraki, M.; Yang, G.; Zakko, Y.; Toma-Dasu, I.; Smedby, Ö.; Wang, C. A Comparative Study of Radiomics and Deep-Learning Based Methods for Pulmonary Nodule Malignancy Prediction in Low Dose CT Images. *Front. Oncol.* **2021**, *11*, 737368. [CrossRef] [PubMed]
34. Li, Y.; Zhang, Y.; Zhang, E.; Chen, Y.; Wang, Q.; Liu, K.; Yu, H.J.; Yuan, H.; Lang, N.; Su, M.Y. Differential diagnosis of benign and malignant vertebral fracture on CT using deep learning. *Eur. Radiol.* **2021**, *31*, 9612–9619. [CrossRef]
35. Kitamura, G.; Chung, C.Y.; Moore, B.E., 2nd. Ankle Fracture Detection Utilizing a Convolutional Neural Network Ensemble Implemented with a Small Sample, De Novo Training, and Multiview Incorporation. *J. Digit. Imaging* **2019**, *32*, 672–677. [CrossRef]
36. He, K.; Zhang, X.; Ren, S.; Sun, J. Deep Residual Learning for Image Recognition. In Proceedings of the 2016 IEEE Conference on Computer Vision and Pattern Recognition (CVPR), Las Vegas, NV, USA, 27–30 June 2016; pp. 770–778. [CrossRef]
37. Li, Y.; Wei, D.; Liu, X.; Fan, X.; Wang, K.; Li, S.; Zhang, Z.; Ma, K.; Qian, T.; Jiang, T.; et al. Molecular subtyping of diffuse gliomas using magnetic resonance imaging: Comparison and correlation between radiomics and deep learning. *Eur. Radiol.* **2022**, *32*, 747–758. [CrossRef]

MDPI AG
Grosspeteranlage 5
4052 Basel
Switzerland
Tel.: +41 61 683 77 34

Bioengineering Editorial Office
E-mail: bioengineering@mdpi.com
www.mdpi.com/journal/bioengineering

www.ingramcontent.com/pod-product-compliance
Lightning Source LLC
Chambersburg PA
CBHW061620210926
51850CB00009B/2385
9783725860890